Periodontitis: Current Status and the Future

Periodontitis: Current Status and the Future

Editor

Susanne Schulz

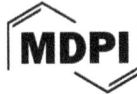

Basel • Beijing • Wuhan • Barcelona • Belgrade • Novi Sad • Cluj • Manchester

Editor
Susanne Schulz
Martin-Luther-Universität
Halle-Wittenberg
Wittenberg
Germany

Editorial Office
MDPI
St. Alban-Anlage 66
4052 Basel, Switzerland

This is a reprint of articles from the Special Issue published online in the open access journal *Journal of Clinical Medicine* (ISSN 2077-0383) (available at: https://www.mdpi.com/journal/jcm/special_issues/Periodontitis_Future).

For citation purposes, cite each article independently as indicated on the article page online and as indicated below:

Lastname, A.A.; Lastname, B.B. Article Title. *Journal Name* **Year**, *Volume Number*, Page Range.

ISBN 978-3-7258-0777-2 (Hbk)
ISBN 978-3-7258-0778-9 (PDF)
doi.org/10.3390/books978-3-7258-0778-9

© 2024 by the authors. Articles in this book are Open Access and distributed under the Creative Commons Attribution (CC BY) license. The book as a whole is distributed by MDPI under the terms and conditions of the Creative Commons Attribution-NonCommercial-NoDerivs (CC BY-NC-ND) license.

Contents

Federica Romano, Stefano Perotto, Sara Elamin Osman Mohamed, Sara Bernardi,
Marta Giraudi, Paola Caropreso, et al.
Bidirectional Association between Metabolic Control in Type-2 Diabetes Mellitus and
Periodontitis Inflammatory Burden: A Cross-Sectional Study in an Italian Population
Reprinted from: *J. Clin. Med.* **2021**, *10*, 1787, doi:10.3390/jcm10081787 1

Tanja Veljovic, Milanko Djuric, Jelena Mirnic, Ivana Gusic, Aleksandra Maletin,
Bojana Ramic, et al.
Lipid Peroxidation Levels in Saliva and Plasma of Patients Suffering from Periodontitis
Reprinted from: *J. Clin. Med.* **2022**, *11*, 3617, doi:10.3390/jcm11133617 15

Magda Aniko-Włodarczyk, Aleksandra Jaroń, Olga Preuss, Anna Grzywacz
and Grzegorz Trybek
Evaluation of the Effect of Surgical Extraction of an Impacted Mandibular Third Molar on the
Periodontal Status of the Second Molar—Prospective Study
Reprinted from: *J. Clin. Med.* **2021**, *10*, 2655, doi:10.3390/jcm10122655 28

Bouchra Sojod, Cibele Pidorodeski Nagano, Glenda Melissa Garcia Lopez, Antoine Zalcberg,
Sophie Myriam Dridi and Fani Anagnostou
Systemic Lupus Erythematosus and Periodontal Disease: A Complex Clinical and
Biological Interplay
Reprinted from: *J. Clin. Med.* **2021**, *10*, 1957, doi:10.3390/jcm10091957 43

Xuanzhi Zhu, Chao-Jung Chu, Weiyi Pan, Yan Li, Hanyao Huang and Lei Zhao
The Correlation between Periodontal Parameters and Cell-Free DNA in the Gingival Crevicular
Fluid, Saliva, and Plasma in Chinese Patients: A Cross-Sectional Study
Reprinted from: *J. Clin. Med.* **2022**, *11*, 6902, doi:10.3390/jcm11236902 55

Ewa Dolińska, Robert Milewski, Maria Julia Pietruska, Katarzyna Gumińska, Natalia Prysak,
Tomasz Tarasewicz, et al.
Periodontitis-Related Knowledge and Its Relationship with Oral Health Behavior among Adult
Patients Seeking Professional Periodontal Care
Reprinted from: *J. Clin. Med.* **2022**, *11*, 1517, doi:10.3390/jcm11061517 67

Elżbieta Dembowska, Aleksandra Jaroń, Aleksandra Homik-Rodzińska,
Ewa Gabrysz-Trybek, Joanna Bladowska and Grzegorz Trybek
Comparison of the Treatment Efficacy of Endo–Perio Lesions Using a Standard Treatment
Protocol and Extended by Using a Diode Laser (940 nm)
Reprinted from: *J. Clin. Med.* **2022**, *11*, 811, doi:10.3390/jcm11030811 79

Ji-Eun Kim, Na-Yeong Kim, Choong-Ho Choi and Ki-Ho Chung
Association between Oral Health Status and Relative Handgrip Strength in 11,337 Korean
Reprinted from: *J. Clin. Med.* **2021**, *10*, 5425, doi:10.3390/jcm10225425 92

Stefan Reichert, Susanne Schulz, Lisa Friebe, Michael Kohnert, Julia Grollmitz,
Hans-Günter Schaller and Britt Hofmann
Is Periodontitis a Predictor for an Adverse Outcome in Patients Undergoing Coronary Artery
Bypass Grafting? A Pilot Study
Reprinted from: *J. Clin. Med.* **2021**, *10*, 818, doi:10.3390/jcm10040818 102

Valentina Cárcamo-España, Nataly Cuesta Reyes, Paul Flores Saldivar,
Eduardo Chimenos-Küstner, Alberto Estrugo Devesa and José López-López
Compromised Teeth Preserve or Extract: A Review of the Literature

Reprinted from: *J. Clin. Med.* **2022**, *11*, 5301, doi:10.3390/jcm11185301 . . . . **114**

Jeong-Hwa Kim, Jae-Woon Oh, Young Lee, Jeong-Ho Yun, Seong-Ho Choi and Dong-Woon Lee
Quantification of Bacteria in Mouth-Rinsing Solution for the Diagnosis of Periodontal Disease
Reprinted from: *J. Clin. Med.* **2021**, *10*, 891, doi:10.3390/jcm10040891 . . . . **129**

Ciprian Roi, Pușa Nela Gaje, Raluca Amalia Ceaușu, Alexandra Roi, Laura Cristina Rusu, Eugen Radu Boia, et al.
Heterogeneity of Blood Vessels and Assessment of Microvessel Density-MVD in Gingivitis
Reprinted from: *J. Clin. Med.* **2022**, *11*, 2758, doi:10.3390/jcm11102758 . . . . **145**

Katrin Nickles, Mischa Krebs, Beate Schacher, Hari Petsos and Peter Eickholz
Long-Term Results after Placing Dental Implants in Patients with Papillon-Lefèvre Syndrome: Results 2.5–20 Years after Implant Insertion
Reprinted from: *J. Clin. Med.* **2022**, *11*, 2438, doi:10.3390/jcm11092438 . . . . **157**

Peter Eickholz, Anne Asendorf, Mario Schröder, Beate Schacher, Gerhard M. Oremek, Ralf Schubert, et al.
Effect of Subgingival Instrumentation on Neutrophil Elastase and C-Reactive Protein in Grade B and C Periodontitis: Exploratory Analysis of a Prospective Cohort Study
Reprinted from: *J. Clin. Med.* **2022**, *11*, 3189, doi:10.3390/jcm11113189 . . . . **167**

Kawaljit Kaur, Shahram Vaziri, Marcela Romero-Reyes, Avina Paranjpe and Anahid Jewett
Phenotypic and Functional Alterations of Immune Effectors in Periodontitis; A Multifactorial and Complex Oral Disease
Reprinted from: *J. Clin. Med.* **2021**, *10*, 875, doi:10.3390/jcm10040875 . . . . **178**

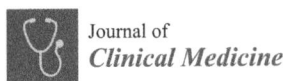

Article

Bidirectional Association between Metabolic Control in Type-2 Diabetes Mellitus and Periodontitis Inflammatory Burden: A Cross-Sectional Study in an Italian Population

Federica Romano [1,†], Stefano Perotto [2,†], Sara Elamin Osman Mohamed [1], Sara Bernardi [3], Marta Giraudi [1], Paola Caropreso [4], Giulio Mengozzi [4], Giacomo Baima [1], Filippo Citterio [1], Giovanni Nicolao Berta [5,*], Marilena Durazzo [3], Gabriella Gruden [3] and Mario Aimetti [1,*]

[1] Department of Surgical Sciences, C.I.R. Dental School, Section of Periodontology, University of Turin, 10126 Turin, Italy; federica.romano@unito.it (F.R.); sara.amosm@gmail.com (S.E.O.M.); marta.giraudi@gmail.com (M.G.); giacomo.baima@unito.it (G.B.); filippo.citterio@unito.it (F.C.)
[2] Postgraduate Program in Periodontology, C.I.R. Dental School, University of Turin, 10126 Turin, Italy; stefanoperotto@libero.it
[3] Department of Medical Sciences, University of Turin, 10126 Turin, Italy; bernardi.sara98@gmail.com (S.B.); marilena.durazzo@unito.it (M.D.); gabriella.gruden@unito.it (G.G.)
[4] Clinical Biochemistry Laboratory, Department of Laboratory Medicine, 10126 Turin, Italy; pcaropreso@cittadellasalute.to.it (P.C.); giulio.mengozzi@unito.it (G.M.)
[5] Department of Clinical and Biological Sciences, University of Turin, 10043 Orbassano, Italy
* Correspondence: giovanni.berta@unito.it (G.N.B.); mario.aimetti@unito.it (M.A.)
† These authors contributed equally to this work.

Abstract: This study assessed the periodontal conditions of type 2 diabetes (T2DM) patients attending an Outpatient Center in North Italy and explored the associations between metabolic control and periodontitis. Periodontal health of 104 T2DM patients (61 men and 43 women, mean age of 65.3 ± 10.1 years) was assessed according to CDC/AAP periodontitis case definitions and Periodontal Inflamed Surface Area (PISA) Index. Data on sociodemographic factors, lifestyle behaviors, laboratory tests, and glycated hemoglobin (HbA1c) levels were collected by interview and medical records. Poor glycemic control (HbA1c ≥ 7%), family history of T2DM, and C-reactive protein levels were predictors of severe periodontitis. An increase in HbA1c of 1% was associated with a rise in PISA of 89.6 mm^2. On the other hand, predictors of poor glycemic control were severe periodontitis, waist circumference, unbalanced diet, and sedentary lifestyle. A rise in PISA of 10 mm^2 increased the odds of having HbA1c ≥ 7% by 2%. There is a strong bidirectional connection between periodontitis and poor glycemic control. The inflammatory burden posed by periodontitis represents the strongest predictor of poor glycemic control.

Keywords: glycated hemoglobin; inflammation; periodontitis; periodontal inflamed surface area (PISA); type-2 diabetes mellitus

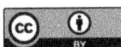

1. Introduction

The prevalence of diabetes mellitus (DM) is increasing worldwide to epidemic proportions: 415 million people suffer from DM and the number is expected to rise to 642 millions by 2040 [1]. DM has two major types: Type 1 (T1DM), characterized by failure to produce insulin, and type 2 (T2DM), in which both insulin resistance and relative insulin deficiency occur. T2DM is the most prevalent form of the disease, accounting for more than 90% of diabetic patients [2].

DM presents a serious challenge to the healthcare system since its complications are the leading causes of morbidity and mortality. According to the World Health Organization, it will be the seventh major cause of death in 2030 [3]. Systemic subclinical inflammation has been proposed as the underlying biological mechanisms of its chronic complications, such as micro vascular and nerve damage [4], with evidence of a strong association between levels of hemoglobin A1c (HbA1c) and risk of complications [5].

Periodontitis is recognized as the sixth most common complication for both DM forms even if most of the studies are related to T2DM [6]. Periodontitis is an infectious disease with a chronic inflammatory response to periodontal pathogens in dental biofilm that leads to the irreversible destruction of the tooth-supporting tissues and eventually to tooth loss. There is consistent and robust evidence supporting the existence of a relationship between T2DM and periodontitis with a dual directionality [7–9]. T2DM enhances the risk for periodontitis initiation and progression, and periodontal inflammation affects both glycemic control and the risk to develop chronic T2DM complications [10–12]. A hyperglycemic status leads to a dysregulated inflammatory response involving immune activity, neutrophil functioning, and cytokine pattern, promoting connective-tissue damage [13,14]. On the other hand, the dissemination of periodontal pathogens and their metabolic products in the bloodstream circulation, results in increased serum levels of inflammatory mediators that can deteriorate blood glucose control via acute-phase (i.e., C-reactive protein, CRP) and neutrophil oxidative response [15,16].

This systemic inflammatory burden has proven to increase with the extent and severity of periodontitis. Conventionally, the overall amount of destruction of tooth-supporting tissues is measured in terms of clinical attachment level (CAL) and probing depth (PD). However, these clinical parameters assess the cumulative effects of periodontal tissue breakdown, but do not measure the amount of inflamed and ulcerated epithelium within the periodontal pocket [17]. The Periodontal Inflamed Surface Area (PISA) Index has been introduced to quantify the amount of bleeding pocket epithelium and it is expected to reflect the inflammatory burden presented by periodontitis [18,19]. PISA values tend to increase consistently as periodontal status worsens, even if they show high variability in studies conducted in different populations [20–23].

Although the association between periodontitis and T2DM has been widely demonstrated, the strength of the relationship seems to differ geographically (based on genetic and lifestyle differences among ethnic groups) [24,25]. Furthermore, little is known on the behavior of PISA in T2DM. A recent study has reported a dose–response relationship between PISA values and HbA1c levels [20].

The aims of the present cross-sectional study were to determine the periodontal health status of T2DM patients attending an Outpatient Diabetes Center in North Italy [26] and to assess the association between glycemic control and periodontitis, as measured clinically and with the PISA Index.

2. Materials and Methods

2.1. Study Design

This cross-sectional study was conducted in accordance with the Helsinki Declaration and approved by the Institutional Ethical Committee of the "AOU Città della Salute e della Scienza", Turin, Italy (No. 0027219, 14 March 2018). Informed consent was obtained from each patient before the study. All participants signed an informed consent to undergo physical and periodontal examination. The study complied with the STROBE guidelines.

Patients with an established diagnosis of T2DM according to World Health Organization criteria [27] were consecutively recruited from among those who came for regular check-ups at the Outpatient Diabetes Center, Turin (Italy) from March 2018 to July 2019.

The following inclusion criteria were considered: (i) at least 40 years of age; (ii) having at least 8 teeth; (iii) availability of measurements of routine diabetes laboratory tests made in the 6 months before enrollment. Exclusion criteria were: (i) T1DM; (ii) intake of drugs known to affect gingival tissues, use of antibiotics, steroidal, and/or non-steroidal anti-inflammatory drugs 3 weeks prior to the visit; (iii) periodontal therapy in the past 6 months; (iv) pregnancy or lactation; and (v) diagnosis of following pathologies: cancer, human immunodeficiency virus/AIDS, chronic infections, liver/kidney failure excluding diabetic nephropathy, chronic obstructive pulmonary disease with acute episodes and/or requiring the use of steroidal inhalator.

2.2. Data Collection

Participants were required to complete a questionnaire to obtain information on socio-demographic characteristics (gender, age, ethnicity, education), general health behavior (leisure-time physical activity level, daily smoking and dietary habits, alcohol consumption), and oral hygiene behavior (toothbrush frequency, use of interdental devices, and frequency of professional oral hygiene sessions).

Data on medical history, parental history of T2DM, T2DM onset and duration, cardiovascular risk factors, chronic T2DM complications, current medications and treatment for T2DM, as well as results of laboratory tests performed in the last diabetic visit (HbA1c level, lipid profile, urine analysis, creatinine, high-sensitivity-CRP (hs-CRP)) were collected.

Two masked Diabetes Specialists reviewed the medical history of the participants and conducted a physical examination including blood pressure levels (average of three blood pressure measurements within 3 min), anthropometric measurements (weight, height, and waist circumference (WC)), palpation, and auscultation. The body mass index (BMI) was calculated as weight/height squared (kg/m^2).

Subsequently, a single dentist conducted a periodontal examination. To ensure inter and intra-examiner reproducibility, measurements of periodontal parameters were repeated in 20% of the sample and compared with those recorded by a gold-standard examiner. The k coefficients (within 1 mm) between examiners ranged from 0.79 to 0.93 in the evaluation of PD and from 0.81 to 0.89 in the evaluation of gingival recession (Rec). The intra-examiner concordance rates for repeated measurements were 0.89 to 0.95 for PD and 0.82 to 0.91 for Rec.

Full-mouth PD, Rec, and CAL were recorded by means of a periodontal probe with 1-mm markings (PCP-UNC 15, Hu-Friedy, Chicago, IL, USA) at six sites per tooth, excluding third molars. The total percentages of sites exhibiting bacterial plaque or bleeding on probing (BoP) were expressed as full mouth plaque score (FMPS) and full mouth-bleeding score (FMBS), respectively. The number of missing teeth was also recorded.

The presence of periodontitis was defined according to the criteria proposed by Centers for Disease Control and Prevention/American Academy of Periodontology (CDC/AAP) for epidemiologic surveys [28,29]. Therefore, moderate periodontitis was defined as at least 2 interproximal sites with attachment loss ≥ 4 mm (not on the same tooth) or at least 2 interproximal sites with PD ≥ 5 mm, also not on the same tooth. The presence of at least 2 interproximal sites with attachment loss ≥ 6 mm (not on the same tooth) and at least 1 interproximal site with PD ≥ 5 mm indicated severe periodontitis. If neither moderate nor severe periodontitis applied, no/mild periodontitis was recorded. Additionally, a recently introduced measure of periodontitis severity, the PISA, was calculated as previously described in the literature [18,19]. It quantifies the amount of bleeding epithelium in mm^2 around individual tooth. The sum of all individual PISAs corresponds to the full-mouth PISA value in mm^2 of each participant and reflects the inflammatory burden posed by periodontitis.

2.3. Statistical Analysis

All data analyses were performed using SPSS software, version 24.0 for MAC (Chicago, IL, USA). Frequency distributions were determined, and descriptive statistics were calculated as means, standard deviations, and ranges. Participants' tobacco use, adherence to balanced diet, and alcohol consumption were classified as dichotomous variables (yes/no). Education was dichotomized according to the years spent in school, considering a cut-off value of 8 years (lower/high school diploma, university bachelor's degree or higher).

Categorical grouping variables included periodontal status (no/mild periodontitis, moderate periodontitis, severe periodontitis) and glycemic control (good: HbA1c < 7%; poor: HbA1c $\geq$ 7%) [30]. Comparisons between groups were performed with chi-square test for categorical variables, unpaired t-test or one-way analysis of variance for normally distributed quantitative variables, and with Mann–Whitney *U*-test or Kruskal–Wallis test for non-normally distributed quantitative variables. Post-hoc tests (Scheffé test and Dunn-test with Bonferroni correction) were used for multiple comparisons.

Because severity of periodontitis was operationalized as both a dichotomous variable (absence or presence) according to the CDC/AAP clinical criteria and a continuous variable (full-mouth PISA value), the associations between severity of periodontitis (outcome variable) and glycemic control (primary explanatory variable) was assessed using logistic and linear regression techniques, respectively. Two sets (each containing two models) of multiple regression analyses were fitted separately to each of the outcomes for a total of four models. In each set, glycemic control was entered as (1) dichotomous variable (poor vs. good) and (2) continuous variable (HbA1c levels). In addition, evaluated covariates included hs-CRP (mg/L), presence of chronic diabetes complications (dichotomous) and family history of T2DM (dichotomous).

The predictors of uncontrolled T2DM (outcome variable) were explored by logistic regression analysis (models 5 and 6) including severity of periodontal damage (as dichotomous or continuous variable), WC, leisure-time physical activity, and balanced diet based on previous literature demonstrating the effect of lifestyle factors on T2DM risk and metabolic control [31]. In the logistic regression analysis, odds ratios (ORs) and 95% confidence intervals (CIs) were calculated. The level of significance was set at 0.05.

3. Results

The study flow-chart is outlined in Figure 1. A total of 104 T2DM patients, 61 men and 43 women, with a mean age of 65.3 ± 10.1 years were consecutively recruited into this study. All participants were Caucasian. Poor glycemic control (HbA1c ≥ 7%) was detected in 63.5% of T2DM patients.

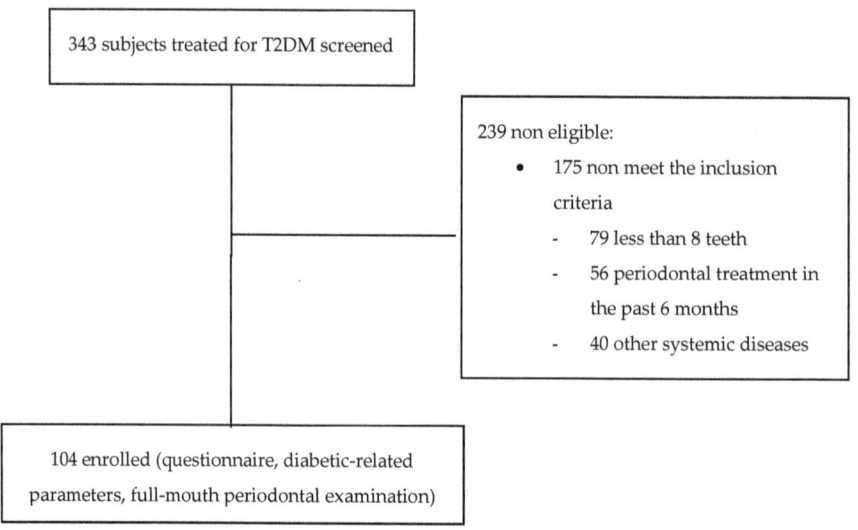

Figure 1. Subject recruitment and participation.

T2DM patients used oral medications, insulin, or a combination of both to treat and control diabetes. Metformin was the oral medication most often prescribed (77.9%), followed by a new generation of DM drugs (59.6%) and other first-generation agents (20.2%). Insulin therapy was prescribed to 54.8% of the patients.

Table 1 summarizes sociodemographic, lifestyle, and periodontal characteristics stratified by glycemic control. Physical activity level, WC, hs-CRP levels, frequency of chronic DM complications, and periodontal status were significantly different between poorly and well-controlled T2DM patients. Patients with poor glycemic control had higher prevalence of severe periodontitis and PISA values than well-controlled T2DM patients.

Table 1. Sociodemographic and clinical characteristics of T2DM patients (mean ± SD (range) or n (%)) according to the glycemic control.

Variable	Poor Glycemic Control (n = 66)	Good Glycemic Control (n = 38)	Total (n = 104)	p Value
Age (years)	65.9 ± 9.7 (43–80)	64.4 ± 10.8 (40–78)	65.3 ± 10.1 (40–80)	0.459
Sex				0.076
Males	43 (70.5)	18 (29.5)	61 (58.7)	
Females	23 (53.5)	20 (46.5)	43 (41.3)	
Education level				0.796
<high school	33 (64.7)	18 (35.3)	51 (48.1)	
high school or higher	33 (62.3)	20 (37.7)	53 (51.9)	
Smoking				0.788
Yes	4 (66.7)	2 (33.3)	6 (5.8)	
No	62 (63.3)	36 (36.7)	98 (94.2)	
Alcohol consumption				0.384
Yes	42 (61.8)	26 (38.2)	68 (64.4)	
No	24 (66.7)	12 (33.3)	36 (34.6)	
Balanced diet				0.105
Yes	4 (40.0)	6 (60.0)	10 (9.6)	
No	62 (66.0)	32 (34.0)	94 (90.4)	
Leisure-time physical activity				0.019
Yes	21 (50.0)	21 (50.0)	42 (40.4)	
No	45 (72.6)	17 (27.4)	62 (59.6)	
Duration of diabetes (years)	15.1 ± 9.9 (1–42)	12.8 ± 11.7 (1–52)	14.2 ± 10.7 (1–52)	0.306
Family history of T2DM				0.395
Yes	47 (66.2)	24 (33.8)	71 (68.3)	
No	19 (57.6)	14 (42.4)	33 (31.7)	
Chronic complications of diabetes				0.009
None	22 (53.7)	19 (46.3)	41 (39.4)	
1	21 (56.8)	16 (43.2)	37 (35.6)	
2 or more	23 (88.5)	3 (11.5)	26 (25.0)	
HbA1c (%)	8.0 ± 1.0 (7.0–11.6)	6.3 ± 0.5 (5.0–6.9)	7.4 ± 1.2 (5.0–11.6)	<0.001
BMI (kg/m^2)	29.6 ± 5.1 (18.8–40.8)	28.1 ± 6.1 (17.0–43.0)	29.1 ± 5.5 (17.0–43.0)	0.162
WC (cm)	104.4 ± 12.6 (71.0–134.0)	94.9 ± 15.2 (60.0–130.0)	100.9 ± 14.3 (60.0–134.0)	0.001
TG (mg/dL)	150.9 ± 81.4 851.0–507.0)	145.0 ± 77.7 (57.0–377.0)	148.8 ± 79.7 (51.0–107.0)	0.719
HDL-C (mg/dL)	47.2 ± 15.1 (23.0–90.0)	53.8 ± 16.7 (31.0–88.0)	49.6 + 15.9 (23.0–80.0)	0.042
LDL-C (mg/dL)	94.9 ± 29.2 (47.6–147.0)	92.8 ± 31.9 (22.4–158.2)	94.1 ± 30.1 (22.4–158.2)	0.738

Table 1. Cont.

Variable	Poor Glycemic Control (n= 66)	Good Glycemic Control (n = 38)	Total (n = 104)	p Value
Total cholesterol (mg/dL)	171.8 ± 31.1 (122.0–227.0)	177.2 ± 31.7 (101.0–224.0)	173.7 ± 31.3 (101.0–227.0)	0.399
hs-CPR (mg/L)	2.9 ± 2.3 (0.2–8.5)	1.8 ± 2.3 (0.0–9.9)	2.5 ± 2.3 (0.0–9.9)	0.030
Number of teeth	21.9 ± 4.9 (6–28)	22.7 ± 4.6 (9–28)	22.2 ± 4.8 (6–28)	0.410
Periodontitis				<0.001
No/mild periodontitis	1 (11.1)	8 (88.9)	9 (8.7)	
Moderate periodontitis	13 (46.4)	15 (53.6)	28 (26.9)	
Severe periodontitis	52 (77.6)	15 (22.4)	67 (64.4)	
Full-mouth PISA (mm^2)	1342.3 ± 487.9 (422.0–2732.0)	946.1 ± 454.1 (229.0–2252.0)	1204.1 ± 507.7 (229.0–2732.0)	<0.001

BMI: Body Mass Index; HbA1c: glycated hemoglobin; WC: waist circumference; TG: triglycerides; HDL-C: High-density-lipoprotein cholesterol; LDL-C: Low-density-lipoprotein cholesterol; hs-CRP: high-sensitivity C-reactive protein; PISA: periodontal inflammation surface area; T2DM: type 2 diabetes.

When we stratified the analysis by periodontal status (Table 2), patients with severe periodontitis showed statistically significant higher frequency of family history of T2DM, higher HbA1c scores, more chronic DM complications, higher hs-CRP and PISA values than moderate, and no/mild periodontitis patients.

Table 2. Sociodemographic and clinical characteristics of T2DM patients (mean ± SD (range) or n (%)) according to the periodontal status.

Variable	No/Mild Periodontitis (n = 9)	Moderate Periodontitis (n = 28)	Severe Periodontitis (n = 67)	Total	p Value
Age (years)	60.1 ± 17.1 (40–79)	66.0 ± 9.7 (47–80)	65.8 ± 8.9 (43–80)	65.3 ± 10.1 (40–80)	0.266
Sex					0.240
Males	3 (4.9)	16 (26.2)	42 (68.9)	61 (58.7)	
Females	6 (14.0)	12 (27.9)	25 (58.1)	43 (41.3)	
Education level					0.902
<high school	5 (9.8)	14 (27.5)	32 (62.7)	51 (48.1)	
high school or higher	4 (7.5)	14 (26.4)	35 (66.0)	53 (51.9)	
Smoking					0.696
Yes	1 (16.7)	1 (16.7)	4 (66.6)	6 (5.8)	
No	8 (8.2)	27 (27.5)	63 (64.3)	98 (94.2)	
Alcohol consumption					0.455
Yes	5 (7.3)	15 (22.1)	48 (70.6)	68 (65.4)	
No	4 (11.1)	13 (36.1)	19 (52.8)	36 (34.6)	
Balanced diet					0.196
Yes	0	1 (10.0)	9 (90.0)	10 (9.6)	
No	9 (9.6)	27 (28.7)	58 (61.7)	94 (90.4)	
Leisure-time physical activity					0.904
Yes	4 (9.5)	12 (28.6)	26 (61.9)	42 (40.4)	
No	5 (8.1)	16 (25.8)	41 (66.1)	62 (59.6)	
Duration of diabetes (yrs)	14.9 ± 11.2 (1–38)	12.9 ± 11.9 (1–52)	14.7 ± 10.1 (1–42)	14.2 ± 10.7 (1–52)	0.754

Table 2. Cont.

Variable	No/Mild Periodontitis (n = 9)	Moderate Periodontitis (n = 28)	Severe Periodontitis (n = 67)	Total	p Value
Family history of T2DM					0.015
Yes	7 (9.9)	13 (18.3)	51 (71.8)	71 (68.3)	
No	2 (6.1)	15 (45.4)	16 (48.5)	33 (31.7)	
Chronic complications of diabetes					0.002
None	5 (12.2)	12 (29.3)	24 (58.5)	41 (39.4)	
1	4 (10.8)	15 (40.5)	18 (48.6)	37 (35.6)	
2 or more	0 (0.0)	1 (3.8)	25 (96.2)	26 (25.0)	
Glycemic control					<0.001
Good	8 (21.1)	15 (39.5)	15 (39.5)	38 (36.5)	
Poor	1 (1.5)	13 (19.7)	52 (78.8)	66 (63.5)	
HbA1c (%)	6.1 ± 0.7 (5.0–7.3)	7.1 ± 1.3 (5.4–10.0)	7.6 ± 1.1 (5.2–11.6)	7.4 ± 1.2 (5.0–11.6)	0.001
BMI (kg/m^2)	31.0 ± 6.3 (23.0–43.0)	27.9 ± 6.0 (18.0–40.3)	29.3 ± 5.1 (17.0–40.8)	29.1 ± 5.5 (17.0–43.0)	0.295
WC (cm)	100.2 ± 11.3 (80.0–115.0)	98.4 ± 16.9 (66.0–130.0)	102.0 ± 13.5 (60.0M–134.0)	100.9 ± 14.3 (60.0–134.0)	0.533
TG (mg/dL)	136.1 ± 92.5 (57.0–374.0)	176.1 ± 109.4 (63.0–107.0)	139.0 ± 59.6 (51.0–358.0)	148.8 ± 79.7 (51.0–107.0)	0.103
HDL-C (mg/dL)	52.2 ± 17.4 (38.0–83.0)	47.1 ± 15.6 (23.0–83.0)	50.3 ± 16.0 (24.0–90.0)	49.6 ± 15.9 (23.0–80.0)	0.592
LDL-C (mg/dL)	94.8 ± 43.6 (22.4–154.0)	91.9 ± 31.9 (38.4–158.2)	95.0 ± 27.7 (47.6–147.0)	94.1 ± 30.1 (22.4–158.2)	0.903
Total cholesterol (mg/dL)	179.1 ± 29.0 (124.0–217.0)	174.6 ± 35.5 (101.0–207.0)	172.6 ± 30.0 (122.0–226.0)	173.7 ± 31.3 (101.0–227.0)	0.832
hs-CPR (mg/L)	0.7 ± 0.06 (0.0–2.0)	1.5 ± 1.2 (0.0–4.7)	3.1 ± 2.5 (0.2–9.9)	2.5 ± 2.3 (0.0–9.9)	<0.001
Number of teeth	24.1 ± 3.8 (18–28)	22.1 ± 4.8 (10–28)	22.0 ± 4.9 (6–28)	22.2 ± 4.8 (6–28)	0.472
Full-mouth PISA (mm^2)	415.5 ± 105.5 (229.0–575.0)	859.4 ± 199.5 (494.0–1298.0)	1454.1 ± 431.3 (585.0–2732.0)	1204.1 ± 507.7 (229.0–2732.0)	<0.001

BMI: Body Mass Index; HbA1c: Glycated hemoglobin; WC: Waist circumference; TG: Triglycerides; HDL-C: High-density-lipoprotein cholesterol; LDL-C: Low-density-lipoprotein cholesterol; hs-CRP: High-sensitivity C-reactive protein; PISA: Periodontal Inflamed Surface Area; T2DM: type 2 diabetes.

In the multiple logistic regression analysis (Table 3, models 1 and 2), hs CRP was a predictor of severe periodontitis with an OR of about 1.7 (for both models). Poor glycemic control and a rise in HbA1c of 1% increased by 4.6-fold and by 1.6-fold, respectively, the odds for having severe periodontitis.

In the multiple linear regression analysis (Table 3, models 3 and 4), hs-CRP levels were shown to be significantly associated with PISA, displaying similar β coefficients in both models (46.0 vs. 49.9). Patients with poor glycemic control had higher PISA values (ß = 297.4) and an increase in HbA1c of 1% was associated with a rise in PISA of 89.6 mm^2. Therefore, the maximum expected area of inflamed epithelium is estimated at 627.2 mm^2 in patients with well-controlled diabetes. A further increase of 412.2 mm^2 is expected in the patient with the highest HbA1c level.

Family history of T2DM was an additional predictor only for severe periodontitis, while the presence of chronic DM complications was associated with a rise in PISA.

Table 3. Association between severe periodontitis and glycemic control.

Model and Variables	Severe Periodontitis (Dichotomous)		
	OR	95% IC	p Value
Model 1			
Glycemic control (poor vs. good)	4.574	1.724 to 12.138	0.002
Family history of T2DM (yes vs. no)	3.323	1.189 to 9.283	0.022
hs-CRP (mg/L)	1.656	1.187 to 2.306	0.003
Model 2			
HbA1c (%)	1.608	1.034 to 2.502	0.035
Family history of T2DM (yes vs. no)	3.257	1.194 to 8.885	0.021
hs-CRP (mg/L)	1.692	1.213 to 2.360	0.002
	PISA (mm^2)		
	ß	95% IC	p Value
Model 3			
Glycemic control (poor vs. good)	297.419	104.887 to 489.951	0.003
Chronic diabetes complications (at least one vs. none)	205.264	19.895 to 390.632	0.030
hs-CRP (mg/L)	46.002	6.136 to 85.868	0.024
Model 4			
HbA1c (%)	89.601	11.265 to 167.937	0.025
Chronic diabetes complications (at least one vs. none)	219.628	30.917 to 408.339	0.023
hs-CRP (mg/L)	49.949	9.412 to 90.486	0.016

HbA1c: Glycated hemoglobin; hs-CRP: High-sensitivity C-reactive protein; PISA: Periodontal Inflames Surface Area; OR: Odds ratio; 95% IC: 95% interval confidence; β: Unstandardized coefficient.

As depicted in Figure 2, patients diagnosed as having severe periodontitis had mean PISA values of 1454.1 mm^2, corresponding to the area of a square having sides 38.1 mm each. Inside this square the surface area attributed to the impact of HbA1c measured on average 681.0 mm^2 (equal to that of a square measuring about 26 mm on each side). The hs-CRP levels accounted for a mean increase in PISA of 154.8 mm^2 (square of 12.4 mm on each side).

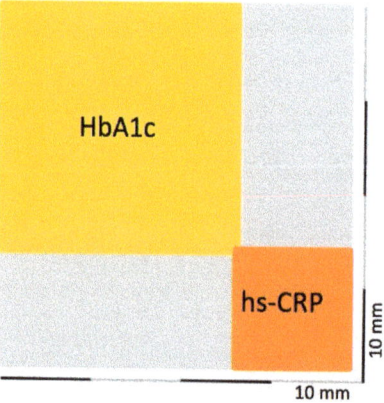

Figure 2. Square in mm^2 representing the mean PISA values for patients diagnosed as having severe periodontitis and depicting the surface area explained by glycated hemoglobin (HbA1c, yellow) and high-sensitivity C reactive Protein (hs-CRP, orange) levels. The grey area identifies the surface area attributable to other unexplored factors that influence the PISA.

In Table 4, the multiple logistic regression analysis (models 5 and 6) showed that poor lifestyle habits were predictors of poor glycemic control. A rise in PISA of 1 mm^2 increased the odds of having HbA1c $\geq$ 7% by 2‰, and patients with severe periodontitis were 8.5-times more likely to have uncontrolled diabetes.

Table 4. Association between poorly controlled T2DM and severe periodontitis.

Model and Variables	Poorly Controlled T2DM (Dichotomous)		
	OR	95% IC	p Value
Model 5			
Severe periodontitis (yes vs. no)	8.509	2.988 to 24.230	<0.001
Leisure-time physical activity (yes vs. no)	0.384	0.143 to 1.033	0.058
Balanced diet (yes vs. no)	0.125	0.027 to 0.580	0.008
WC (cm)	1.057	1.018 to 1.096	0.004
Model 6			
PISA (mm^2)	1.002	1.001 to 1.003	<0.001
Leisure-time physical activity (yes vs. no)	0.397	0.150 to 1.051	0.063
Balanced diet (yes vs. no)	0.140	0.027 to 0.725	0.019
WC (cm)	1.062	1.023 to 1.103	0.002

PISA: Periodontal Inflamed Surface Area; WC: Waist circumference; OR: Odds ratio; 95% IC: 95% interval confidence.

4. Discussion

This cross-sectional study aimed to assess the periodontal conditions of T2DM adult patients attending an Outpatient Clinic in the North of Italy, and to examine predictors of the association between periodontitis and glycemic control. In spite of the large number of studies investigating this latter aspect, only a few of them focused on the impact of the inflammatory burden of periodontitis assessed using the PISA Index and none referred to the CDC/AAP periodontitis case definition [18–20]. The present study used a full-mouth examination protocol and applied this classification system [28,29]. These criteria have been recommended when investigating systemic periodontal linkages [32].

Previous investigations on T2DM reported largely variable percentages of periodontitis, ranging between 13.6% and 97.7%, as a result of differences in both ethnic background and measures of periodontitis severity [25,33–37]. In an epidemiologic survey on our Caucasian population, 52% of all adults over 60 of age, irrespective of their diabetes status, suffered from severe periodontitis based on CDC/AAP algorithms [38]., Futhermore, the percentage of periodontitis was 91% with 63.4% of the severe form, reflecting an urgent need for treatment and preventive oral care programs.

Although the two-way relationship between periodontitis and T2DM has been long established, multivariable modelling procedures have rarely been applied to explore such an association from both perspectives. We used two methods to operationalize severe periodontitis: the first method relied on clinical examination of PD and CAL based on CDC/AAP case definition, and the second one measured the surface area of bleeding periodontal epithelium according to the PISA Index [18,19]. This parameter, recently introduced in periodontal medicine research, is based on mathematical algorithms difficult to apply during the routine clinical practice but it could be a valid method to numerically represent the active inflammatory status of periodontium.

When periodontitis was entered as a dependent variable in the multivariate analysis, family history of T2DM, glycemic control, and serum hs-CRP levels were found to be significantly associated with an increased odds for having poorer periodontal health. These findings were irrespective of the definitions used for periodontitis and corroborate with those documented in the literature [9,39]. Familiarity was reported by approximately 70% of patients with severe periodontitis compared with 20% and 10% of individuals with moderate and no/mild periodontitis, respectively.

Individuals suffering from uncontrolled T2DM were at least four times more likely to have severe periodontitis than those with better-controlled diabetes. About 63.5%

of T2DM patients had poor glycemic control, with a trend to suggest higher HbA1c levels with increasing periodontitis severity. This percentage is high compared with data previously published in the literature, reporting that one-third to half of diabetics having an HbA1c level $\geq 7\%$ [36,40,41]. Our study population derives from a specialized diabetic center where severe cases are referred to. Patients had a mean duration of T2DM of 14.2 ± 10.7 years, long enough for chronic complications of the disease to appear.

Interestingly, the strength of the association of HbA1c levels with severe periodontitis was comparable to that of serum hs-CRP, a marker of systemic inflammation [42]. A one-unit rise in both serum HbA1c and hs-CRP could increase the odds for having severe periodontitis by approximately 60%. Serum reactive oxygen species, interleukin (IL)-1, IL-6, tumor necrosis factor (TNF)-α, and CRP have been found to be elevated in the bloodstream of patients with established T2DM and may play an important role in tissue breakdown in periodontitis [43]. This suggests that as the severity and duration of chronic hyperglycemia increase, the periodontal inflammatory response is also expected to rise.

When considering the PISA Index as dependent variable, the mean surface area of ulcerated epithelium was estimated 288.33 mm^2 higher in uncontrolled than that in well-controlled T2DM, and an increase in HbA1c of 1% was associated with a rise in PISA of 89.6 mm^2. The PISA increased by 46 mm^2 for every one-unit increase in hs-CRP concentration. To date, only one study reported data on this outcome and found PISA as a predictor of periodontitis severity with an expected increase of 275.29 mm^2 in T2DM compared to non-diabetics [44].

On the other hand, we explored the relationship between glycemic control, dependent variable, and periodontitis. Predictors of poor glycemic control were periodontitis, WC, unbalanced diet, and sedentary lifestyle habits. Patients affected by severe periodontitis were eight times more likely to have uncontrolled T2DM than those with moderate or no periodontitis. Odds were increased by 2% for a $\times 10$ mm^2 PISA raise. Only two studies investigated the association between periodontitis and HbA1c with conflicting results [20,34]. Susanto et al. did not find any association in Indonesians with T2DM, but they identified PISA as predictor of HbA1c together with CRP in non-diabetic controls [34]. Conversely, a dose–response relationship was previously reported between PISA and HbA1c in T2DM patients living in Carribean island Curaçao [20].

An interesting finding in this study was the absence of any statistically significant association of plasma lipid profile and overweight/obesity (BMI ≥ 25 kg/m^2) with severity of periodontitis in both the bivariate and multivariate analysis. It cannot rule out the possibility that the effects of obesity and low HDL levels, that are major components of the metabolic syndrome, may be masked by the hyperglycemic status [45]. The present data support a relationship between inadequate glycemic control and poor lifestyle habits. Although regular exercise improves insulin sensitivity and regulates blood glucose levels, it is often difficult for T2DM patients to maintain regular exercise habits [46,47]. In our study, only one-third of poorly controlled diabetics reported that they exercised regularly.

Biological mechanisms explaining the effect of periodontitis on the metabolic control have been proposed in the literature, but the actual evidence is moderate [8]. Local inflammation can affect systemic health through this ulcerated interface, allowing bacteria and inflammatory mediators to access to the bloodstream [48–52]. The amount of ulcerated epithelial area, according to the study by Leira et al. [21], was between 934 and 3274 mm^2 in patients with severe periodontitis. These values are higher than those observed in the present severe periodontitis group ranging between 585 and 2732 mm^2 (mean value 1454 mm^2). In recent years, the surface area of ulcerated epithelium in contact with the subgingival biofilm, previously estimated to be large as the palm of an adult hand (about 7000 mm^2) [53], has been resized to values ranging between 800 and 2000 mm^2 in patients diagnosed with periodontitis [18]. The present data confirm these previous findings.

There is evidence of reduced pancreatic beta-cell function and increased low-grade inflammatory burden in individuals suffering from periodontitis, which in turn affects lipid metabolism and contributes to increased insulin resistance and poor glycemic control [54–57].

This has relevant implications because chronic inflammation represents the biological linking mechanism between periodontitis, T2DM, and its complications [8,9]. A recent systematic review associated diabetes-related retinopathy, nephropathy, and neuropathic foot ulceration to the severity of the periodontal damage [15]. Consistently, effective non-surgical periodontal treatment has resulted in statistically significant reduction of HbA1c levels of about 0.40% at 3 months in T2DM patients [58].

This study has some limitations. A cause–effect interpretation cannot be determined in a cross-sectional survey limiting the strength of the conclusions. The sample size was also limited owing to the use of restricted enrollment criteria. A notably high number of patients were excluded because they had less than eight remaining teeth. As reported by Susanto et al. [34], the application of the PISA Index requires the presence of at least eight natural teeth. Accordingly, a minimum number of four to six natural teeth is needed when using CDC/AAP algorithms to ensure the measurements necessary to diagnose periodontitis and to minimize its misclassification [59,60]. Therefore, the association between periodontitis and T2DM cannot be generalized to almost and completely edentulous persons even though they may have had a past history of periodontal disease.

Furthermore, in spite of the well-established correlation of smoking habits with both poor glycemic control and periodontitis, the number of smokers was small and unable to be included in the statistical analysis [61,62]. Last, we selected a non-random convenience sample of diabetics from an Outpatient Diabetic Center that probably provided medical care to more severely affected T2DM people than the community-based diabetic population. This may limit the generalizability of the present findings.

5. Conclusions

There is a strong association between severe periodontitis and poor glycemic control. The predictors were different when considering the relationship between the two diseases in both directions. The inflammatory burden posed by periodontitis, as measured by the PISA score, represents the strongest predictor of poor glycemic control in T2DM. To the best of our knowledge, this is the first study addressing these clinically relevant aspects using the PISA Index and the CDC/AAP periodontitis case definition. This finding is in line with the prominent role played by poorly controlled T2DM in the progression rate of periodontitis as recently emphasized in the International Workshop on Classification of Periodontal Diseases [30] and by the Joint Workshop of the International Diabetes Federation and the European Federation of Periodontology [8].

Author Contributions: Conceptualization, F.R., S.P., G.G. and M.A.; methodology, F.R., G.B., F.C., M.D., G.G. and M.A.; formal analysis, F.R. and S.P.; investigation, S.E.O.M., M.G., S.B., P.C. and G.M.; resources, F.C. and G.N.B.; data curation, F.R, S.P., S.E.O.M. and S.B.; writing—original draft preparation, F.R. and S.P.; writing—review and editing, G.N.B., G.G. and M.A.; supervision, M.D., G.G. and M.A. All authors have read and agreed to the published version of the manuscript.

Funding: This research received no external funding.

Institutional Review Board Statement: The study was conducted according to the guidelines of the Declaration of Helsinki, and approved by the Institutional Ethics Committee of the "AOU Città della Salute e della Scienza", Turin, Italy (No. 0027219, Date of Approval 14 March 2018).

Informed Consent Statement: Informed consent was obtained from all subjects involved in the study.

Data Availability Statement: The data presented in this study are available on request from the corresponding author.

Conflicts of Interest: The authors declare no conflict of interest.

References

1. Ogurtsova, K.; da Rocha Fernandes, J.D.; Huang, Y.; Linnenkamp, U.; Guariguata, L.; Cho, N.H.; Cavan, D.; Shaw, J.E.; Makaroff, L.E. IDF Diabetes Atlas: Global estimates for the prevalence of diabetes for 2015 and 2040. *Diabetes Res. Clin. Pr.* **2017**, *128*, 40–50. [CrossRef]
2. American Diabetes Association. Classification and diagnosis of diabetes. *Diabetes Care* **2017**, *40* (Suppl. 1), S11–S24. [CrossRef] [PubMed]
3. Mathers, C.D.; Loncar, D. Projections of global mortality and burden of disease from 2002 to 2030. *PLoS Med.* **2006**, *3*, e442. [CrossRef] [PubMed]
4. Forbes, J.M.; Cooper, M.E. Mechanisms of diabetic complications. *Physiol. Rev.* **2013**, *93*, 137–188. [CrossRef] [PubMed]
5. Lind, M.; Odén, A.; Fahlén, M.; Eliasson, B. A systematic review of HbA1c variables used in the study of diabetic complications. *Diabetes Metab. Syndr.* **2008**, *2*, 282–293. [CrossRef]
6. Löe, H. Periodontal disease: The sixth complication of diabetes mellitus. *Diabetes Care* **1993**, *16*, 329–334. [CrossRef]
7. Chee, B.; Park, B.; Barthold, P.M. Periodontitis and type II diabetes: A two-way relationship. *Int. J. Evid. Based Healthc.* **2013**, *11*, 317–329. [CrossRef] [PubMed]
8. Sanz, M.; Ceriello, A.; Buysschaert, M.; Chapple, I.; Demmer, R.T.; Graziani, F.; Herrera, D.; Jepsen, S.; Lione, L.; Madianos, P.; et al. Scientific evidence on the links between periodontal diseases and diabetes: Consensus report and guidelines of the joint workshop on periodontal diseases and diabetes by the International Diabetes Federation and the European Federation of Periodontology. *J. Clin. Periodontol.* **2018**, *45*, 138–149. [CrossRef] [PubMed]
9. Wu, C.-Z.; Yuan, Y.-H.; Liu, H.-H.; Li, S.-S.; Zhang, B.-W.; Chen, W.; An, Z.-J.; Chen, S.-Y.; Wu, Y.-Z.; Han, B.; et al. Epidemiologic relationship between periodontitis and type 2 diabetes mellitus. *BMC Oral Health* **2020**, *20*, 204. [CrossRef]
10. Chavarry, N.G.; Vettore, M.V.; Sansone, C.; Sheiham, A. The relationship between diabetes mellitus and destructive periodontal disease: A meta-analysis. *Oral Health Prev. Dent.* **2009**, *7*, 107–127.
11. Lalla, E.; Papapanou, P.N. Diabetes mellitus and periodontitis: A tale of two common interrelated diseases. *Nat. Rev. Endocrinol.* **2011**, *7*, 738–748. [CrossRef] [PubMed]
12. Chapple, I.L.; Genco, R. Working group 2 of the joint EFP/AAP workshop. Diabetes and periodontal diseases: Consensus report of the joint EFP/AAP Workshop on Periodontitis and Systemic Diseases. *J. Periodontol.* **2013**, *40* (Suppl. 14), 106–112. [CrossRef]
13. Stumvoll, M.; Goldstein, B.J.; van Haeften, T.W. Type 2 diabetes: Principles of pathogenesis and therapy. *Lancet* **2005**, *365*, 1333–1346. [CrossRef]
14. Graves, D.T.; Ding, Z.; Yang, Y. The impact of diabetes on periodontal diseases. *Periodontology 2000* **2020**, *82*, 214–224. [CrossRef]
15. Graziani, F.; Gennai, S.; Solini, A.; Petrini, M. A systematic review and meta-analysis of epidemiologic observational evidence on the effect of periodontitis on diabetes an update of the EFP-AAP review. *J. Clin. Periodontol.* **2018**, *45*, 167–187. [CrossRef]
16. Aral, C.A.; Nalbantoğlu, Ö.; Nur, B.G.; Altunsoy, M.; Aral, K. Metabolic control and periodontal treatment decreases elevated oxidative stress in the early phases of type 1 diabetes onset. *Arch. Oral Biol.* **2017**, *82*, 115–120. [CrossRef]
17. Armitage, G.C. The complete periodontal examination. *Periodontolology 2000* **2004**, *34*, 22–33. [CrossRef] [PubMed]
18. Nesse, W.; Abbas, F.; van der Ploeg, I.; Spijkervet, F.K.; Dijkstra, P.U.; Vissink, A. Periodontal inflamed surface area: Quantifying inflammatory burden. *J. Clin. Periodontol.* **2008**, *35*, 668–673. [CrossRef]
19. Hujoel, P.P.; White, B.A.; Garcia, R.I.; Listgarten, M.A. The dentogingival epithelial surface area revisited. *J. Periodont. Res.* **2001**, *36*, 48–55. [CrossRef] [PubMed]
20. Nesse, W.; Linde, A.; Abbas, F.; Spijkervet, F.K.; Dijkstra, P.U.; de Brabander, E.C.; Gerstenbluth, I.; Vissink, A. Dose–response relationship between periodontal inflamed surface area and HbA1c in type 2 diabetics. *J. Clin. Periodontol.* **2009**, *36*, 295–300. [CrossRef]
21. Leira, Y.; Martín-Lancharro, P.; Blanco, J. Periodontal inflamed surface area and periodontal case definition classification. *Acta Odontol. Scand.* **2018**, *76*, 195–198. [CrossRef]
22. Park, S.Y.; Ahn, S.; Lee, J.T.; Yun, P.Y.; Lee, Y.J.; Lee, J.Y.; Song, Y.W.; Chang, Y.S.; Lee, H.J. Periodontal inflamed surface area as a novel numerical variable describing periodontal conditions. *J. Periodontal Implant. Sci.* **2017**, *47*, 328–338. [CrossRef]
23. Balaji, S.K.; Lavu, V.; Rao, S. Chronic periodontitis prevalence and the inflammatory burden in a sample population from South India. *Indian J. Dent. Res.* **2018**, *29*, 254. [CrossRef] [PubMed]
24. Novak, M.J.; Potter, R.M.; Blodgett, J.; Ebersole, J.L. Periodontal disease in Hispanic Americans with type 2 diabetes. *J. Periodontol.* **2008**, *79*, 629–636. [CrossRef] [PubMed]
25. Wang, T.T.; Chen, T.H.; Wang, P.E.; Lai, H.; Lo, M.T.; Chen, P.Y.C.; Chiu, S.Y.H. A population-based study on the association between type 2 diabetes and periodontal disease in 12,123 middle-aged Taiwanese (KCIS No. 21). *J. Clin. Periodontol.* **2009**, *36*, 372–379. [CrossRef]
26. Bonora, E.; Cataudella, S.; Marchesini, G.; Miccoli, R.; Vaccaro, O.; Fadini, G.P.; Martini, L.; Rossi, E. Under te mandate of the Italian Diabetes Society. Clinical burden of diabetes in Italy in 2018: A look at a systemic disease from the ARNO Diabetes Observatory. *BMJ Open Diab. Res. Care* **2020**, *8*, e001191. [CrossRef]
27. Alberti, K.G.; Zimmet, P.Z. Definition, diagnosis and classification of diabetes mellitus and its complications. Part 1: Diagnosis and classification of diabetes mellitus provisional report of a WHO consultation. *Diabet. Med.* **1998**, *15*, 539–553. [CrossRef]
28. Page, R.C.; Eke, P.I. Case definitions for use in population-based surveillance of periodontitis. *J. Periodontol.* **2007**, *78*, 1387–1399. [CrossRef]

29. Eke, P.I.; Page, R.C.; Wei, L.; Thornton-Evans, G.; Genco, R.J. Update of the case definitions for population-based surveillance of periodontitis. *J. Periodontol.* **2012**, *83*, 1449–1454. [CrossRef]
30. Tonetti, M.S.; Greenwell, H.; Kornman, K.S. Staging and grading of periodontitis: Framework and proposal of a new classification and case definition. *J. Clin. Periodontol.* **2018**, *89* (Suppl. 20), S159–S172. [CrossRef]
31. Kolb, H.; Martin, S. Environmental/lifestyle factors in the pathogenesis and prevention of type 2 diabetes. *BMC Med.* **2017**, *15*, 131. [CrossRef] [PubMed]
32. Holtfreter, B.; Albandar, J.M.; Dietrich, T.; Dye, B.A.; Eaton, K.A.; Eke, P.I.; Papapanou, P.N.; Kocher, T.; Joint EU/USA Periodontal Epidemiology Working Group. Standards of reporting chronic periodontitis prevalence and severity in epidemiological studies: Proposed standards from the Joint EU/USA Periodontal Epidemiology Working Group. *J. Clin. Periodontol.* **2015**, *42*, 407–412. [CrossRef] [PubMed]
33. Preshaw, P.M.; de Silva, N.; McCracken, G.I.; Fernando, D.J.S.; Dalton, C.F.; Steen, N.D.; Heasman, P.A. Compromised periodontal status in an urban Sri Lankan population with type 2 diabetes. *J. Clin. Periodontol.* **2010**, *37*, 165–171. [CrossRef] [PubMed]
34. Susanto, H.; Nesse, W.; Dijkstra, P.U.; Hoedemaker, E.; van Reenen, Y.H.; Agustina, D.; Vissink, A.; Abbas, F. Periodontal inflamed surface area and C-reactive protein as predictors of HbA1c: A study in Indonesia. *Clin. Oral. Investig.* **2012**, *16*, 1237–1242. [CrossRef]
35. Kim, E.-K.; Lee, S.G.; Choi, Y.-H.; Won, K.-C.; Moon, J.S.; Merchant, A.T.; Lee, H.-K. Association between diabetes-related factors and clinical periodontal parameters in type-2 diabetes mellitus. *BMC Oral Health* **2013**, *13*, 64. [CrossRef]
36. Mohamed, H.G.; Idris, S.B.; Ahmed, M.F.; Bøe, O.E.; Mustafa, K.; Ibrahim, S.O.; Åstrøm, A.N. Association between oral health status and type 2 diabetes mellitus among Sudanese adults: A matched case-control study. *PLoS ONE* **2013**, *8*, e82158. [CrossRef] [PubMed]
37. Hong, J.W.; Noh, J.H.; Kim, D.-J. The prevalence and associated factors of periodontitis according to fasting plasma glucose in the Korean adults. *Medicine* **2016**, *95*, e3226. [CrossRef]
38. Aimetti, M.; Perotto, S.; Castiglione, A.; Mariani, G.M.; Ferrarotti, F.; Romano, F. Prevalence of periodontitis in an adult population from an urban area in North Italy: Findings from a cross-sectional population-based epidemiological survey. *J. Clin. Periodontol.* **2015**, *42*, 622–631. [CrossRef] [PubMed]
39. Abduljabbar, T.; Al-sahaly, F.; Al-kathami, M.; Afza, S.; Vohra, F. Comparison of periodontal and peri-implant inflammatory parameters among patients with prediabetes, type 2 diabetes mellitus and non-diabetic controls. *Acta Odontol. Scand.* **2017**, *75*, 319–324. [CrossRef] [PubMed]
40. Kowall, B.; Holtfreter, B.; Volzke, H.; Schipf, S.; Mundt, T.; Rathmann, W.; Kocher, T. Pre-diabetes and well-controlled diabetes are not associated with periodontal disease: The SHIP Trend Study. *J. Clin. Periodontol.* **2015**, *42*, 422–430. [CrossRef]
41. Campus, G.; Salem, A.; Uzzau, S.; Baldoni, E.; Tonolo, G. Diabetes and periodontal disease. A case-control study. *J. Periodontol.* **2005**, *76*, 418–425. [CrossRef] [PubMed]
42. Ioannidou, E.; Malekzadeh, T.; Dongari-Bagtzoglou, A. Effect of periodontal treatment on serum C-reactive protein levels: A systematic review and meta-analysis. *J. Periodontol.* **2006**, *77*, 1635–1642. [CrossRef] [PubMed]
43. Polak, D.; Sanui, T.; Nishimura, F.; Shapira, L. Diabetes as a risk factor for periodontal disease-Plausible mechanisms. *Periodontology 2000* **2020**, *83*, 46–58. [CrossRef]
44. Susanto, H.; Nesse, W.; Dijkstra, P.U.; Agustina, D.; Vissink, A.; Abbas, F. Periodontitis prevalence and severity in Indonesians with type 2 diabetes. *J. Periodontol.* **2011**, *82*, 550–557. [CrossRef]
45. Sora, N.D.; Marlow, N.M.; Bandyopadhyay, D.; Leite, R.S.; Slate, E.H.; Fernandes, J.K. Metabolic syndrome and periodontitis in Gullah African Americans with type 2 diabetes mellitus. *J. Clin. Periodontol.* **2013**, *40*, 599–606. [CrossRef] [PubMed]
46. Kirwan, J.P.; Sacks, J.; Nieuwoudt, S. The essential role of exercise in the management of type 2 diabetes. *Cleve. Clin. J. Med.* **2017**, *84* (7 Suppl. 1), S15–S21. [CrossRef]
47. Janiiszewski, P.M.; Janssen, I.; Ross, R. Does waist circumference predict diabetes and cardiovascular disease beyond commonly evaluated cardio metabolic risk factors? *Diabetes Care* **2007**, *30*, 3105–3109. [CrossRef]
48. Romano, F.; Bongiovanni, L.; Bianco, L.; Di Scipio, F.; Yang, Z.; Sprio, A.E.; Berta, G.N.; Aimetti, M. Biomarker levels in gingival crevicular fluid of generalized aggressive periodontitis patients after non-surgical periodontal treatment. *Clin. Oral Invest.* **2018**, *22*, 1083–1092. [CrossRef] [PubMed]
49. Romano, F.; Del Buono, W.; Bianco, L.; Arana, M.; Mariani, G.M.; Di Scipio, F.; Berta, G.N.; Aimetti, M. Gingival crevicular fluid cytokines in moderate and deep pocket sites of Stage III periodontitis patients in different rated of clinical progression. *Biomedicines* **2020**, *8*, 515. [CrossRef]
50. Loos, B.G. Systemic markers of inflammation of periodontitis. *J. Periodontol.* **2006**, *76*, 2106–2115. [CrossRef] [PubMed]
51. Polak, D.; Shapira, L. An update of the evidence for pathogenic mechanisms that may link periodontitis and diabetes. *J. Clin. Periodontol.* **2018**, *45*, 150–166. [CrossRef] [PubMed]
52. Cecoro, G.; Annunziata, M.; Iuorio, M.T.; Nastri, L.; Guida, L. Periodontitis, low-grade inflammation and systemic health: A scoping review. *Medicina* **2020**, *56*, 272. [CrossRef]
53. Page, R.C. The pathobiology of periodontal diseases may affect systemic diseases: Inversion of a paradigm. *Ann. Periodontol.* **1998**, *3*, 108–120. [CrossRef] [PubMed]
54. Preshaw, P.M.; Foster, N.; Taylor, J.I. Cross-susceptibility between periodontal disease and type 2 diabetes mellitus: An immunobiological perspective. *Periodontology 2000* **2007**, *45*, 138–157. [CrossRef]

55. Nishimura, F.; Soga, Y.; Iwamoto, Y.; Kudo, C.; Murayama, Y. Periodontal disease as part of the insulin resistance syndrome in diabetic patients. *J. Int. Acad. Periodontol.* **2005**, *7*, 16–20.
56. Shoelson, S.E.; Lee, J.; Goldfine, A.B. Inflammation and insulin resistance. *J. Clin. Investig.* **2006**, *116*, 793–1801. [CrossRef] [PubMed]
57. Engebretson, S.; Chertog, R.; Nichols, A.; Hey-Hadavi, J.; Celenti, R.; Grbic, J. Plasma levels of tumour necrosis factor-alpha in patients with chronic periodontitis and type 2 diabetes. *J. Clin. Periodontol.* **2007**, *34*, 18–24. [CrossRef]
58. Madianos, P.M.; Koromantzos, P.A. An update of the evidence on the potential impact of periodontal therapy on diabetes outcomes. *J. Clin. Periodontol.* **2018**, *45*, 188–195. [CrossRef] [PubMed]
59. Pérez, C.; Muñoz, F.; Andriankaja, O.M.; Ritchie, C.S.; Martínez, S.; Vergara, J.; Vivaldi, J.; Lòpez, L.; Campos, M.; Joshipura, K.J. Cross-sectional associations of impaired glucose metabolism measures with bleeding on probing and periodontitis. *J. Clin. Periodontol.* **2017**, *44*, 142–149. [CrossRef] [PubMed]
60. Romano, F.; Perotto, S.; Castiglione, A.; Aimetti, M. Prevalence of periodontitis: Misclassification, under-recognition or over-diagnosis using partial and full-mouth periodontal examination protocols. *Acta Odontol. Scand.* **2019**, *77*, 189–196. [CrossRef] [PubMed]
61. Nilsson, P.M.; Gudbjörnsdottir, S.; Eliasson, B.; Cederholm, J.; Steering Committee of the Swedish National Diabetes Register. Smoking is associated with increased HbA1c values and microalbuminuria in patients with diabetes-data from the National Diabetes Register in Sweden. *Diabetes Metab.* **2004**, *30*, 261–268. [CrossRef]
62. Leite, F.R.M.; Nascimento, G.G.; Scheutz, F.; Lòpez, R. Effect of smoking on periodontitis: A systematic review and meta-regression. *Am. J. Prev. Med.* **2018**, *54*, 831–841. [CrossRef] [PubMed]

Journal of Clinical Medicine

Article

Lipid Peroxidation Levels in Saliva and Plasma of Patients Suffering from Periodontitis

Tanja Veljovic [1,*], Milanko Djuric [1,2], Jelena Mirnic [1], Ivana Gusic [1,2], Aleksandra Maletin [1], Bojana Ramic [1], Isidora Neskovic [1,2], Karolina Vukoje [1] and Snezana Brkic [1,3]

1. Department of Dental Medicine, Faculty of Medicine, University of Novi Sad, 21000 Novi Sad, Serbia; milanko.djuric@mf.uns.ac.rs (M.D.); jelena.mirnic@mf.uns.ac.rs (J.M.); ivana.gusic@mf.uns.ac.rs (I.G.); aleksandra.maletin@mf.uns.ac.rs (A.M.); bojana.ramic@mf.uns.ac.rs (B.R.); isidora.neskovic@mf.uns.ac.rs (I.N.); karolina.vukoje@mf.uns.ac.rs (K.V.); snezana.brkic@mf.uns.ac.rs (S.B.)
2. Dentistry Clinic of Vojvodina, 21000 Novi Sad, Serbia
3. Clinic for Infectious Diseases, Clinical Centre of Vojvodina, 21000 Novi Sad, Serbia
* Correspondence: tanja.veljovic@mf.uns.ac.rs; Tel.: +381-643-037-449

Abstract: Lipid peroxidation (LPO) participates in the development of various diseases, including periodontitis, and malondialdehyde (MDA) is its terminal product. Therefore, in the present study, salivary and plasma MDA levels in 30 periodontitis patients were compared to those in 20 healthy controls, as well as in relation to periodontal therapy in order to assess its effectiveness. Periodontal status was assessed via plaque index, gingival index, papilla bleeding index, probing depth and clinical attachment level, while salivary and plasma MDA levels were determined by the ELISA method. The periodontitis group had a significantly greater salivary (2.99 pmol/μL) and plasma (0.50 pmol/μL) MDA levels relative to the healthy controls (1.33 pmol/μL and 0.40 pmol/μL, respectively). Three months after the periodontal therapy completion, although salivary MDA levels were significantly lower than those measured at the baseline ($p < 0.001$), the reduction in plasma MDA was not statistically significant ($p > 0.05$). These findings indicate that, while inflammatory processes in periodontium may increase local and systemic lipid peroxidation, periodontal therapy can result in a significant decrease in salivary, but not plasma, MDA levels.

Keywords: malondialdehyde; oxidative stress; periodontitis; plasma

1. Introduction

Periodontitis is an inflammatory disease of tooth-supporting structures, which leads to tissue destruction and tooth loss as a result of the interaction of dental plaque microorganisms and the host's immune response. According to the World Health Organization (WHO) data, the global incidence of a more severe form of periodontal disease is estimated at 10–15% [1]. Therefore, this disease is a serious medical, economic and social problem. The significance of periodontitis is increased further due to its potential impact on systemic health. Although the exact mechanism of this relationship has not been fully elucidated, in recent years, increasing importance has been attached to oxidative stress arising in the course of periodontal disease as a potential risk factor in the development of some systemic diseases [2,3].

Oxidative stress arises due to an imbalance between the reactive oxygen species (ROS) and the antioxidant defense system, which results in damage to important cellular macromolecules, such as lipids, proteins and DNA. Lipid peroxidation (LPO) is the process of oxidative lipid damage. Due to the significant presence of lipids in the cell membrane and its subcellular organelles, they are the site of peroxidation onset. The LPO outcome is a marked change in the membrane permeability, which contributes to the degradation of cellular metabolism and homeostasis and may ultimately result in cell death [4].

ROS are unstable molecules with a short half-life, making them difficult to detect. This issue is overcome by using the terminal products of macromolecule oxidative damage, one of which is malondialdehyde (MDA), as it results from lipid oxidative damage. An extensive body of empirical data indicates that the MDA level in bodily fluids may be a reliable indicator of the extent of oxidative damage to cells in the body [5]. Available research indicates that MDA levels are increased due to cancer [6], atherosclerosis [7], diabetes [8], liver disease [9] and preeclampsia [10], as well as in smokers, while recent data suggest a strong link with periodontal disease [11–15].

Previously, the LPO level in saliva was believed to be predominantly affected by the extent of this process in blood. However, recent evidence indicates that locally induced oxidative stress plays a more important role. Namely, in the course of periodontal disease, free radical production by polymorphonuclear leukocytes increases as a defense mechanism against periodontopathogens. Existing studies indicate that, in the course of periodontal disease, LPO products such as MDA are released and participate in the progress of periodontal tissue inflammation and destruction [13–18]. However, periodontal therapy is believed to induce a reduction in this marker.

Furthermore, available research findings suggest that LPO products diffuse from the initial inflammation site and can be registered in the bloodstream [19]. This process could result in the emergence of certain systemic diseases. Tests conducted on laboratory animals have shown that experimentally induced periodontal disease can cause oxidative damage to the liver, thus increasing oxidative stress in the blood [20–23]. In addition, oxidative stress due to damage to periodontal tissues is posited to be involved in the development of atherosclerosis in laboratory animals [24]. As the number of such studies involving humans is limited, further research is required in order to reach more definitive conclusions about the impact of periodontal disease on systemic oxidative stress.

The objectives of the present investigation were to: (1) compare the level of LPO in plasma and saliva of patients with and without periodontal disease; (2) examine the impact of periodontal therapy on the salivary and blood LPO levels in patients with periodontitis; and (3) examine the link between the level of LPO and clinical markers of periodontal status.

The overall aim of the study was to determine if periodontitis can result in an increase in local and systemic oxidative stress levels, which would potentially provide a link between periodontitis and systemic diseases.

2. Materials and Methods

2.1. Subjects

This research involved 50 patients. All participants were informed in writing about the study aims, the nature of their involvement and the intended use of the results obtained, after which they signed the consent form. The study was approved by the local ethics committee. All procedures performed in the study involving human participants were in accordance with the Declaration of Helsinki.

The study inclusion criteria were being 30–70 years old, having at least 20 teeth and being systemically healthy. Patients were excluded from the study if they met any of the following criteria: periodontal therapy in the previous six months, use of antibiotics in the last three months, use of any vitamin supplementation and pregnancy.

2.2. Periodontal Examination

In all study participants, periodontal status was assessed via plaque index (PI) [25], gingival index (GI) [26], papilla bleeding index (PIB) [27], probing depth (PD) and clinical attachment level (CAL). We utilized the same indices in our earlier studies, as empirical evidence indicated that they are most representative of periodontium conditions [28–30]. Measurements were performed on mesio-buccal, disto-buccal, mid-buccal and mid-lingual tooth surfaces using Michigan 'O' probe with William's markings. All measurements were performed by the same periodontist.

2.3. Study Groups

Criteria for inclusion in the group of patients with periodontal disease were as follows: at least two sites per quadrant with PD ≥ 4 mm, 30% bone loss and gingival inflammation [31]. Thirty periodontitis patients formed the experimental group, designated as Group A. The control group (Group B) consisted of 20 patients with no signs of damage to periodontal supporting structures. Before commencing the study, we used power analysis, which indicated that 18 participants would be sufficient for achieving a 95% power and 95% significance level. As our study design involved pre- and post-treatment evaluations, to account for possible attrition, we included 20 and 30 patients in the control and the experimental group, respectively.

In order to assess the influence of the GI, PD and CAL on the MDA levels, periodontitis patients were divided into six subgroups. The GI levels allowed a further division into two subgroups, comprising of individuals with moderate (Loë–Silness 0.1–2) and severe (Loë–Silness 2.1–3) inflammation. Similarly, two subgroups were formed based on the PD, with patients with PD ≥ 5 mm on more than 20% of sites forming one subgroup and those with PD ≥ 5 mm on fewer than 20% of sites forming the other. Finally, CAL was used to separate patients into a subgroup with the mean value of CAL ≥ 3 mm and CAL < 3 mm, respectively.

2.4. Sample Collection and Preparation

Determination of oxidative stress markers was conducted in mixed unstimulated saliva samples taken in the morning from patients who were instructed not to drink or eat prior to attending the appointment. Salivary samples were centrifuged at 3000× g for 10 min at room temperature, after which time the supernatant was isolated and stored at −80 °C until required for analysis.

Blood samples were taken from a fingertip and collected in special tubes coated with EDTA (Kabe Labotechnik, Nümbrecht-Elsenroth, Germany) and were transported to the laboratory, where they were immediately centrifuged at 3000× g for 10 min. The thus obtained plasma samples were stored at −80 °C until required for analysis.

2.5. MDA Assay

The salivary and blood MDA values were determined using the commercial OxiSelect MDA Adduct ELISA Kit (Cell Biolabs' OxiSelect, San Diego, CA, USA) according to the manufacturer's instructions. The kit had a sensitivity limit of 2 pmol/mg MDA adduct. All samples were tested in duplicate. MDA concentration was expressed in pmol/μL.

2.6. Treatment

Patients with periodontal disease were subjected to periodontal therapy comprising of scaling and root planing using Gracey curettes and ultrasonic scalers (Mini Piezon, Electro-Medical Systems, Nyon, Switzerland). The therapy was carried out in the form of 1–2 visits within 7 days without the use of antibiotics or antiseptics.

2.7. Follow-Up

Patients included in the experimental group underwent periodontal status assessment and had their saliva and blood samples taken during the first visit prior to commencing periodontal therapy, as well as three months after therapy completion, while the control group was subjected to the same procedure at the baseline only.

2.8. Statistical Analysis

Data collected as a part of the study were analyzed using the statistical package SPSS 16 for Windows. All values are presented as mean ± SD. Pearson χ^2 test was used for testing relationships between individual pairs of observed attribute characteristics (gender). On the other hand, a *t*-test was performed to determine the differences in the mean values of numerical characteristics (age, number of teeth present, periodontal indices, comparison of index levels before and after the treatment, level of lipid peroxidation in the two groups, comparison of oxidative stress marker values obtained before and after treatment). The correlation between lipid peroxidation markers in saliva and blood was determined by Spearman's rank correlation coefficient. We adopted the factorial ANOVA test to assess the influence of the confounding factors (sex, age and smoking status) on MDA values. The results for which the level of significance met the $p < 0.05$ criterion were interpreted as statistically significant.

3. Results

As can be seen from the flow chart of the experimental design presented in Figure 1, 87 individuals were initially eligible for participation in the study. However, eleven were excluded because they did not meet the inclusion criteria, while a further six refused to participate. After full-mouth periodontal clinical parameters examination, further 13 patients were excluded because they did not meet either Group A or Group B criteria. The remaining 57 patients were divided into Group A (37 patients) and Group B (20 patients). However, as seven patients from Group A did not return for the 3-month visit, their data were excluded from statistical analyses.

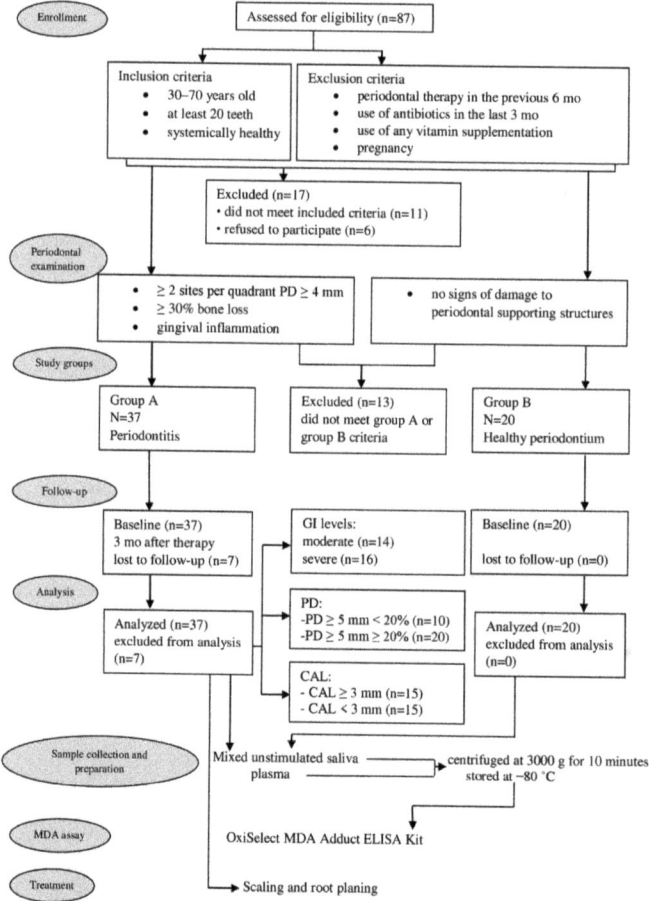

Figure 1. Flow chart of clinical study. GI—gingival index; PD—probing depth; CAL—clinical attachment level; MDA—malondialdehyde.

Therefore, the study sample comprised 50 patients, 30 of whom suffered from periodontitis (10 men and 20 women, average age 48.70 ± 9.68), while the remaining 20 had a healthy periodontium (9 men and 11 women, average age 46.25 ± 9.25).

The demographic characteristics of the patients are shown in Table 1. No statistically significant differences in age, gender and number of teeth present in the two groups were noted.

Table 1. Patients' demographic characteristics.

	Group A (n = 30)	Group B (n = 20)	p-Value
Gender, n (%)			0.553
Male	10 (33.3%)	9 (45%)	
Female	20 (66.7%)	11 (55%)	
Age in years (mean ± SD)	48.70 ± 9.68	46.25 ± 9.25	0.472
Number of teeth (mean ± SD)	22.54 ± 2.14	25.34 ± 3.94	0.487
Smoking, n (%)			1.000
Yes	10 (33.3%)	7 (35%)	
No	20 (66.7%)	13 (65%)	

The mean values of the examined clinical parameters obtained before and after periodontal treatment are shown in Table 2. At baseline, the mean values of all periodontal indices were statistically significantly higher in the experimental group compared to the controls. Periodontal therapy led to a significant reduction in these indices in the group of patients with periodontitis.

Table 2. Periodontal indices and MDA levels at baseline and three months upon therapy completion (mean ± SD, minimum−maximum).

	Group A Baseline	Group A Three Months after Therapy	Group B
PI	1.40 ± 0.43 (0.83−1.97)	0.35 ± 0.22 (0.08−1.12) [a]	0.32 ± 0.28 (0.04−1.01) [b]
GI	1.79 ± 0.64 (1.08−2.79)	0.25 ± 0.33 (0.02−1.31) [a]	0.19 ± 0.37 (0.00−0.50) [b]
PBI	1.57 ± 0.81 (0.64−3.47)	0.71 ± 0.43 (0.08−1.73) [a]	0.28 ± 0.39 (0.00−1.78) [b,c]
PD (mm)	3.14 ± 0.56 (2.87−4.42)	2.59 ± 0.45 (1.95−3.81) [a]	1.45 ± 0.18 (1.13−1.71) [b,c]
CAL (mm)	2.70 ± 1.03 (1.76−5.50)	2.19 ± 0.81 (0.59−4.08) [a]	0.43 ± 0.56 (0.00−1.09) [b,c]
MDA-saliva (pmol/μL)	2.99 ± 1.21 (1.11−4.80)	2.14 ± 0.95 (1.11−4.80) [a]	1.33 ± 0.92 (0.23−3.70) [b,c]
MDA-plasma (pmol/μL)	0.50 ± 0.13 (0.29−0.70)	0.47 ± 0.11 (0.29−0.70)	0.40 ± 0.13 (0.13−0.62) [b]

[a] Statistically significant difference compared with the baseline values ($p < 0.05$) [b] The difference between Group A and Group B was significant at the baseline ($p < 0.05$). [c] Statistically significant difference compared with the values after therapy ($p < 0.05$).

The salivary level of the tested LPO marker (MDA) in the experimental group was significantly higher at baseline than in the control group, and its values were significantly reduced three months upon periodontal therapy completion (Table 2). Further, in patients with periodontal disease, markedly higher MDA values in plasma were noted relative to those measured in subjects with healthy periodontium (Table 2). Periodontal therapy, however, did not yield a statistically significant reduction in the MDA levels in plasma of patients with periodontal disease.

Patients with severe gingival inflammation had significantly higher MDA levels in saliva compared to patients with moderate gingival inflammation (Table 3). However, no statistically significant differences in the level of this marker in saliva were noted between the subgroups with PD $\geq$ 5 mm $\geq$ 20% and PD $\geq$ 5 mm < 20% (Table 4) or between those with CAL $\geq$ 3 mm and CAL < 3 mm (Table 5). The results obtained from plasma analysis indicate that the MDA level in patients with severe gingival inflammation was significantly higher compared to that in patients with moderate gingival inflammation (Table 3). When the patients were divided into subgroups based on the PD and CAL values, the differences noted between MDA values in plasma were found not to be statistically significant (Tables 4 and 5).

Table 3. Periodontal indices and MDA levels at baseline and three months upon therapy completion in groups with moderate and severe gingival inflammation (GI).

	GI Moderate (n = 14)	GI Severe (n = 16)
PI—baseline	1.08 ± 0.27	1.76 ± 0.11 [a]
PI—3 mo after therapy	0.31 ± 0.10 [b]	0.67 ± 0.35 [b]
GI—baseline	1.37 ± 0.26	2.28 ± 0.21 [a]
GI—3 mo after therapy	0.41 ± 0.20 [b]	0.68 ± 0.52 [b]
PBI—baseline	1.89 ± 0.39	2.01 ± 0.77 [a]
PBI—3 mo after therapy	0.56 ± 0.27 [b]	0.88 ± 0.53 [b]
PD (mm)—baseline	2.88 ± 0.40	3.30 ± 0.57 [a]
PD (mm)—3 mo after therapy	2.40 ± 0.31 [b]	2.81 ± 0.49 [b]
CAL (mm)—baseline	2.48 ± 0.78	2.96 ± 1.32
CAL (mm)—3 mo after therapy	1.69 ± 0.73 [b]	1.91 ± 1.03 [b]
MDA-saliva (pmol/µL)—baseline	2.42 ± 1.10	3.62 ± 1.22 [a]
MDA-saliva (pmol/µL)—3 mo after therapy	1.83 ± 0.73 [b]	2.50 ± 1.07 [b]
MDA-plasma (pmol/µL)—baseline	0.45 ± 0.12	0.55 ± 0.13 [a]
MDA-plasma (pmol/µL)—3 mo after therapy	0.43 ± 0.12	0.51 ± 0.09

[a] The difference between subgroups with moderate and severe inflammation was significant at baseline ($p < 0.05$).
[b] Statistically significant difference compared with the baseline values ($p < 0.05$).

At baseline, MDA levels in saliva showed a significant positive correlation with MDA levels in the plasma of patients with periodontal disease (r = 0.451, p = 0.012) (Figure 2).

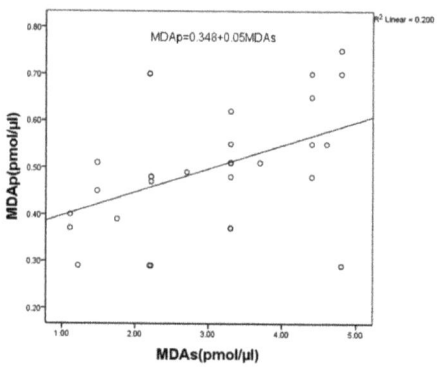

Figure 2. Correlation between MDA levels in saliva and plasma in periodontitis patients. Statistically significant at $p < 0.05$. MDAp—malondialdehyde in plasma; MDAs—malondialdehyde in saliva.

Table 4. Periodontal indices and MDA levels at baseline and three months upon therapy completion in groups with PD ≥ 5 mm < 20% and PD ≥ 5 mm ≥ 20%.

	PD ≥ 5 mm < 20% (n = 10)	PD ≥ 5 mm ≥ 20% (n = 20)
PI—baseline	1.24 ± 0.32	1.49 ± 0.43
PI—3 mo after therapy	0.37 ± 0.23 [b]	0.54 ± 0.33 [b]
GI—baseline	1.55 ± 0.54	1.93 ± 0.45
GI—3 mo after therapy	0.48 ± 0.34 [b]	0.59 ± 0.44 [b]
PBI—baseline	1.41 ± 0.74	1.67 ± 0.71
PBI—3 mo after therapy	0.59 ± 0.40 [b]	0.78 ± 0.45 [b]
PD (mm)—baseline	2.58 ± 0.21	3.46 ± 0.41 [a]
PD (mm)—3 mo after therapy	2.21 ± 0.21 [b]	2.81 ± 0.40 [b]
CAL (mm)—baseline	2.22 ± 0.91	2.99 ± 1.01 [a]
CAL (mm)—3 mo after therapy	1.45 ± 0.75 [b]	1.98 ± 0.90 [b]
MDA-saliva (pmol/µL)—baseline	2.62 ± 1.11	3.21 ± 1.23
MDA-saliva (pmol/µL)—3 mo after therapy	2.09 ± 0.88 [b]	2.15 ± 1.03 [b]
MDA-plasma (pmol/µL)—baseline	0.44 ± 0.12	0.53 ± 0.12
MDA-plasma (pmol/µL)—3 mo after therapy	0.42 ± 0.12	0.45 ± 0.11 [b]

[a] The difference between subgroups with PD ≥ 5 mm < 20% and PD ≥ 5 mm ≥ 20% was significant at baseline ($p < 0.05$). [b] Statistically significant difference compared with the baseline values ($p < 0.05$).

Table 5. Periodontal indices and MDA levels at baseline and three months upon therapy completion in groups with CAL < 3 mm and CAL ≥ 3 mm.

	CAL < 3 mm (n = 15)	CAL ≥ 3 mm (n = 15)
PI—baseline	1.22 ± 0.37	1.58 ± 0.36 [a]
PI—3 mo after therapy	0.43 ± 0.28 [b]	0.53 ± 0.33 [b]
GI—baseline	1.65 ± 0.50	1,94 ± 0.43
GI—3 mo after therapy	0.49 ± 0.34 [b]	0.60 ± 0.46 [b]
PBI—baseline	1.38 ± 0.78	1.77 ± 0.62
PBI—3 mo after therapy	0.53 ± 0.33 [b]	0.88 ± 0.46 [b]
PD (mm)—baseline	3.05 ± 0.61	3.23 ± 0.50
PD (mm)—3 mo after therapy	2.42 ± 0.31 [b]	2.75 ± 0.52 [b]
CAL (mm)—baseline	1.99 ± 0.72	3.42 ± 0.77 [a]
CAL (mm)—3 mo after therapy	1.35 ± 0.69 [b]	2.23 ± 0.83 [b]
MDA-saliva (pmol/µL)—baseline	2.80 ± 0.91	3.18 ± 1.45
MDA-saliva (pmol/µL)—3 mo after therapy	2.09 ± 0.74 [b]	2.18 ± 1.15 [b]
MDA-plasma (pmol/µL)—baseline	0.46 ± 0.13	0.54 ± 0.13
MDA-plasma (pmol/µL)—3 mo after therapy	0.44 ± 0.08	0.49 ± 0.14

[a] The difference between subgroups with CAL < 3 mm and CAL ≥ 3 mm was significant at baseline ($p < 0.05$). [b] Statistically significant difference compared with the baseline values ($p < 0.05$).

The results yielded by the *t*-test and correlation analysis indicate the absence of statistically significant differences in the MDA levels in blood and saliva with respect to patients' sex or age in either study group (Table 6).

Table 6. The influence of sex, age and smoking status on the salivary and plasma MDA levels.

Parameter	MDA-Plasma		MDA-Saliva	
Variable	Statistics	p-Value	Statistics	p-Value
Group	2.593 [a]	0.013	5.226 [a]	<0.001
Smoking	−3.077 [a]	0.003	−4.543 [a]	<0.001
Gender	0.073 [a]	0.942	−1.249 [a]	0.218
Age	0.155 [b]	0.283	0.014 [b]	0.926

[a] Independent t-test, [b] Correlation coefficient.

Given the well-established prooxidative effect of tobacco smoke, the salivary and plasma MDA values in relation to the smoking status were analyzed in both study groups. In the group comprising patients with periodontitis, there were 10 smokers and 20 non-smokers, while in the control group, the ratio was 7 to 13 (Table 1). In smokers with periodontitis, the MDA value in saliva and plasma was 4.06 pmol/μL and 0.57 pmol/μL, respectively, while 2.46 pmol/μL and 0.46 pmol/μL were measured for non-smokers with periodontitis. In the control group, these values were 2.34 pmol/μL and 0.49 pmol/μL for smokers and 0.77 pmol/μL and 0.35 pmol/μL for non-smokers (Figures 3 and 4).

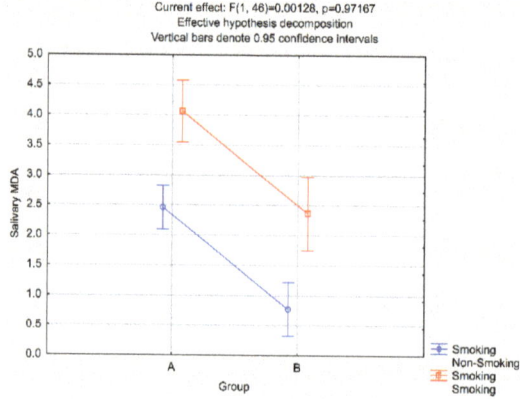

Figure 3. Salivary MDA and smoking interaction.

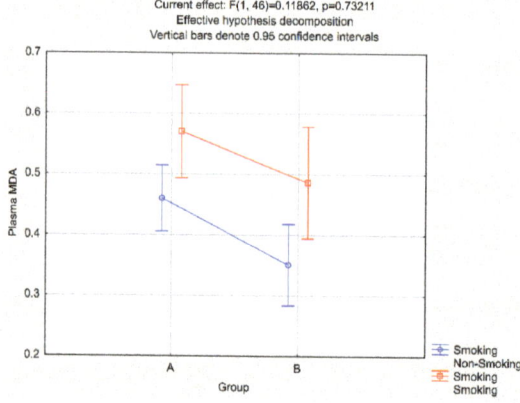

Figure 4. Plasma MDA and smoking interaction.

The salivary and plasma MDA levels in smokers were statistically significantly higher than those measured for non-smokers in both groups. Therefore, a factorial ANOVA test was conducted to analyze the average salivary and plasma MDA levels according to study groups and smoking status. The obtained p-values suggest the presence of statistically significant differences in both salivary and plasma MDA between groups, as well as between smokers and non-smokers, but that there is no statistically significant interaction between groups or between smokers and non-smokers (Figures 3 and 4).

4. Discussion

Misbalance between the production of free radicals and antioxidant protection leads to oxidative stress in the oral cavity. Existing studies show that the LPO terminal product concentrations in the gingival crevicular fluid and saliva of patients with periodontal disease are significantly higher compared to patients with healthy periodontium [16,18,32–36]. For example, Canakci et al. recorded an MDA concentration of 7.35 nmol/mL in the saliva of periodontitis patients, compared to 5.41 nmol/mL in subjects with healthy periodontium [13]. The results yielded by our investigation also indicate an increase in the salivary MDA levels in the presence of periodontal tissue inflammation. The value of this marker in patients with periodontal disease at baseline was 2.99 pmol/µL, which is significantly greater than 1.33 pmol/µL measured in healthy subjects. Higher MDA values obtained in the study conducted by Canakci et al. can be attributed to a greater degree of destruction to the periodontal supporting structures than was observed in our patients, as well as differences in methodology [13]. Specifically, this group of authors used stimulated saliva, whereas unstimulated saliva was utilized in our study. It is known that, during the sampling of stimulated saliva, greater quantities of gingival crevicular fluid are exerted into the saliva, which can significantly increase the values of the tested markers.

Empirical evidence supports the view that LPO marker levels can be used to estimate the extent of periodontium destruction [37]. This is confirmed by the findings reported by Khalili et al., who noted higher MDA values in patients with periodontal disease relative to healthy controls [11]. In addition, these authors found differences in the values of this marker in patients with mild, moderate and severe forms of the disease and reported a significant correlation between MDA and papilla bleeding index, probing depth and clinical attachment level. On the other hand, based on a comparison of the clinical parameters of periodontal disease with the MDA levels in saliva, Dakovic reported the presence of a link between the level of this marker and the degree of inflammation, but not periodontal probing depth [12]. As periodontitis is a cyclical process, whereby periods of remission alternate with periods of exacerbation, marked by the activation of all signs of inflammation, this author postulated that high MDA levels in patients with periodontal disease might be a sign of active processes in the periodontium. The results obtained in our study are consistent with the findings reported by Dakovic [12]. The salivary MDA levels in our patients were primarily influenced by gingival inflammation. Specifically, patients with severe gingival inflammation had significantly higher MDA values (3.62 pmol/µL) compared to patients with moderate inflammation (2.42 pmol/µL) ($p = 0.045$). The impact of probing depth, and clinical attachment level in particular, was not statistically significant.

In our study, periodontal therapy led to a significant reduction in the LPO levels in the saliva of patients with periodontal disease. Dakovic also reported a 58% reduction in the MDA levels in saliva of patients with the periodontal disease following treatment and concluded that, along with the elimination of gingival inflammation, the products of cell oxidative damage are also neutralized by periodontal therapy [12]. Based on the analysis of the salivary MDA values obtained after treatment in relation to the extent of gingival inflammation, probing depth and clinical attachment level, we can conclude that the reduction in MDA was primarily caused by the reduction in probing depth. Specifically, in the group of patients with greater PD, the difference in the MDA values before and after treatment was 1.06 pmol/µL, compared to only 0.53 pmol/µL measured for the group with lower PD ($p < 0.05$).

Presently, there is no consensus on the effect of periodontal disease on the occurrence of systemic oxidative stress. While some authors report higher levels of LPO markers in the blood of patients with periodontal disease relative to healthy controls [14,17,38], other studies reveal no significant differences [16,35,39,40]. The results yielded by our study show statistically significantly higher MDA levels in the blood of patients with periodontal disease compared to the levels measured in healthy subjects. Although it is possible that the increased MDA plasma concentration is due to some other pathological processes in the body, we nonetheless postulate that it is indeed the result of periodontal disease. This assertion is based on the fact that all our patients were systemically healthy and the presence of a statistically significant positive correlation between the MDA levels in saliva and in the blood (Figure 2).

Upon examining the process of LPO in patients with periodontal disease, Bastos et al. reported a significant correlation between the MDA levels in the blood and locally produced inflammatory cytokines (IL-10 and TNFα), highlighting that this marker is a valid indicator of the inflammatory process severity [41]. Our results also show that gingival inflammation was the primary factor in the high MDA value in the blood of patients with periodontal disease. Specifically, in patients with severe inflammation (0.55 pmol/μL), this marker was statistically significantly higher than in patients with moderate gingivitis (0.45 pmol/μL) ($p = 0.047$).

The periodontal therapy, however, did not result in a decline in the MDA concentration in the blood of our patients. Although the MDA value in the blood of our patients with periodontal disease at baseline was primarily affected by the extent of gingival inflammation, marked improvement in this condition after the therapy was not accompanied by a significant reduction in MDA. In fact, based on our findings, the decrease in MDA that was observed three months after therapy completion was mainly influenced by the reduction in probing depth in patients with the initially greater PD. This finding could point to the conclusion that periodontal therapy may have a greater benefit for patients with severe periodontal disease, as it results in a more pronounced reduction in circulating LPO. This conclusion is supported by the findings reported by Ambati et al. based on a sample of patients with higher PD values, in whom periodontal therapy resulted in statistically significantly lower serum MDA levels [42].

As a part of this research, we examined the influence of smoking on the level of lipid peroxidation in patients with and without periodontitis, given that smoking increases exposure to free radicals while also reducing the body's antioxidant protection [43]. Moreover, smoking is one of the main contributing factors in the development of periodontitis, as it affects many aspects of the host's immune response. The results yielded by our analyses indicate that the salivary and plasma MDA levels were much higher in smokers, irrespective of their periodontal status. These findings concur with the results published by other authors. For example, Guentsch et al. [44] reported a progressive increase in the salivary MDA values from healthy non-smokers to healthy smokers and further to non-smokers and smokers with periodontitis. Garg et al. [45] similarly noted that the MDA levels in gingival tissue are affected by the number of cigarettes smoked. Similar to our results, these authors recorded significantly higher MDA values in the blood of smokers compared to non-smokers with periodontitis.

We deliberately chose not to exclude smokers from our research, as our aim was to assess oxidative stress levels in the general population, and in our country, a significant proportion of adults smoke. For the same reason, we did not exclude obesity and physical activity as the risk factors for the emergence of oxidative stress. As the control and the experimental group were comparable and both included smokers, any influence of smoking on our findings would be minimized, as confirmed by the factorial ANOVA test results (Figures 3 and 4).

5. Conclusions

Based on the results reported here, it can be concluded that salivary and plasma MDA (as a final LPO product) levels were significantly higher in patients with periodontal disease compared to healthy subjects. The level of this marker was most significantly impacted by the severity of gingival inflammation. However, only the salivary MDA levels were significantly reduced by periodontal therapy. Therefore, even though these findings are based on a relatively small sample, they point to the potential link between periodontitis and local and systemic oxidative stress, as well as highlight the benefits of periodontal therapy in mitigating this issue. Further research based on larger patient samples and examining a greater number of oxidative stress markers is nonetheless needed to confirm our results and expand our findings.

Author Contributions: Conceptualization and methodology, T.V., M.D. and S.B.; validation, A.M.; formal analysis, K.V. and I.N.; investigation, T.V.; data curation, A.M.; writing—original draft preparation, T.V.; writing—review and editing, J.M. and I.G.; supervision, M.D. and B.R. All authors have read and agreed to the published version of the manuscript.

Funding: This research received no external funding.

Institutional Review Board Statement: The study was conducted according to the guidelines of the Declaration of Helsinki and approved by the Ethics Committee of Clinic for Dentistry, Novi Sad, Serbia (protocol no. 01-3/14-10).

Informed Consent Statement: Informed consent was obtained from all subjects involved in the study.

Conflicts of Interest: The authors declare no conflict of interest.

References

1. Peterson, P.E.; Ogawa, H. Strengthening the Prevention of Periodontal Disease: The WHO Approach. *J. Periodontol.* **2005**, *76*, 2187–2193. [CrossRef] [PubMed]
2. Żukowski, P.; Maciejczyk, M.; Waszkiel, D. Sources of free radicals and oxidative stress in the oral cavity. *Arch. Oral Biol.* **2018**, *92*, 8–17. [CrossRef] [PubMed]
3. Wang, Y.; Andrukhov, O.; Rausch-Fan, X. Oxidative Stress and antioxidant system in periodontitis. *Front. Physiol.* **2017**, *8*, 910. [CrossRef] [PubMed]
4. Gaschler, M.M.; Stockwell, B.R. Lipid peroxidation in cell death. *Biochem. Biophys. Res. Commun.* **2017**, *482*, 419–425. [CrossRef]
5. Tsikas, D. Assessment of lipid peroxidation by measuring malondialdehyde (MDA) and relatives in biological samples: Analytical and biological challenges. *Anal. Biochem.* **2017**, *524*, 13–30. [CrossRef]
6. Chole, R.H.; Patil, R.N.; Basak, A.; Palandurkar, K.; Bhowate, R. Estimation of serum malondialdehyde in oral cancer and precancer and its association with healthy individuals, gender, alcohol, and tobacco abuse. *J. Cancer Res. Ther.* **2010**, *6*, 487–491. [CrossRef]
7. Rašić, S.; Rebić, D.; Hasić, S.; Rašić Šarac, M.D. Influence of malondialdehyde and matrix metalloproteinase-9 on progression of carotid atherosclerosis in chronic renal disease with cardiometabolic syndrome. *Mediat. Inflamm.* **2015**, *2015*, 614357. [CrossRef]
8. Kaefer, M.; De Carvalho, J.A.; Piva, S.J.; da Silva, D.B.; Becker, A.M.; Sangoi, M.B.; Almeida, T.C.; Hermes, C.L.; Coelho, A.C.; Tonello, R.; et al. Plasma malondialdehyde levels and risk factors for the development of chronic complications in type 2 diabetic patients on insulin therapy. *Clin. Lab.* **2012**, *58*, 973–978. [CrossRef]
9. Almaeen, A.H.; Alduraywish, A.A.; Mobasher, M.A.; Almadhi, O.I.M.; Nafeh, H.N.; El-Metwally, T.H. Oxidative stress, immunological and cellular hypoxia biomarkers in hepatitis C treatment-naïve and cirrhotic patients. *Arch. Med. Sci.* **2021**, *17*, 368–375. [CrossRef]
10. Rumopa, H.; Wagey, F.W.; Supaarman, E. Malondialdehyde levels in preeclampsia before and after delivery. *Obstet. Ginekol. Indones.* **2018**, *6-3*, 143–148. [CrossRef]
11. Khalili, J.; Biloklytska, H.F. Salivary malondialdehyde levels in clinically healthy and periodontal diseased individuals. *Oral Dis.* **2008**, *14*, 754–760. [CrossRef] [PubMed]
12. Dakovic, D. Malondialdehyde as an Indicator of Local Oxidative Cell Damage in Periodontitis Patients. Master's Thesis, Military Medical Academy, Belgarde, Serbia, 2005.
13. Canakci, C.F.; Cicek, Y.; Yildirim, A.; Sezer, U.; Canakci, A. Increased levels of 8-hydroxydeoxyguanosine and malondialdehyde and its relationship with antioxidant enzymes in saliva of periodontitis patients. *Eur. J. Dent.* **2009**, *3*, 100–106. [CrossRef] [PubMed]
14. Trivedi, S.; Lal, N.; Mahdi, A.A.; Mittal, M.; Singh, B.; Pandey, S. Evaluation of antioxidant enzymes activity and malondialdehyde levels in patients with chronic periodontitis and diabetes mellitus. *J. Periodontol.* **2014**, *85*, 713–720. [CrossRef]

15. Skutnik-Radziszewska, A.; Zalewska, A. Salivary redox biomarkers in the course of caries and periodontal disease. *Appl. Sci.* **2020**, *10*, 6240. [CrossRef]
16. Akalın, F.A.; Baltacıoğlu, E.; Alver, A.; Karabulut, E. Lipid peroxidation levels and total oxidant status in serum, saliva and gingival crevicular fluid in patients with chronic periodontitis. *J. Clin. Periodontol.* **2007**, *34*, 558–565. [CrossRef] [PubMed]
17. Dhotre, P.S.; Suryaker, A.N.; Bhogade, R.B. Oxidative stress in periodontitis. *Eur. J. Gen. Med.* **2012**, *9*, 81–84. [CrossRef]
18. Cherian, D.A.; Peter, T.; Narayanan, A.; Madhavan, S.S.; Achammana, S.; Vynat, G.P. Malondialdehyde as a marker of oxidative stress in periodontitis patients. *J. Pharm. Bioallied Sci.* **2019**, *11* (Suppl. S2), 297–300. [CrossRef] [PubMed]
19. Sobaniec, H.; Sobaniec-Lotowska, M.E. Morphological examinations of hard tissues of periodontium and evaluation of selected processes of lipid peroxidation in blood serum of rats in the course of experimental periodontitis. *Med. Sci. Monit.* **2000**, *6*, 875–881. [PubMed]
20. Cesaratto, L.; Vascotto, C.; Calligaris, S.; Tell, G. The importance of redox state in liver damage. *Ann. Hepatol.* **2004**, *3*, 86–92. [CrossRef]
21. Ekuni, D.; Tomofuji, T.; Tamaki, N.; Sanbe, T.; Azuma, T.; Yamanaka, R.; Yamamoto, T.; Watanabe, T. Mechanical stimulation of gingiva reduces plasma 8-OHdG level in rat periodontitis. *Arch. Oral Biol.* **2008**, *53*, 324–329. [CrossRef]
22. Tomofuji, T.; Sanbe, T.; Ekuni, D.; Azuma, T.; Irie, K.; Maruyama, T.; Tamaki, N.; Yamamoto, T. Oxidative damage of rat liver induced by ligature-induced periodontitis and chronic ethanol consumption. *Arch. Oral Biol.* **2008**, *53*, 1113–1118. [CrossRef] [PubMed]
23. Albano, E. Oxidative mechanisms in the pathogenesis of alcoholic liver disease. *Mol. Asp. Med.* **2008**, *29*, 9–16. [CrossRef] [PubMed]
24. Ekuni, D.; Tomofuji, T.; Sanbe, T.; Irie, K.; Azuma, T.; Maruyama, T.; Tamaki, N.; Murakami, J.; Kokeguchi, S.; Yamamoto, T. Periodontitis-induced lipid peroxidation in rat descending aorta is involvedin initiation of atherosclerosis. *J. Periodontal Res.* **2009**, *44*, 434–442. [CrossRef] [PubMed]
25. Silness, J.; Löe, H. Periodontal disease in pregnancy (II). Correlation between oral hygiene and periodontal condition. *Acta Odontol. Scand.* **1964**, *22*, 121–135. [CrossRef]
26. Löe, H.; Silness, P. Periodontal disease in pregnancy I. Prevalence and severity. *Acta Odontol. Scand.* **1963**, *21*, 533–551. [CrossRef]
27. Saxer, U.P.; Mühlemann, H.R. Motivation und Aufklarung. *Schweiz. Mon. Für Zahnmed.* **1975**, *85*, 905–919.
28. Predin, T.; Djuric, M.; Nikolic, N.; Mirnic, J.; Gusic, I.; Petrovic, D.J.; Milasin, J. Clinical and microbiological effects of quadrant versus full-mouth root planing—A randomized study. *J. Dent. Sci.* **2014**, *9*, 400–406. [CrossRef]
29. Mirnic, J.; Djuric, M.; Predin, T.; Gusic, I.; Petrovic, D.; Andjelkovic, A.; Bajkin, B. Impact of the level of metabolic control on the non-surgical periodontal therapy outcomes in diabetes mellitus type 2 patients: Clinical effects. *Srp. Arh. Celok. Lek.* **2013**, *141*, 738–743. [CrossRef]
30. Veljović, T.; Đurić, M.; Gušić, I.; Mirnić, J.; Čakić, S.; Maletin, A.; Brkić, S. The Influence of Periodontal Disease Treatment on 8-Hydroxy-Deoxyguanosine Concentrations in Saliva and Plasma of Chronic Periodontitis Patients. *Acta Clin. Croat.* **2020**, *59*, 615–622. [CrossRef]
31. Armitage, G.C. Development of a classification system for periodontal diseases and conditions. *Ann. Periodontol.* **1999**, *4*, 1–6. [CrossRef]
32. Tsai, C.C.; Chen, H.S.; Chen, S.L.; Ho, Y.P.; Ho, K.Y.; Wu, Y.M.; Hung, C.C. Lipid peroxidation: A possible role in the progression of the chronic periodontitis. *J. Periodontal Res.* **2005**, *40*, 378–384. [CrossRef] [PubMed]
33. Takane, M.; Sugano, N.; Ezawa, T.; Uchiyama, T.; Ito, K. A marker of oxidative stress in saliva: Association with periodontally-involved teeth of a hopeless prognosis. *J. Oral Sci.* **2005**, *47*, 53–57. [CrossRef] [PubMed]
34. Takane, M.; Sugano, N.; Iwasaki, H.; Iwano, Y.; Shimizu, N.; Ito, K. New biomarker evidence of oxidative DNA damage in whole saliva from clinically healthy and periodontally diseased individuals. *J. Periodontol.* **2002**, *73*, 551–554. [CrossRef] [PubMed]
35. Önder, C.; Kurgan, S.; Altıngöz, M.; Bağış, N.; Uyanık, M.; Serdar, M.A.; Kantarcı, A.; Günhan, M. Impact of non-surgical periodontal therapy on saliva and serum levels of markers of oxidative stress. *Clin. Oral Investig.* **2017**, *2*, 1961–1969. [CrossRef]
36. Warad, S.B.; Pattanashetti, J.; Kalburgi, N.; Koregol, A.; Rao, S. Estimation of salivary malondialdehyde levels in smokeless tobacco chewers with chronic periodontitis-A cross sectional clinico biochemical study. *Odovtos-Int. J. Dental. Sci.* **2021**, *23*, 137–146. [CrossRef]
37. Gutteridge, J.M.C. Lipid peroxidation and antioxidants as biomarkers of tissue damage. *Clin. Chem.* **1995**, *41*, 1819–1828. [CrossRef]
38. Aziz, A.S.; Kalekar, M.G.; Benjamin, T.; Suryakar, A.N.; Prakashan, M.M.; Bijle, M.N.A. Effect of nonsurgical periodontal therapy on some oxidative stress markers in patients with chronic periodontitis: A biochemical study. *World J. Dent.* **2013**, *4*, 17–23. [CrossRef]
39. Wei, D.; Zhang, X.L.; Wang, Y.Z.; Yang, C.X.; Chen, G. Lipid peroxidation levels, total oxidant status and superoxide dismutase in serum, saliva and gingival crevicular fluid inchronic periodontitis patients before and after periodontal therapy. *Aust. Dent. J.* **2010**, *55*, 70–78. [CrossRef]
40. Tripathi, V.; Singh, S.T.; Sharma, V.; Verma, A.; Singh, C.D.; Gill, J.S. Assessment of lipid peroxidation levels and total antioxidant status in chronic and aggressive periodontitis patients: An in vivo study. *J. Contemp. Dent. Pract.* **2018**, *19*, 287–291. [CrossRef]

41. Bastos, A.S.; Graves, D.T.; de Melo Loureiro, A.P.; Júnior, C.R.; Abdalla, D.S.P.; Faulin, T.E.S.; Câmara, N.O.; Andriankaja, O.M.; Orrico, S.R.P. Lipid peroxidation is associated with the severity of periodontal disease and local inflammatory markers in patients with type 2 diabetes. *J. Clin. Endocr. Metab.* **2012**, *97*, 1353–1362. [CrossRef]
42. Ambati, M.; Rani, K.R.; Reddy, P.V.; Suryaprasanna, J.; Dasari, R.; Gireddy, H. Evaluation of oxidative stress in chronic periodontitis patients following systemic antioxidant supplementation: A clinical and biochemical study. *J. Nat. Sci. Biol. Med.* **2017**, *8*, 99–103. [CrossRef] [PubMed]
43. Naresh, K.C.; Subramaniam, M.R.; Prashanth, R.S.; Ranganath, V.; Abhilasha, S.P.; Anu, A.J. Salivary antioxidant enzymes and lipid peroxidation product malondialdehyde and sialic acid levels among smokers and non-smokers with chronic periodontitis—A clinico-biochemical study. *J. Fam. Med. Prim. Care* **2019**, *8*, 2960–2964. [CrossRef]
44. Guentsch, A.; Preshaw, P.M.; Bremer, S.S.; Klinger, G.; Glockmann, E.; Sigusch, B.W. Lipid peroxidation and antioxidant activity in saliva of periodontitis patients: Effect of smoking and periodontal treatment. *Clin. Oral Investig.* **2008**, *12*, 345–352. [CrossRef] [PubMed]
45. Garg, N.; Singh, R.; Dixit, J.; Jain, A.; Tewari, V. Levels of lipid peroxides and antioxidants in smokers and nonsmokers. *J. Periodontal Res.* **2006**, *41*, 405–410. [CrossRef]

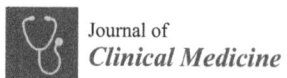

Article

Evaluation of the Effect of Surgical Extraction of an Impacted Mandibular Third Molar on the Periodontal Status of the Second Molar—Prospective Study

Magda Aniko-Włodarczyk [1,†], Aleksandra Jaroń [1,†], Olga Preuss [1], Anna Grzywacz [2] and Grzegorz Trybek [1,*]

1. Department of Oral Surgery, Pomeranian Medical University in Szczecin, 72 Powstańców Wlkp. St., 70-111 Szczecin, Poland; dominika.wlodarczyk@pum.edu.pl (M.A.-W.); jaronola@gmail.com (A.J.); olga.preuss@pum.edu.pl (O.P.)
2. Independent Laboratory of Health Promotion, Pomeranian Medical University in Szczecin, 11 Chlapowskiego St., 70-204 Szczecin, Poland; anna.grzywacz@pum.edu.pl
* Correspondence: g.trybek@gmail.com
† These authors made equal contributions as first author.

Abstract: Dental injury to the second molar (SM) caused by the surgical extraction of the impacted third molar tends to be underestimated. The necessity of assessment of the impact of the removal of the wisdom tooth in the mandible on the second molar arose. The study group ($n = 60$) was the one with the second molar on the surgical side, and the control group ($n = 60$) was the one with the tooth on the opposite side of the alveolar arch. Before the surgery, the difficulty level was assessed according to the Pederson scale. The periodontal status of the SM was assessed by probing depth (PD), gingival index (GI), tooth mobility (TM) examination by the percussion method and resonance frequency. Measurements were taken before and after the surgery, 7 days and 8 weeks after the surgery. The study demonstrated the significant impact of the surgical removal of the wisdom tooth on the PD, GI and TM of the SM. The predicted degree of difficulty of the very difficult surgery had an influence on the increase in PD on the distal buccal and lingual surface of the SM, and on the GI in the proximity of the examined tooth. The results of the presented research confirm the necessity of the clinical assessment of the lower SM before and after the surgical removal of the impacted wisdom tooth in the mandible.

Keywords: third molar; mandibular third molar; impaction; periodontal status; complications

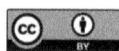

1. Introduction

The presence of a partially or completely impacted wisdom tooth can cause a deepening of the gingival sulcus and periodontal changes in the distal region of the mandibular second molar [1]. These changes may be asymptomatic and only involve deepening of the gingival sulcus—in addition, there may be redness or a tendency to bleed [2]. A change in the periodontal status of a mandibular second molar may also be a consequence of surgical intervention—this occurs only after surgical removal of an impacted wisdom tooth [3]. The removal of an impacted wisdom tooth carries the risk of traumatizing the second molar, causing it to become more mobile or dislocated during the anteroposterior extraction movements during the procedure. The pressure force generated by the operator using an elevator on the second molar during the removal of the impacted tooth is equal to the resistance that this tooth presents during the final phase of extraction. Despite the frequent coverage of complications associated with surgical removal of wisdom teeth in the scientific literature, increased mobility of the second molar, which can affect the clinical status of the pulp, is often downplayed or overlooked [4]. Clinical and population-based data on the periodontal pathophysiology of the third molar are limited. Information is not collected or even excluded from studies due to the high variability in the morphology and physiology of the wisdom tooth concerning teeth located in the anterior segment of the dental arch. The unclear periodontal status is reflected in the periodontal status of the adjacent tooth, which is the second molar in the mandible. Surgical removal of an impacted mandibular third molar involves soft tissue incision, full-thickness flap dehiscence, alveotomy, or separation, which may adversely affect the periodontal tissues adjacent to the surgical area of the second molar. The data in the literature are not consistent. Surgical intervention on the distal surface of the second lower molar may result in bone loss, periodontal pocket development, or root cement exposure [5,6]. However, some studies confirm an improvement in the level of connective tissue attachment and a reduction in probing depth [7,8]. The analysis of the impact of surgery can be based on the clinical assessment of the pocket depth (PD) and gingival index (GI). The complications of surgical extraction of impacted wisdom teeth in the form of ligamentous damage to the second molar and impaired blood supply to the pulp, which can lead to pulp necrosis, have been overlooked in the literature. In particular, there are no data on the effect of the surgical procedure on changes in the threshold of excitability of the pulp of the second molar, and, thus, its clinical status.

This study aimed to:

1. Evaluate the effect of surgical removal of an impacted third molar on:
   a. Clinical probing depth of the mandibular second molar.
   b. Gingival condition of the mandibular second molar.
   c. Mobility of the mandibular second molar.
2. To determine if there is a relationship between the degree of difficulty of surgical removal of an impacted wisdom tooth and the postoperative probing depth, gingival condition, and mobility of the mandibular second molar.

2. Materials and Methods

The study was conducted after obtaining consent from the Bioethics Committee with the number KB-0012/89/16.

The study included 60 consecutive patients with indications for surgical removal of the third mandibular molar. Adult patients, generally healthy, not taking any permanent medication, and non-smokers, who declared their willingness to participate in the study, were eligible for the procedure. The exclusion criteria were the absence of a second and third mandibular molar in the operated quadrant and on the opposite side in the mandible, the presence of a fixed orthodontic appliance, malocclusions such as distocclusion, mesiocclusion, crowding of teeth, scissor bite, crossbite, tobacco smoking and age below 18 years, and an implanted cardiac electro stimulator. In each patient, the second lower molars were examined—a total of 120 teeth in all patients. We identified two groups:

1. Study group ($n = 60$)—second and third molars in the mandible in the operated quadrant;
2. Control group ($n = 60$)—mandibular second and third molars on the side opposite to the operated side.

Before the study, patients were informed about the study. All participants gave their informed consent to participate in the study and confirmed it with their signature on the form. All patients had a pantographic X-ray taken before the surgery. The degree of impaction was assessed according to Winter [9] and Pell and Gregory [10]. The degree of difficulty of surgical removal of impacted third molars in the mandible was assessed using the Pederson index. All mandibular 2nd molars were vital before surgery, with no prosthetic restoration, only small fillings, and no fractures.

All procedures were performed by three oral surgery specialists with a similar (extensive) level of surgical experience. Tooth extraction was performed under local anesthesia: block anesthesia and infiltration anesthesia 2% with norepinephrine 0.00125% in the amount of 4–6 mL. The first incision was performed with a #15 scalpel at the top of the mandibular alveolar region behind the second molar, and the second releasing incision was performed in the oral vestibule in the distal third of the crown of the second molar. The full-thickness flap was deflected with Molt's elevator to the level of the external oblique line and stabilized with Langenbeck's long retractor, resting it on the bone at a ninety-degree angle. With the use of a rubella drill and/or a Lindemann bur, mounted on a surgical handpiece and cooled with a sterile 0.9% sodium chloride solution, the bone was removed from the impacted molar to the level of its neck. Depending on the angle of inclination, the tooth was cut with a drill, and, using elevators and/or forceps, the tooth was removed in whole or in parts. The last stage of the surgical procedure was the wound toilet, which consisted of the removal of bone resulting from the drill cutting, removal of the tooth follicle, possibly inflammatory tissue of granuloma, smoothing of the sharp bone edges, and copious rinsing with a saline solution. The mucoperiosteal flap was then repositioned and stabilized with single knotted sutures using 3-0 silk sutures and left in place for seven days. After surgery, compression with a sterile gauze tampon was applied for 20 min. Patients were advised to maintain postoperative wound hygiene. Patients brushed their teeth after each meal, used a 0.1% chlorhexidine-based rinse and were advised to use nonsteroidal anti-inflammatory drugs in the form of ketoprofen 100 mg twice daily.

2.1. Clinical Examination

Clinical examination of the mandibular second molars in both the study and control groups was performed immediately before surgery, seven days after surgery, and eight weeks after surgery. The following parameters were used for clinical evaluation: gingival index, probing depth, impaction, and resonance frequency mobility measurement.

2.1.1. Gingival Assessment

The evaluation was performed using the gingival index (GI) according to Loe and Silness [11]. The index was assessed using a periodontal probe at four measurement points: mesially, distally, vestibularly, and lingually.

2.1.2. Probing Depth (PD) Measurement

The measurement was carried out using a Williams periodontal probe calibrated every 1 mm with an accuracy of 0.5 mm at six measurement points of each second molar—distally, centrally, and mesially on the buccal side and similarly on the lingual side. The probe was inserted into the gingival crevice until gentle resistance, parallel to the long axis of the tooth, and the measurement obtained was archived.

2.1.3. Tooth Mobility Measurement

The mobility of the mandibular second molars was measured using the Periotest M (Medizintechnik Gulden, Bensheim, Germany) and Osstell (Osstell, Gothenburg, Sweden). In addition to the time sequence appropriate for all other clinical parameters (seven days after surgery and eight weeks after surgery), mobility was also measured immediately after surgery.

2.1.4. Measurement with Periotest M

The mobility was measured on the buccal surface of the second molar based on the percussion method. The head of the device was applied perpendicularly to the buccal surface of the tested tooth at a distance of approximately 2 mm. Correct orientation of the head was indicated by a low tone. To obtain repeatable measurements, the Periotest M was always positioned in the same way in relation to the tooth under test. The test was performed twice for each tooth of the test and control groups. The results expressed on the PTV (Periotest value) scale, displayed on the instrument panel, were recorded in a prepared sheet—the mean value from the two measurements was used in the statistical analysis.

2.1.5. Measurement Using Osstell

The measurement was performed based on resonance frequency analysis. With the mouth wide open, a magnetic sensor (SmartPeg; Osstell, Gothenburg, Sweden) was attached using a composite cured with a polymerization lamp to the chewing surface of the tooth from the test and control groups. The pulse probe was brought approximately one millimeter parallel and perpendicular to the dental arch. The magnetic sensor, along with the polymerized composite, was then removed using light pressure. The readings expressed on the ISQ scale, archived in the memory of the device, were transferred to the developed test card, where their mean value was recorded.

2.2. Methodology of Statistical Analysis

Statistical analysis was performed using the statistical package R—version 3.4.2 (R Foundation for Statistical Computing: Vienna, Austria). Qualitative variables were described by the number and percentage of occurrences of each value. Standard measures of position and measures of variability were used to describe quantitative variables. Arithmetic means, standard deviation, median, quartiles, and minimum and maximum values were calculated.

Qualitative variables that did not have a normal distribution were compared using the Kruskal–Wallis test. The chi-square test was used to compare qualitative variables in the study and control groups. To make a more accurate comparison between the groups, the method of multiple comparisons, i.e., post-hoc analysis (Dunn's test), was used.

In the case of small expected values, the Fisher's exact test was used. The analysis was used to evaluate the effect of the anticipated difficulty of the procedure on the clinical status of the second molar. Quantitative variables were analyzed using the Wilcoxon paired t-test and Student's t-test. These were used in the comparison of the clinical status of the 2nd molar from the test and control groups and in the comparative analysis of individual parameters of the clinical status of second molars from the test group between time points. Sequential analysis was used to interpret the change in the clinical status of the second molar teeth between time intervals.

A value of 0.05 was taken as the level of significance (p). All p values that were below 0.05 were interpreted as indicating significant relationships.

3. Results

3.1. Characteristics of the Study Group

Sixty patients, consecutively presenting for surgical removal of impacted wisdom teeth in the mandible, were included in the clinical study. Among them, there were 17 males and 34 women. Table 1 summarizes the detailed results for the study sample. A total of 60 surgical removals of impacted mandibular third molars were performed with a mean angle of 63.47 degrees (29.34) to the occlusal plane. The spatial position was determined by the position of the wisdom tooth relative to the second molar and mandibular branches. Table 2 shows the detailed characteristics of the position of the third molars and the expected difficulty of the procedure.

Table 1. Characteristics of the study patients.

		Mean (SD)	Median (Quartil)	IQR
Age		24.82 (5.51)	23 (21–28)	27
		n	(%)	
Sex	Woman	43	71.67	
	Man	17	28.33	

Explanations: SD—standard deviation; n—number of subjects.

Table 2. Characteristics of the position of lower wisdom teeth.

		Mean (SD)	Median (Quartil)	IQR
Angultion		63.47 (29.34)	74.45 (40–87.75)	47.75
		n	(%)	
Winter	Mesioangular	30	50.00	
	Horizontal	7	11.67	
	Vertical	16	26.67	
	Distoangular	7	11.67	
Pell and Gregory	Level A	30	50.00	
	Level B	19	31.67	
	Level C	11	18.33	
Pell and Gregory	Class 1	9	15.00	
	Class 2	40	66.67	
	Class 3	11	18.33	
Difficulty of the procedure (Pederson)	Slightly difficult	10	16.67	
	Moderately difficult	36	60.00	
	Very difficult	14	23.33	

Explanations: SD—standard deviation; n—number of patients.

3.2. Comparative Analysis of Clinical Status Parameters of Second Molars of the Study and Control Groups before the Procedure, after the Procedure, Seven Days after the Procedure, and Eight Weeks after the Procedure

3.2.1. Comparative Analysis of the Gingival Index (GI) at Second Molars of the Study and Control Groups

Analyses of the GI were performed before surgical removal of the mandibular wisdom tooth, seven days after surgery, and eight weeks after surgical intervention. The mean GI value in the study group before surgery was 0.69 ($\pm$0.47), seven days after surgery was 1.65 ($\pm$0.47), and eight weeks after surgery was 0.28 ($\pm$0.47). There was a significant difference in GI values before surgery compared to seven days after surgical intervention ($p < 0.001$). The results are summarized in Table 3.

Table 3. Comparison of the GI before surgery, 7 days after surgery, and 8 weeks after surgery.

GI	Group	n	Mean	SD	Median	Min	Max	Q1	Q3	IQR	p *
Before the procedure	Study	60	0.69	0.47	0.5	0	2	0.5	0.81	0.31	0.002
	Control	60	0.5	0.42	0.5	0	2	0.25	0.75	0.5	
After 7 days	Study	60	1.65	0.47	1.75	0.5	2.5	1.5	2	0.5	<0.001
	Control	60	0.62	0.46	0.5	0	2.5	0.25	1	0.75	
After 8 weeks	Study	60	0.28	0.33	0.25	0	1.25	0	0.5	0.5	0.081
	Control	60	0.4	0.43	0.25	0	2.25	0	0.5	0.5	

* Wilcoxon test for dependent (repeated) measurements. Explanations: n—number of teeth; SD—standard deviation; Min—minimum value; Max—maximum value; Q1—first quartile; Q3—third quartile; p—significance level.

3.2.2. Comparative Analysis of Probing Depth at Second Molars of the Study and Control Groups

Measurement of Probing Depth before Treatment

Before treatment, the pocket depth in the study group was greatest at the distal–buccal surface, averaging 3.67 mm (1.39). Similar values were also recorded in the control group at 3 mm (1.26). There were significant differences in measurements on the mesial–buccal surface ($p = 0.003$) and distal ($p = 0.002$) and central–lingual surfaces ($p = 0.046$). The results of the full analysis are summarized in Table 4.

Table 4. Comparison of probing depth at the second molar in the study and control groups before treatment.

PD (mm)	Group	n	Mean	SD	Median	Min	Max	Q1	Q3	IQR	p*
Buccal—m	Study	60	1.52	0.67	1.5	0.5	3.5	1	2	0.5	0.003
	Control	60	1.31	0.58	1	0.5	4	1	1.5	0.5	
Buccal—c	Study	60	1.62	0.69	1.5	0.5	3	1	2	1	0.077
	Control	60	1.47	0.58	1.5	0.5	3	1	2	1	
Buccal—d	Study	60	3.67	1.39	3.5	1	8	3	4.62	1.62	0.002
	Control	60	3	1.26	3	1	5.5	2	3.5	1.5	
Lingual—m	Study	60	1.54	0.61	1.5	0.5	3.5	1	2	1	0.667
	Control	60	1.48	0.68	1	0.5	4	1	2	1	
Lingual—c	Study	60	1.71	0.63	1.5	0.5	3.5	1	2	1	0.046
	Control	60	1.51	0.6	1.5	0.5	3	1	2	1	
Lingual—d	Study	60	3.38	1.21	3.5	1	5.5	2.88	4	1.12	0.16
	Control	60	3.17	1.14	3.5	1	5.5	2	3.5	1.5	

* Wilcoxon test for dependent (repeated) measurements. Notes: n—number of teeth; SD—standard deviation; Min—minimum value; Max—maximum value; Q1—first quartile; Q3—third quartile; p—significance level; m—mesially; c—centrally; d—distally.

Measurement of Probing Depth Seven Days after Treatment

All probing depth values seven days after surgery were significantly greater in the study group compared to the control group ($p < 0.05$). As preoperatively, the highest scores in the study and control groups were recorded on the distal–buccal surface with mean measurements of 7.68 mm (2.44) in the study group and 3.13 (1.29) in the control group. The results of the analysis are summarized in Table 5.

Table 5. Comparison of probing depth at the second molar of the study and control groups measured 7 days after treatment.

PD (mm)	Group	n	Mean	SD	Median	Min	Max	Q1	Q3	IQR	p*
Buccal—m	Study	60	2.08	0.84	2	1	5	1.5	2.5	1	<0.001
	Control	60	1.52	0.74	1	0.5	4	1	2	1	
Buccal—c	Study	60	2.91	1.33	3	1	8	2	3.62	1.62	<0.001
	Control	60	1.57	0.63	1.5	0.5	3.5	1	2	1	
Buccal—d	Study	60	7.68	2.44	8	3	12	5.5	9.62	4.12	<0.001
	Control	60	3.13	1.29	3	1	5.5	2	3.62	1.62	
Lingual—m	Study	60	1.95	0.82	2	0.5	4	1	2	1	0.007
	Control	60	1.62	0.7	1.5	1	4	1	2	1	
Lingual—c	Study	60	2.28	1.01	2	1	5	1.5	3	1.5	<0.001
	Control	60	1.62	0.67	1.5	1	3.5	1	2	1	
Lingual—d	Study	60	4.68	1.78	4	2	10.5	3.5	5.62	2.12	<0.001
	Control	60	3.18	1.12	3	1	5.5	2	4	2	

* Wilcoxon test for dependent (repeated) measurements. Explanations: n—number of teeth; SD—standard deviation; Min—minimum value; Max—maximum value; Q1—first quartile; Q3—third quartile; p—significance level.

Probing Depth Measurement Eight Weeks after Treatment

The greatest probing depth eight weeks after treatment was 6 mm distally buccally and lingually in the study group, while the lowest depth was 0.5 mm. Statistical analysis revealed a significant difference in probing depth measurements performed buccally mesially and centrally and lingually mesially, centrally, and distally at second molars between the study and control groups ($p < 0.05$). Eight weeks after the procedure, the mean probing depth in both groups was still greatest on the distal buccal surface. The data are summarized in Table 6.

Table 6. Comparison of probing depth at the second molar of the study and control groups measured 8 weeks after the procedure.

PD (mm)	Group	n	Mean	SD	Median	Min	Max	Q1	Q3	IQR	p *
Buccal—m	Study	60	1.69	0.58	2	0.5	3	1	2	1	0.009
	Control	60	1.43	0.71	1	0.5	4	1	2	1	
Buccal—c	Study	60	1.79	0.59	2	1	4	1	2	1	0.001
	Control	60	1.5	0.74	1.25	0.5	5.5	1	2	1	
Buccal—d	Study	60	3.05	0.94	3	1.5	6	2	3.5	1.5	0.202
	Control	60	2.83	1.16	2.5	1	5.5	2	3.5	1.5	
Lingual—m	Study	60	1.73	0.65	2	1	4	1	2	1	0.017
	Control	60	1.47	0.71	1	0.5	4	1	2	1	
Lingual—c	Study	60	1.82	0.73	2	1	4	1	2	1	0.007
	Control	60	1.5	0.62	1.5	0.5	3	1	2	1	
Lingual—d	Study	60	2.62	0.95	2.5	1	6	2	3	1	0.319
	Control	60	2.85	1.14	2.75	1	5.5	2	3.5	1.5	

* Wilcoxon test for dependent (repeated) measurements. Explanations: n—number of teeth; SD—standard deviation; Min—minimum value; Max—maximum value; Q1—first quartile; Q3—third quartile; p—significance level.

3.2.3. Comparative Analysis of the Mobility of Second Molars of the Study Group and the Control Group before the Procedure, Seven Days after the Procedure, and Eight Weeks after the Procedure

Measurement with Periotest M

The differences in the seventh tooth mobility seven days after treatment in the study and control groups were significant ($p < 0.001$). The study group had higher values averaging 2.27 (−2.55–6.2). No statistically significant differences were observed at the other time points. Preoperatively, and eight weeks postoperatively, both the seventh teeth of the study and control groups were not significantly different in terms of mobility. The remaining results of the statistical analysis are summarized in Table 7.

Table 7. Comparison of the mobility of second molars of the study and control groups at different time points as measured by Periotest M.

Periotest	Group	n	Mean	SD	Median	Min	Max	Q1	Q3	IQR	p *
Before the procedure	Study	60	−0.68	2.18	−1	−5.85	5.7	−1.8	0.54	−1.26	0.965
	Control	60	−0.7	1.97	−0.78	−5.35	4.15	−1.8	0.66	−1.14	
After 7 days	Study	60	1.2	2.27	0.95	−2.55	6.2	−0.4	3.01	2.61	<0.001
	Control	60	−0.46	1.85	−0.62	−4.25	4.05	−1.61	0.74	−0.87	
After 8 weeks	Study	60	−0.18	2.46	−0.4	−8	4.9	−1.51	1.27	−0.24	0.096
	Control	60	−0.6	1.82	−0.62	−4.3	3.95	−1.56	0.65	−0.91	

* Wilcoxon test for dependent (repeated) measurements. Explanations: n—number of teeth; SD—standard deviation; Min—minimum value; Max—maximum value; Q1—first quartile; Q3—third quartile; p—significance level.

Osstell Measurement

Similar to the mobility measurements performed with the Periotest—the Osstell—after seven days, mobility was significantly higher in the study group compared to the control group ($p < 0.001$). The mean Osstell readings were 46.47 (10.51) and 55.65 (10.56), respectively. The measurement values in the control group decreased, indicating an increase in the seventh tooth mobility. After eight weeks, no significant differences were observed between the study group and the control group. The remaining values were summarized in Table 8.

Table 8. Comparison of mobility of second molars of the study and control groups at different time points as measured by Osstell.

Osstell	Group	n	Mean	SD	Median	Min	Max	Q1	Q3	IQR	p *
Before the procedure	Study	60	55.26	11.47	54	23.5	84	48.25	64	15.75	0.471
	Control	60	56.28	10.54	59.75	27	73.5	48.38	64.5	16.12	
After 7 days	Study	60	46.47	10.51	48.5	19.5	66.5	39.75	54	14.25	<0.001
	Control	60	55.65	10.56	57.75	27.5	70.5	49.5	64.5	15	
After 8 weeks	Study	60	59.98	9.23	63	34.5	72.5	55.38	66.62	11.24	0.604
	Control	60	58.49	11.86	62.75	−1.3	71.5	52	66.5	14.5	

* Wilcoxon test for dependent (repeated) measurements. Explanations: n—number of teeth; SD—standard deviation; Min—minimum value; Max—maximum value; Q1—first quartile; Q3—third quartile; p—significance level.

3.2.4. Gingival Index (GI)

There was a significant relationship between predicted procedure difficulty and gingival index before surgery and seven days after surgery ($p < 0.05$). The GI in patients who were predicted to have a very difficult procedure was statistically significantly higher before surgery than in patients who were predicted to have a moderate or minor procedure ($p = 0.01$). The rate of gingivitis seven days after surgery was significantly higher in patients with a very difficult procedure than in patients after a slightly difficult procedure ($p = 0.047$). The details of the statistical analysis are summarized in Table 9.

Table 9. Comparison of the relationship of predicted procedure difficulty and the gingival index of the second molar before surgery, 7 days after surgery, and 8 weeks after surgery.

GI	Difficulty of the Procedure	n	Mean	SD	Median	Min	Max	Q1	Q3	IQR	p *
Before the procedure	Slightly difficult	10	0.48	0.14	0.5	0.25	0.75	0.5	0.5	0	0.01
	Moderately difficult	36	0.64	0.49	0.5	0	2	0.44	0.81	0.37	B >
	Very difficult	14	0.98	0.46	0.75	0.5	1.75	0.56	1.5	0.94	U. N
After 7 days	Slightly difficult	10	1.35	0.5	1.25	0.5	2.25	1.06	1.5	0.44	0.047
	Moderately difficult	36	1.68	0.45	1.62	0.5	2.5	1.5	2	0.5	B >
	Very difficult	14	1.79	0.45	2	0.75	2.5	1.75	2	0.25	N
After 8 weeks	Slightly difficult	10	0.2	0.33	0	0	0.75	0	0.38	0.38	0.527
	Moderately difficult	36	0.28	0.33	0.25	0	1.25	0	0.5	0.5	
	Very difficult	14	0.32	0.36	0.25	0	1.25	0	0.5	0.5	

* Kruskal–Wallis test + post-hoc analysis (Dunn's test). Explanations: n—number of teeth; SD—standard deviation; Min—minimum value; Max—maximum value; Q1—first quartile; Q3—third quartile; p—significance level; N—slightly difficult procedure; U—moderately difficult procedure; B—very difficult procedure.

3.2.5. Probing Depths: Before Surgery, Seven Days after Surgery, and Eight Weeks after Surgery

The clinical probing depths obtained at each time point are presented later in the chapter in paragraph four. Statistical analysis revealed that the probing depth on the distal surface of the second molar before the procedure, measured on both the buccal and lingual sides, was significantly different in patients qualified for the procedure with different degrees of difficulty ($p < 0.005$; Kruskal–Wallis test). Using post-hoc analysis, the above relationship was further described. The probing depth of the distal–buccal side in patients who were scheduled for a very difficult procedure was significantly greater before the procedure than in patients who were scheduled for a slightly difficult procedure ($p = 0.042$). Moreover, patients with an anticipated very difficult procedure had a greater probing depth on the distal surface on the lingual side than those with an anticipated procedure with moderate difficulty ($p = 0.041$). Seven days after the procedure, the highest probing depth measurement of 11.5 mm was recorded distally on the buccal surface where the wisdom tooth removal procedure was characterized as moderately difficult. The lowest preoperative PD value recorded was 0.5 mm. The probing depth eight weeks after the procedure showed no significant relationship with the difficulty of the procedure ($p > 0.05$). The details of the analysis performed are summarized in Table 10.

Table 10. Comparison of the relationship of predicted treatment difficulty and probing depth before treatment, 7 days after treatment, and 8 weeks after treatment.

	PD (mm)	Difficulty of the Procedure	n	Mean	SD	Median	Min	Max	Q1	Q3	IQR	p *
Before the procedure	Buccal—m	Slightly difficult	10	1.2	0.54	1	0.5	2.5	1	1.38	0.38	0.162
		Moderately difficult	36	1.6	0.72	1.5	1	3.5	1	2	1	
		Very difficult	14	1.57	0.58	1.75	0.5	2.5	1	2	1	
	Buccal—c	Slightly difficult	10	1.15	0.53	1	0.5	2	1	1.38	0.38	0.058
		Moderately difficult	36	1.71	0.67	1.75	1	3	1	2	1	
		Very difficult	14	1.71	0.75	1.75	1	3	1	2	1	
	Buccal—d	Slightly difficult	10	3	1.2	3	1	5.5	2.25	3.5	1.25	0.042
		Moderately difficult	36	3.61	1.44	3.5	1	8	3	4	1	B > N
		Very difficult	14	4.29	1.16	4.25	2	5.5	3.5	5.5	2	
	Lingual—m	Slightly difficult	10	1.45	0.86	1	0.5	3.5	1	1.88	0.88	0.445
		Moderately difficult	36	1.6	0.58	1.5	1	3.5	1	2	1	
		Very difficult	14	1.46	0.5	1.5	1	2.5	1	1.88	0.88	
	Lingual—c	Slightly difficult	10	1.75	0.86	1.75	0.5	3.5	1.12	2	0.88	0.237
		Moderately difficult	36	1.78	0.55	2	1	3	1.5	2	0.5	
		Very difficult	14	1.5	0.65	1.25	1	3	1	1.88	0.12	
	Lingual—d	Slightly difficult	10	2.95	1.26	3	1	5.5	2.25	3.5	1.25	0.041
		Moderately difficult	36	3.26	1.17	3.5	1	5.5	2.38	4	1.62	B > U
		Very difficult	14	3.96	1.13	4	2	5.5	3.5	4.75	1.25	
After 7 days	Buccal—m	Slightly difficult	10	2.15	1.08	2	1	5	1.62	2	0.38	0.454
		Moderately difficult	36	2.12	0.74	2	1	3.5	1.88	2.5	0.62	
		Very difficult	14	1.89	0.92	2	1	4	1	2	1	
	Buccal—c	Slightly difficult	10	3.2	2.24	2	1	8	1.62	4.75	3.13	0.964
		Moderately difficult	36	2.86	1.08	3	1	5	2	3.5	1.5	
		Very difficult	14	2.82	1.17	2.75	1	5	2	3	1	
	Buccal—d	Slightly difficult	10	7.35	1.76	8	4	10	6.25	8	1.75	0.075
		Moderately difficult	36	7.26	2.44	7	3	11.5	5	9.5	4.5	
		Very difficult	14	9	2.56	8.5	4	12	8	11	3	
	Lingual—m	Slightly difficult	10	1.55	0.6	1.5	1	2.5	1	2	1	0.068
		Moderately difficult	36	2.17	0.86	2	1	4	1.88	3	1.12	
		Very difficult	14	1.68	0.7	2	0.5	3	1	2	1	
	Lingual—c	Slightly difficult	10	1.8	1.01	1.25	1	3.5	1	2.75	1.75	0.165
		Moderately difficult	36	2.44	1.05	2	1	5	2	3	1	
		Very difficult	14	2.21	0.85	2	1	4	2	2.5	0.5	
	Lingual—d	Slightly difficult	10	4.1	1.43	4	2	6	3.5	5	1.5	0.55
		Moderately difficult	36	4.61	1.46	4.25	2	8	3.88	5.5	1.62	
		Very difficult	14	5.29	2.55	4.5	2	10.5	3.62	6.75	3.13	

Table 10. Cont.

PD (mm)		Difficulty of the Procedure	n	Mean	SD	Median	Min	Max	Q1	Q3	IQR	p *
After 8 weeks	Buccal—m	Slightly difficult	10	1.7	0.54	2	1	2.5	1.12	2	0.88	0.975
		Moderately difficult	36	1.67	0.46	2	1	2	1	2	1	
		Very difficult	14	1.75	0.85	2	0.5	3	1	2	1	
	Buccal—c	Slightly difficult	10	1.9	0.61	2	1	3	1.62	2	0.38	0.759
		Moderately difficult	36	1.75	0.42	2	1	2	1.5	2	0.5	
		Very difficult	14	1.82	0.91	2	1	4	1	2	1	
	Buccal—d	Slightly difficult	10	2.8	0.98	2.75	1.5	4.5	2	3.38	1.38	0.481
		Moderately difficult	36	3.03	0.86	3	2	5	2.38	3.12	0.74	
		Very difficult	14	3.29	1.12	3.25	2	6	2.25	4	1.75	
	Lingual—m	Slightly difficult	10	1.7	0.54	2	1	2.5	1.12	2	0.88	0.397
		Moderately difficult	36	1.78	0.61	2	1	4	1.38	2	0.62	
		Very difficult	14	1.61	0.81	1.25	1	3.5	1	2	1	
	Lingual—c	Slightly difficult	10	1.9	1.07	1.75	1	4	1	2	1	0.615
		Moderately difficult	36	1.88	0.71	2	1	4	1.5	2	0.5	
		Very difficult	14	1.64	0.46	2	1	2	1.12	2	0.88	
	Lingual—d	Slightly difficult	10	2.9	1.2	2.5	2	5	2	3.25	1.25	0.266
		Moderately difficult	36	2.44	0.75	2	1	5	2	3	1	
		Very difficult	14	2.89	1.15	3	1	6	2.12	3	0.88	

* Kruskal–Wallis test + post-hoc analysis (Dunn's test). Explanations: n—number of teeth; SD—standard deviation; Min—minimum value; Max—maximum value; Q1—first quartile; Q3—third quartile p—significance level; m—mesial; c—central; d—distally; N—slightly difficult procedure; U—moderately difficult procedure; B—very difficult procedure.

3.2.6. Second Molar Mobility before the Procedure, after the Procedure, Seven Days after the Procedure, and Eight Weeks after the Procedure

Periotest M Measurement

The highest values were recorded seven days after the slightly difficult procedure: mean—1.99 (2.55); maximum—6.2. Before the procedure, the mobility of second molars did not differ significantly in terms of the difficulty of the procedure. The mobility immediately after surgery increased significantly and depended on the anticipated difficulty of surgical removal of the third molar ($p < 0.05$; Kruskal–Wallis Test). Post-hoc analysis showed that, in patients after a slightly difficult procedure, the mobility of the second molar was significantly higher than in patients after a moderately difficult procedure ($p = 0.043$).

There were no significant differences in second molar mobility according to the difficulty of the procedure at seven days and eight weeks after the procedure. The results are presented in Table 11.

Osstell Measurement

Osstell readings, obtained at particular time points, are presented. Statistical analysis showed no significant correlation between the mobility of the seventh tooth measured with the Osstell and the anticipated difficulty of wisdom tooth removal surgery. The highest mean measurement value was 60.3 (8.38) eight weeks after the slightly difficult procedure. The results of the statistical analysis were summarized in Table 12.

Table 11. Comparison of the relationship of predicted procedure difficulty and second molar mobility before the procedure, immediately after the procedure, 7 days after the procedure, and 8 weeks after the procedure (measured by Periotest M).

Periotest	Difficulty of the Procedure	n	Mean	SD	Median	Min	Max	Q1	Q3	IQR	p *
Before the procedure	Slightly difficult	10	0.82	2.31	−0.05	−1.55	4.15	−0.99	3.15	2.16	0.091
	Moderately difficult	36	−0.91	2.12	−1.23	−5.85	5.7	−2.06	0.19	−1.87	
	Very difficult	14	−1.15	1.91	−1.1	−5.45	1.4	−1.79	0.14	−1.65	
After the procedure	Slightly difficult	10	1.99	2.55	1.82	−0.55	6.2	−0.49	3.79	3.3	0.044
	Moderately difficult	36	−0.07	1.77	−0.32	−3.4	4.55	−1.42	0.86	−0.56	N >
	Very difficult	14	0.43	2.5	1.1	−5.2	4.6	−0.51	1.85	1.34	U
After 7 days	Slightly difficult	10	1.94	1.87	2.27	−0.75	4.3	0.48	3.09	2.61	0.433
	Moderately difficult	36	1.08	2.38	0.8	−2.55	5.85	−0.85	2.51	3.36	
	Very difficult	14	0.98	2.28	0.85	−2.35	6.2	0.11	1.71	1.6	
After 8 weeks	Slightly difficult	10	0.74	2.24	0.02	−1.65	4.9	−0.87	2.22	1.35	0.529
	Moderately difficult	36	−0.46	2.44	−0.45	−8	4.5	−1.6	1.02	−0.58	
	Very difficult	14	−0.15	2.66	−0.57	−5	4.25	−1.11	1.66	0.55	

* Kruskal–Wallis test + post-hoc analysis (Dunn's test). Explanations: n—number of teeth; SD—standard deviation; Min—minimum value; Max—maximum value; Q1—first quartile; Q3—third quartile; p—significance level; N—slightly difficult procedure; U—moderately difficult procedure; B—very difficult procedure.

Table 12. Comparison of the relationship of predicted treatment difficulty and second molar mobility before treatment, immediately after treatment, 7 days after treatment, and 8 weeks after treatment (Osstell measurement).

Osstell	Difficulty of the Procedure	n	Mean	SD	Median	Min	Max	Q1	Q3	IQR	p *
Before the procedure	Slightly difficult	10	58.25	13.48	61.5	33.5	80	57.25	64	6.75	0.394
	Moderately difficult	36	55.75	11.35	53.75	23.5	84	49.25	63.62	14.37	
	Very difficult	14	51.86	10.19	52.5	38.5	67.5	42.5	56.25	13.75	
After the procedure	Slightly difficult	10	48.45	15.48	54.75	24	64	34.38	59.62	25.24	0.135
	Moderately difficult	36	46.94	13.37	49.5	12	66	38	59	21	
	Very difficult	14	40.43	9.81	41.25	24.5	58	32	45.38	13.38	
After 7 days	Slightly difficult	10	48.95	12.57	52	25.5	64.5	43.5	54	10.5	0.624
	Moderately difficult	36	46.4	10.22	47	19.5	66.5	41.5	53.12	11.62	
	Very difficult	14	44.86	10.16	47.75	27.5	57.5	35.25	53.5	18.25	
After 8 weeks	Slightly difficult	10	60.3	8.38	60.75	44	72.5	56	65.62	9.62	0.877
	Moderately difficult	36	59.76	9.97	64.75	34.5	70.5	52.88	67	14.12	
	Very difficult	14	60.29	8.39	63	42.5	72.5	57.12	65.62	8.5	

* Kruskal–Wallis test. Explanations: n—number of teeth; SD—standard deviation; Min—minimum value; Max—maximum value; Q1—first quartile; Q3—third quartile; p—significance level.

4. Discussion

Surgical removal of the impacted third molar is a commonly performed procedure by dental surgery specialists. It is estimated that 16.7–73% of the world population presents at least one impacted molar, most commonly in the mandible [12–14]. Parafunctions and abnormal eating habits, such as the consumption of soft textured foods by children, lead to abnormal oral development and consequently malocclusion [15,16]. The most common cause of tooth impaction is a deficit of space in the dental arch, impaction can also be the result of an abnormal position and path of eruption of the bud, tooth morphology, or function of the dental follicle, and genetic causes [17–19]. Over the last 40 years, there has been an increase in the incidence of tooth impaction, which is a consequence of the development of civilization. It should be predicted that health needs in this area will continue to increase.

Surgical removal of an impacted lower wisdom tooth requires interference into the soft and hard tissues. The procedure involves incision of tissues, often with the performance of vestibular alveotomy, distal–lingual, or crown–root separation of the removed tooth. The surgical removal of wisdom teeth carries a variable risk of complications, and their occurrence depends on factors such as the location of the tooth, the age and general condition of the patient, the difficulty of the procedure, as well as the knowledge and experience of the operator. Complications associated with the surgical removal of wisdom teeth can be divided into those arising during and after the procedure. During the procedure, complications may arise in connection with the impacted or adjacent tooth, soft and hard tissues, inferior alveolar nerve, or lingual nerve. However, postoperatively, pain, swelling, trismus, infection, bleeding, delayed healing, and wound edge dehiscence may occur [20,21]. There are many methods to reduce non-invasive post-surgical complications, which include kinesio taping (KT). KT application is an effective method for reducing postoperative edema, pain, and trismus after impacted mandibular wisdom teeth surgery [22].

There are many papers available in the literature regarding perioperative complications associated with surgical removal of wisdom teeth [20,21,23–28]. However, the impact of surgical removal of wisdom teeth in the mandible on the postoperative status of the second lower molar is marginalized or completely ignored. Consequently, no algorithm has been developed to evaluate the clinical status of the second molar after surgery. Thus, there is a need to develop a useful scheme for its monitoring. This would allow us to predict the potential risk of complications associated with perioperative trauma suffered by the second lower molar.

The probing depth (PD) measurement of the mandibular second molar was adapted from a scenario by the team of Faria et al. [29], in which measurements were taken on the distal surface of the tooth buccally and lingually. In addition, in our work, PD measurements on the mentioned surfaces were supplemented by four additional surfaces with the following locations: centrally buccal and lingual and mesially buccal and lingual, examining both second lower molars. The six-surface examination scheme allowed for a more complete assessment of the periodontal status, especially in conjunction with mobility, as PD has a direct impact on it [30]. Authors Chou et al. [31] included patients in the study group of similar age, with a mean of 45.12 years, ranging from 26 to 73 years of age. The study included second molars in 42 patients who underwent surgical removal of wisdom teeth in the mandible. Each tooth was classified into the appropriate group based on its position relative to the occlusal plane. However, the authors did not provide information on the time elapsed since tooth extraction, which was strictly defined in our study. The probing depth measured in the distal part of the buccal surface of the second molar was significantly greater after wisdom tooth removal compared to the tooth on the opposite side of the arch where the procedure was not performed ($p = 0.004$) [31]. Similar correlations, that is, a significant deepening of probing on the distal surface, were obtained in our study seven days after treatment ($p < 0.001$). Our study, in the assumptions evaluating the clinical condition of second molars, was extended to evaluate the probing depth at additional points on the buccal and lingual surfaces of second molars, unlike the study by Tabrizi et al. [32], who probed only the distal part of the tooth. Measurements were taken at three points on the distal surface, arguing that this was the greatest tissue traumatization during the procedure in the mentioned area. The age of the patients was similar to the age in the present study and a mean of 20.9 (18 to 25 years). Forty-two patients who underwent surgical removal of an impacted third molar were included in the study. All teeth were in a mesioangular position and belonged to group C1 according to the Pell and Gregory classification. In our study, a greater variety of teeth qualifying for surgery was observed, with mesial angle teeth accounting for 50%. The intraoperative procedure and the type of flap created were similar to the study by Tabrizi et al. [32]. The authors compared all measurements with the preoperative state, without a control group. A significant increase in pocket depth was observed after 26 weeks compared to the preoperative status ($p = 0.012$). The mean pocket depth before surgery was 2.71 mm (± 0.59) [32]. In our study, at a shorter time after eight weeks, a significant reduction in depth was observed in the distal part of the buccal ($p = 0.007$) and lingual ($p < 0.001$) surfaces compared to the pre-treatment condition. Tooth mobility, due to trauma and/or periodontal disease, is defined as the movement of the tooth in the horizontal and/or vertical planes under the influence of forces applied by the examiner [33]. An increase in tooth mobility can be caused by the loss of one of the alveolar bone walls that provides support for the tooth embedded in it [34]. The above situation often occurs after surgical removal of a lower impacted tooth, where the distal bony support of the second molar is lost.

Czechowska et al. [24] described a case of partial dislocation of the second molar—47—during surgical removal of an impacted wisdom tooth in the mandible—48. Radiological analysis revealed horizontal impaction of the third molar and, according to Pell–Gregory, it was classified as group B. Surgical intervention resulted in the subluxation of tooth 47, which required immobilization. The consequence was pulp necrosis and the need for endodontic treatment [24].

There are no data in the literature on what percentage of second molars the ligamentous apparatus weakens. Studies conducted show that there is a transient increase in mobility shortly after surgical removal of wisdom teeth but within the physiological range.

Ye et al. [4], based on the analysis of cone-beam tomography images, performed a preoperative computer simulation of the procedure, adequate to the position and impaction of the lower wisdom tooth. The developed method allowed the successful removal of the impacted wisdom tooth in different degrees of impaction. According to the authors, adequate osteotomy and separation of the tooth can reduce the potential risk of injury to the adjacent tooth. However, despite such careful preoperative diagnosis and individualized surgical planning, the researchers were unable to prevent partial dislocation of the second molar, which is near the operated area. Subluxation occurred in one of 136 mandibular second molars studied. The article does not state how the degree of tooth mobility was assessed (Ye et al., 2016) [4]. Monitoring the mobility of the second molar before and after surgical removal of the wisdom tooth in the mandible allows us to indirectly assess the loss of bone support and the forces that acted on the tooth during the surgical intervention. According to some authors, the increase in tooth mobility caused by surgical intervention has a direct bearing on the magnitude of the pulp excitability threshold tested by the electrical test [35–37]. In our study, the last measurements after eight weeks, performed with Osstell and Periotest M, differed. Second molars showed a lower degree of mobility as measured with Osstell than with Periotest M. The method of testing probably underlies this discrepancy. The specificity of Periotest M only allows mobility to be tested in the vestibulo-lingual direction. Osstell, on the other hand, is a composite of vestibulo-lingual and mesiodistal mobility. The results of the present study indicate the need for evaluation of the clinical condition of the second molar before surgery and periodic monitoring after removal of the impacted third molar in the mandible. The evaluation should be based on the study of parameters such as probing depth, mobility, and gingival index. This management algorithm, augmented by Pederson's degree of difficulty assessment, helps minimize complications associated with the clinical condition of the second molar and is often overlooked in the diagnosis and treatment of complications after surgical removal of an impacted wisdom tooth in the mandible. It is important to emphasize the significant impact of tobacco smoking on oral health, particularly the periodontal status. Therefore, we excluded all smokers from the study [38].

It should be emphasized that this study has limitations. It was short—only an 8-week follow-up—; however, it is conditioned by the healing time of soft tissues (24–35 days) [39] and hard tissues (8 weeks) [40] in the oral cavity. In addition, the study included subjects with varying degrees of retention and difficulty, which may have had different effects on the 2nd molar. Sixty consecutively enrolled patients who met the inclusion and exclusion criteria were included in the study, regardless of the anticipated difficulty of the procedure or degree of retention. Because the control group was the tooth on the opposite side of the mandible, different degrees of retention and difficulty of surgery were considered. Another limitation of the study is the fact that teeth from the opposite quadrant were not included in the study, due to the lack of a control group in this case (because the operator had already removed the third molar on one side of the mandible). It should also be noted that in the literature there are also new scales for assessing the difficulty of the procedure, e.g., taking into account the time of the procedure [41,42].

5. Conclusions

The surgical removal of an impacted third molar in the mandible significantly affects the clinical probing depth of the second lower molar, causes a significant increase in the gingivitis index shortly after the procedure, and significantly increases the mobility of the second molar shortly after the procedure. There is a relationship between the degree of difficulty of removal of an impacted third molar in the mandible and the postoperative probing depth and mobility of the second molar and the gingivitis index value. The results of the present study support the need for a clinical evaluation of the second lower molar before and after surgical removal of an impacted wisdom tooth in the mandible.

Author Contributions: Conceptualization, M.A.-W. and G.T.; methodology, M.A.-W. and G.T.; software, A.J.; validation, M.A.-W. and G.T.; formal analysis, M.A.-W. and G.T.; investigation, M.A.-W. and G.T.; resources, A.J., O.P. and A.G.; data curation, M.A.-W. and G.T.; writing—original draft preparation, M.A.-W., G.T. and A.J.; writing—review and editing, G.T. and A.J.; visualization, A.J.; supervision, G.T.; project administration, G.T. All authors have read and agreed to the published version of the manuscript.

Funding: This research received no external funding.

Institutional Review Board Statement: The study was conducted according to the guidelines of the Declaration of Helsinki and approved by the Ethics Committee KB-0012/89/16.

Informed Consent Statement: Informed consent was obtained from all subjects involved in the study.

Data Availability Statement: Data available on request.

Conflicts of Interest: The authors declare no conflict of interest.

References

1. Richardson, D.T.; Dodson, T.B. Risk of periodontal defects after third molar surgery: An exercise in evidence-based clinical decision-making. *Oral Surg. Oral Med. Oral Pathol. Oral Radiol. Endod.* **2005**, *100*, 133–137. [CrossRef]
2. Román-Malo, L.; Bullon, P. Influence of the periodontal disease, the most prevalent inflammatory event, in peroxisome proliferator—Activated receptors linking nutrition and energy metabolism. *Int. J. Mol. Sci.* **2017**. [CrossRef]
3. Sammartino, G.; Tia, M.; Bucci, T.; Wang, H.L. Prevention of mandibular third molar extraction-associated periodontal defects: A comparative study. *J. Periodontol.* **2009**, *80*, 389–396. [CrossRef]
4. Ye, Z.X.; Yang, C.; Ge, J. Adjacent tooth trauma in complicated mandibular third molar surgery: Risk degree classification and digital surgical simulation. *Sci. Rep.* **2016**, *6*, 1–7. [CrossRef]
5. Peng, K.Y.; Tseng, Y.C.; Shen, E.C.; Chiu, S.C.; Fu, E.; Huang, Y.W. Mandibular second molar periodontal status after third molar extraction. *J. Periodontol.* **2001**, *72*, 1647–1651. [CrossRef]
6. Kugelberg, C.F.; Ahlstrom, U.; Ericson, S.; Hugoson, A. Periodontal healing after impacted lower third molar surgery. A retrospective study. *Int. J. Oral Surg.* **1985**, *14*, 29–40. [CrossRef]
7. Kugelberg, C.F.; Ahlstrom, U.; Ericson, S.; Hugoson, A.; Thilander, H. The influence of anatomical, pathophysiological and other factors on periodontal healing after impacted lower third molar surgery. A regression analysis. *J. Clin. Periodontol.* **1991**, *18*, 37–43. [CrossRef]
8. Dodson, T.B. Management of mandibular third molar extraction sites to prevent periodontal defects. *J. Oral Maxillofac. Surg.* **2004**, *62*, 1213–1224. [CrossRef]
9. Winter, G.B. *Impacted Mandibular Third Molars*; American Medical Book Company: St. Louis, MO, USA, 1926.
10. Pell, G.J.; Gregory, G.T. Impacted mandibular third molars: Classification and modified technique for removal. *Dent. Dig.* **1933**, *39*, 330–338.
11. Silness, J.; Löe, H. Periodontal disease in pregnancy (II). Correlation between oral hygiene and periodontal condition. *Acta Odontol. Scand.* **1964**, *22*, 121–135. [CrossRef]
12. Kaapoglu, C.; Brkic, A.; Gurkan-Koseoglu, B.; Kocak-Berberoglu, H. Complications following surgery of impacted teeth and their management. In *A Textbook of Advanced Oral and Maxillofacial Surgery*; IntechOpen: London, UK, 2013. [CrossRef]
13. Juodzbalys, G.; Povilas, D. Mandibular third molar impaction: Review of literature and a proposal of a classification. *J. Oral Maxillofac. Res.* **2013**, *4*, 1–11.
14. Trybek, G.; Chruściel-Nogalska, M.; Machnio, M.; Smektała, T.; Malinowski, J.; Tutak, M.; Sporniak-Tutak, K. Surgical extraction of impacted teeth in elderly patients. A retrospective analysis of perioperative complications—The experience of a single institution. *Gerodontology* **2016**, *33*, 410–415. [CrossRef] [PubMed]
15. Kaczmarek, M. Poznańskie badania długofalowe. Wzorce i dynamika wyrzynania zębów stałych a ocena dojrzałości biologicznej organizmu. *Przegląd Antropol.* **1995**, *58*, 9–31.

16. Osmólska-Bogucka, A.; Buczek, O.; Bilińska, M.; Zadurska, M. Parafuncje niezwarciowe u dzieci i rodziców oraz ich wpływ na występowanie wad zgryzu u dzieci na podstawie badania ankietowego i klinicznego. *Nowa Stomatol.* **2014**, *2*, 63–69.
17. Huang, G.J.; Cruz-Cunha, J.; Rothen, M.; Spiekerman, C.; Drangsholt, M.; Anderson, L.; Rosent, G.A. A prospective study of clinical outcomes treated to third molar removal or retention. *Am. J. Public Health* **2014**, *104*, 728–734. [CrossRef]
18. Perillo, L.; Esposito, M.; Caprioglio, A.; Attanasio, S.; Santini, A.C.; Carotenuto, M. Orthodontic treatment need for adolescents in the Campania region: The malocclusion impact on self-concept. Orthodontic treatment need for adolescents in the Campania region: The malocclusion impact on self-concept. *Patient Prefer Adherence* **2014**, *19*, 353–359.
19. Trybek, G.; Jaroń, A.; Grzywacz, A. Association of Polymorphic and Haplotype Variants of the MSX1 Gene and the Impacted Teeth Phenomenon. *Genes* **2021**, *12*, 577. [CrossRef]
20. Brauer, H.U.; Green, R.A.; Pynn, R.B. Complications during and after surgical removal of third molars. *Mag. Oral Health* **2009**, *40*, 565–572.
21. Deliverska, E.G.; Petkova, M. Complication after extraction of impacted third molars-literature review. *J. IMAB* **2016**, *22*, 1202–1211. [CrossRef]
22. Jaroń, A.; Preuss, O.; Grzywacz, E.; Trybek, G. The Impact of Using Kinesio Tape on Non-Infectious Complications after Impacted Mandibular Third Molar Surgery. *Int. J. Environ. Res. Public Health* **2021**, *18*, 399. [CrossRef]
23. Pitekova, L.; Satko, I.; Novotnakova, D. Complications after third molar surgery. *Quintessence Int.* **2010**, *111*, 296–298.
24. Czechowska, E.; Rydzewska-Lipińska, M.; Szubert, P.; Sokalski, J. Komplikacje podczas zabiegu usuwania zęba mądrości—opis przypadku. *Dent. Forum* **2013**, *31*, 119–122.
25. Guerrouani, A.; Zeinoun, T.; Vervaet, C.; Legrand, W. A four monocentric study of the complications of third molars extractions under general anesthesia: About 2112 patients. *Int. J. Dent.* **2013**. [CrossRef]
26. Jaroń, A.; Trybek, G. The Pattern of Mandibular Third Molar Impaction and Assessment of Surgery Difficulty: A Retrospective Study of Radiographs in East Baltic Population. *Int. J. Environ. Res. Public Health* **2021**, *18*, 6016. [CrossRef]
27. Osunde, O.D.; Saheeb, B.D. Effect of age, sex and level of surgical difficulty on inflammatory complications after third molar surgery. *J. Maxillofac. Oral Surg.* **2015**, *14*, 7–12. [CrossRef] [PubMed]
28. Szubert, P.; Jankowski, M.; Krajecki, M.; Jankowska-Wik, A.; Sokalski, J. Analiza czynników predysponujących do powikłań po chirurgicznym usunięciu zębów mądrości w żuchwie. *Dent. Forum* **2015**, *63*, 45–50.
29. Faria, A.I.; Gallas-Torreira, M.; Gallas-Torreira, M.; López-Ratón, M. Mandibular second molar periodontal healing after impacted third molar extraction in young adults. *J. Maxillofac. Oral Surg.* **2012**, *70*, 2732–2741. [CrossRef] [PubMed]
30. Zawada, Ł.; Konopka, T. Nowe wskaźniki periodontologiczne. *Dent. Med. Probl.* **2011**, *48*, 243–250.
31. Chou, Y.H.; Ho, P.S.; Ho, K.Y.; Wang, W.C.; Hu, K.F. Association between the eruption of the third molar and caries and periodontitis distal to the second molars in elderly patients. *Kaohsiung J. Med. Sci.* **2017**, *33*, 246–251. [CrossRef] [PubMed]
32. Tabrizi, R.; Arabion, H.; Gholami, M. How will mandibular third molar surgery affect mandibular second molar periodontal parameters? *Dent. Res.* **2013**, *19*, 523–526.
33. Azodo, C.C.; Erhabor, P. Management of tooth mobility in the periodontology clinic: An overview and experience from a tertiary healthcare setting. *Afr. J. Med. Health Sci.* **2016**, *15*, 50–57. [CrossRef]
34. Purkait, S.; Bandyopadhyaya, P.; Mallick, B.; Das, I. Classification of tooth mobility—Concept Revisited. *Int. J. Rec. Advan. Multidiscip. Res.* **2016**, *3*, 1510–1522.
35. Andreasen, J.O.; Andreasen, F.M.; Skeie, A.; Hjørting-Hansen, E.; Schwartz, O. Effect of treatment delay upon pulp and periodontal healing of traumatic dental injuries -a review article. *Dent. Traumatol.* **2002**, *18*, 116–128. [CrossRef] [PubMed]
36. Abbot, P.V.; Salgado, J.C. Strategies to minimise the consequences of trauma to the teeth. *Oral Health Dent. Manag.* **2014**, *13*, 229–242.
37. Arun, A.; Mythri, H.; Chachapan, D. Pulp vitality test—An overwiew on comparison of sensitivity and vitality. *Indian J. Oral Sci.* **2015**, *6*, 41–46.
38. Suchanecka, A.; Chmielowiec, K.; Chmielowiec, J.; Trybek, G.; Masiak, J.; Michałowska-Sawczyn, M.; Nowicka, R.; Grocholewicz, K.; Grzywacz, A. Vitamin D Receptor Gene Polymorphisms and Cigarette Smoking Impact on Oral Health: A Case-Control Study. *Int. J. Environ. Res. Public Health* **2020**, *17*, 3192. [CrossRef]
39. Adeyemo, W.L.; Ladeinde, A.L.; Ogunlewe, M.O. Clinical evaluation of post-extraction site wound healing. *J. Contemp. Dent. Pract.* **2006**, *7*, 40–49. [CrossRef] [PubMed]
40. Rever, L.J.; Manson, P.N.; Randolph, M.A.; Yaremchuk, M.J.; Weiland, A.; Siegel, J.H. The Healing of Facial Bone Fractures by the Process of Secondary Union. *Plast. Reconstr. Surg.* **1991**, *87*, 451–458. [CrossRef] [PubMed]
41. Ku, J.K.; Chang, N.H.; Jeong, Y.K.; Baik, S.H.; Choi, S.K. Development and validation of a difficulty index for mandibular third molars with extraction time. *J. Korean Assoc. Oral Maxillofac. Surg.* **2020**, *46*, 328–334. [CrossRef] [PubMed]
42. Kim, J.Y.; Yong, H.S.; Park, K.H.; Huh, J.K. Modified difficult index adding extremely difficult for fully impacted mandibular third molar extraction. *J. Korean Assoc. Oral Maxillofac. Surg.* **2019**, *45*, 309–315. [CrossRef]

Review

Systemic Lupus Erythematosus and Periodontal Disease: A Complex Clinical and Biological Interplay

Bouchra Sojod [1,2], Cibele Pidorodeski Nagano [3], Glenda Melissa Garcia Lopez [1,2], Antoine Zalcberg [1,2], Sophie Myriam Dridi [4] and Fani Anagnostou [1,2,3,*]

1. Service d'Odontologie, Hôpital Universitaire Pitié Salpêtrière (AP-HP), 75013 Paris, France; bouchrasojod@gmail.com (B.S.); m.e.l.i.843@gmail.com (G.M.G.L.); pbca@hotmail.fr (A.Z.)
2. Faculté de Chirurgie Dentaire-Garancière, Université de Paris, 75006 Paris, France
3. B3OA, CNRS UMR 7052-INSERM U1271, Université de Paris, 75010 Paris, France; cibele.nagano@gmail.com
4. Faculté de Chirurgie Dentaire, Université Côte d'Azur, 06300 Nice, France; dr.sm.dridi@free.fr
* Correspondence: fani.anagnostou@univ-paris-diderot.fr

Abstract: Reports on the association of periodontal disease (PD) with systemic lupus erythematosus (SLE) have regularly been published. PD is a set of chronic inflammatory conditions linked to a dysbiotic microbial biofilm, which affects the periodontal tissues, resulting eventually in their destruction and contributing to systemic inflammation. SLE is a multi-system chronic inflammatory autoimmune disease that has a wide range of clinical presentations, touching multiple organ systems. Many epidemiological studies have investigated the two-way relationship between PD and SLE, though their results are heterogeneous. SLE and PD are multifactorial conditions and many biological-based hypotheses suggest common physiopathological pathways between the two diseases, including genetics, microbiology, immunity, and environmental common risk factors. By focusing on recent clinical and translational research, this review aimed to discuss and give an overview of the relationship of SLE with PD, as well as looking at the similarities in the immune-pathological aspects and the possible mechanisms connecting the development and progression of both diseases.

Keywords: systematic lupus erythematosus; periodontal disease; risk factors; autoimmune and inflammatory diseases; periodontitis; periopathogens

1. Introduction

Systematic lupus erythematosus (SLE) is an autoimmune disease, which is characterized by the loss of self-tolerance and immune complex-mediated inflammation, and can affect almost every system in the body, with varying degrees of severity [1,2]. The clinical course of the disease is described by recurrent acute or chronic inflammation episodes, leading to the dysfunction of several organs, for example, kidneys, joints, and the skin. In this respect, the oral cavity is not spared. Patients with SLE may present with some oral manifestations, including a wide spectrum of oral mucosal ulceration, such as cheilitis, erythematous patches, honeycomb plaques, discoid lesions, lichen planus (LP)-like lesions, hyposalivation, and xerostomia [3,4]. SLE patients also exhibit a high prevalence of dental caries [5] and an increased number of missing teeth. The aforementioned clinical manifestations result in a negative impact of patients' oral condition on their quality of life [6]. Moreover, several recent literature have reported that patients with SLE present also a higher risk of periodontitis [7], suggesting a potential association between the two conditions.

Periodontal diseases (PD) comprising gingivitis and periodontitis are highly prevalent diseases worldwide. The prevalence of gingivitis was reported to range from 38% to 85% [8], while severe forms of periodontitis affect ~11% of the global adult population [9]. Gingivitis, the mildest form of periodontal disease, is caused by bacterial biofilms deposited on dental surfaces, subsequent to inadequate self-performed oral hygiene procedures. Gingivitis is characterized by a reversible inflammatory response confined in the gingiva. Its onset and progression may be modified by local factors and/or systemic conditions [8]. Periodontitis, on the other hand, a multifactorial chronic disease caused by polymicrobial synergy of dysbiotic biofilms in susceptible hosts [10], is characterized by the inflammatory destruction of the periodontium, resulting in the irreversible loss of the supporting tooth apparatus, including alveolar bone and, eventually, tooth loss [11]. The effects of periodontitis are not constrained to the oral cavity. Numerous epidemiological, interventional and experimental studies show that periodontitis is associated with several non-communicable pathologies [12], as well as with an increased risk of mortality [13]. It is associated with cardiovascular disease, stroke [14], diabetes [15], adverse pregnancy outcomes [16], pulmonary disease [17]. In addition to these pathologies, periodontitis has been shown recently to be also associated with several other diseases, including metabolic disease and obesity, Alzheimer's disease [18], certain cancers [12], inflammatory bowel disease [19], and immunoinflammatory diseases, such as rheumatoid arthritis [20–22]. Growing evidence suggests that oral dysbiosis, as well as pathogens associated with periodontitis could be involved in the pathophysiology of autoimmune inflammatory diseases, including the SLE.

As aforementioned, the complex multifactorial disease of SLE, characterized by an excessive autoimmune response in the body, represents a major diagnostic and therapeutic clinical challenge [23]. This disease is of unknown etiology and genetic and environmental factors contribute to its susceptibility [24]. Studies on SLE patients (and on mouse models of lupus) have implied the contribution of almost every cell type of the immune system in either the induction or amplification of the autoimmune response, as along with the promotion of an inflammatory environment that exacerbates tissue damage (arthritis, glomerulonephritis, etc.) [25]. Pathogenic autoantibodies mediate the cell damage, which is directed against nucleic acids and protein complexes [1]. Infection is regarded as a trigger for autoimmune diseases and is responsible for controlling the SLE systemic activity. Periodontitis, and specifically oral dysbiosis, could be a contributing factor in sustaining the inflammatory response observed in SLE.

Considering the aforementioned, it was hypothesized that there is an interplay between PD and SLE; the environmental and genetic factors involved in SLE may also contribute to PD pathogenesis while PD may critically act in the initiation and/or the maintenance of the immune-inflammatory response that occurs in SLE. The objective of this article was, therefore, to identify and discuss the evidence regarding the two-way relationship between PD and SLE. The present review was conducted through the PubMed/MEDLINE database, searching for articles written in English and published from 1990 to 2020. The keywords were searched in MeSh (Medical Subject Headings), and the terms used to target peer-reviewed articles were: (systematic lupus erythematosus) AND ((periodontitis) OR (periodontal disease)).

2. Epidemiological Evidence for the Association between PD Parameters and SLE

2.1. The Impact of SLE Activity on PD

The first literature article dealing with the association between PD and SLE published in 1981 was a case report presenting a 17-year-old female who exhibited edematous gingiva and spontaneous bleeding, and thus was diagnosed with SLE and megakaryocytic thrombocytopenia [26]. Another publication reported the case of an 18-year-old female with SLE who presented severe periodontal involvement manifested by generalized gingival recession [27]. In this case, lack of predisposing aspects for chronic periodontitis was interpreted by the authors in favor of direct association between SLE and the periodontal status. A case of acute necrotizing ulcerative gingivitis (ANUG) was also reported in a patient with SLE in 1985 [28]. A higher incidence of gingivitis was also observed in juvenile SLE patients in contrast to that observed in healthy children and adolescents [29].

The prevalence and severity of PD, specifically periodontitis, in the SLE patients have been the subject of several studies (summarized in Table 1). The most studied clinical parameters of PD were pocket depth, bleeding on probing, gingival recession, and clinical attachment loss, which is the representative of cumulative periodontal destruction. According to literature reports, the prevalence of periodontitis in SLE patients varies between 60% and 94% [30]. Other studies have also reported the increased prevalence of PD in the SLE patients compared to the healthy controls [31–35]. In agreement with these studies, compared to adult population, higher prevalence (almost 70%) was observed in the SLE patients.

However, data regarding the severity of clinical parameters of periodontitis in the SLE patients compared to either healthy volunteers, or patients with PD without SLE are conflicting. Recent controlled studies have reported greater severity of PD in the patients with SLE, exhibiting more clinical attachment loss [34], and/or increased pocket depth [36]. Moreover, reduced periodontal probing depths in the SLE patients (compared to the control group) was noticed [32,37–40]. Severity of the periodontal parameters monitored was similar in the SLE patients and the control subjects; however, chronic periodontitis occurred earlier in the SLE patients [30]. Absence of a statistically significant difference between the results from controls and SLE cases could be ascribed to the use of various anti-inflammatory drugs. This could also raise the question around the impact of the immunosuppressive treatment of SLE on the PD parameters. Moreover, in a meta-analysis, it was shown that the overall risk of periodontitis was significantly increased by 1.76 (95% CI 1.29–2.41, $p = 0.0004$) in the patients with SLE, compared to the respective controls. However, there was no statistically significant difference in individual parameters of periodontitis such as probing depth ($p = 0.06$) and clinical attachment loss ($p = 0.08$) between the SLE cases and healthy cases [7]. Likewise, a recent meta-analysis involving 80,633 subjects showed a significant increase in the prevalence of periodontitis (odds ratio = 5.32, 95% CI 1.69–16.78, $p = 0.004$), while no significant difference was observed in the incidence of severe periodontitis between the patients with SLE and healthy controls [41]. In the SLE patients, a higher prevalence of bleeding on probing, higher mean clinical attachment loss, and similar values of mean pocket depth, gingival index, and plaque index were observed [41]. These conflicting findings might be attributed to many factors, including (i) differences in the definition and the clinical measurement of PD; (ii) differences in the scoring of SLE activity and damage; (iii) the presence of potential confounding factors of comorbidity (e.g., smoking and stress); (iv) the use of anti-inflammatory drugs for the treatment of SLE; and (v) differences in the genetic and environmental backgrounds of the studied populations; as well as (vi) the clinical study design (e.g., sample size, type of study, etc.).

2.2. Impact of PD on the Pathogenesis of SLE

Recent clinical evidence has demonstrated the implication of PD in the pathogenesis of SLE. A nationwide, population-based, retrospective case-control study explained the association between the history of PD and newly diagnosed SLE (OR, 1.21; 95% CI, 1.14–1.28; $p < 0.001$), which was both dose- and time-dependent [42]. Given that smoking is a common risk factor for both PD and SLE, the aforementioned association is weak and attributed to the lack of information on the individual smoking status of patients. Nevertheless, in another recent randomized clinical trial, the influence of periodontitis treatment on the manifestation of SLE was investigated. The authors reported that PD treatment improved response to immunosuppressive therapy, suggesting that PD may be a modifiable risk factor for SLE [31]. The strength of this association is weak due to the cross-sectional nature of this study, the limited information collected on the progression of SLE, and the use of immunosuppressive treatment. On the other hand, Wang et al. [34] reported that patients with periodontitis had 26.94 times higher risk of having SLE than the patients without periodontitis; these results highlighted the role of periodontal interventions in the prevention and risk assessment of SLE. Moreover, Bae and Lee [43], in a recent study, analyzed the associations from genome-wide association studies on European population, using PD as an exposure and SLE as an outcome with Mendelian randomization. Interestingly, they found a weak but significant evidence that periodontitis is causally related with an elevated risk of SLE incidence in line with the published epidemiological studies.

Table 1. Epidemiologic observational studies investigating the association between PD and SLE.

Reference	Design	Quality Rating	Demographics	Periodontal Assessment Methodology	Results
Rutter-Locher et al. 2017 (England) [7]	Systematic review and meta-analysis	Good	487 SLE patients 896 controls	PI BOP PD CAL Residual teeth	Statistically significant increased risk of periodontitis in patients with SLE compared to controls.
Voger et al. 1981 (USA) [26]	Case report	Poor	A 17-year old black female	BOP, PD	The patient was diagnosed with a generalized severe gingivitis associated with SLE and amegakaryocytic thrombocytopenia.
Nagler et al. 1999 (Israel) [27]	Case report	Poor	An 18-year old female	BOP, PD, Recession	Severe periodontal loss was manifested by gingival recession. Focal lymphoepithelial lesion was found in the gingival subepithelium. Periodontitis was found in the SLE patient.
Jaworski et al. 1985 (Korea) [28]	Case report	Poor	A 35-year old Korean female	Gingival aspect Pain Swelling Adenopathy	The patient presented ANUG. SLE and the therapeutic amounts of steroids may have contributed to the increased severity of the oral disease.
Fernandes et al. 2007 (Brazil) [29]	Case control study	Fair	48 children and adolescents with SLE, 48 children and adolescents as controls	PI GI	Patients with SLE presented poor oral hygiene. Higher incidence of gingivitis
Fabbri et al. 2014 (Brazil) [31]	Randomized controlled trial	Fair	32 SLE/ periodontitis-treated patients 17 SLE/ periodontitis-untreated patients	PD CAL GBI	Prevalence of periodontitis among SLE patients initially selected for the study was 89%. PD treatment improved response to immunosuppressive therapy in SLE patients.
Kobayashi et al. 2007 (Japan) [32]	Case control study	Fair	46 SLE/periodontitis patients 25 SLE patients 58 periodontitis patients 44 controls	Number of missing teeth PD CAL BOP PI	64.8% of SLE patients had periodontitis. The combination of stimulatory FcγRIIa and inhibitory FcγRIIb genotypes was associated with the risk of periodontitis in SLE patients in the Japanese population.

Table 1. *Cont.*

Reference	Design	Quality Rating	Demographics	Periodontal Assessment Methodology	Results
Novo et al. 1999 (Venezuela) [33]	Comparative study	Fair	30 patients with SLE 30 patients with RA 20 controls	PD BOP Bone loss (estimated in a periapical Rx)	60% of SLE patients had periodontitis. An association was found between ANCA and periodontitis in SLE patients.
Wang et al. 2015 (Japan) [34]	Case-control study	Fair	53 SLE patients 56 controls	PD CAL Pg and Td levels in gingival sulcus Levels of serum anti-CL and anti-β2GPI antibodies	Prevalence of periodontitis among SLE patients was 79%. Periodontitis was associated with an increased production of anti-β2GPI-dependent anti-CL antibodies in patients with SLE.
De Pablo et al. 2015 (England) [35]	Case-control study	Fair	105 SLE patients 484 controls	PD	Periodontal disease was more common among individuals with SLE.
Correa et al. 2017 (Brazil) [36]	Case-control study	Fair	52 SLE patients 52 controls	PD CAL BOP PI Dental personal hygiene Subgingival bacterial composition	Prevalence of periodontitis among SLE patients was 53%.
Zhang et al. 2017 (Chine) [37]	Case-control study	Fair	108 SLE patients 108 controls	PI BOP GI Bone loss PD CAL	Chinese SLE patients were likely to suffer from higher odds of PD.
Figueredo et al. 2008 (Brazil) [38]	Case-control study	Fair	16 JSLE patients 14 controls	PD PI GBI CAL Expression of IL-18, IL-1β, elastase activity in GCF	Higher levels of active elastase in GCF from inflamed sites in JSLE patients. Greater risk of tissue degradation and periodontal attachment loss of JSLE patients compared to healthy juvenile controls.

Table 1. Cont.

Reference	Design	Quality Rating	Demographics	Periodontal Assessment Methodology	Results
Kobayashi et al. 2003 (Japan) [39]	Case control study	Fair	42 SLE/periodontitis patients 18 SLE patients 42 periodontitis patients 42 controls	Number of missing teeth PD CAL BOP, PI	70% of SLE patients had periodontitis. FcγRIIa -R131 allele was associated with the risk of periodontitis in SLE patients in the Japanese population.
Mutlu et al. 1993 (England) [40]	Case-control study	Fair	27 SLE patients 25 controls	PD	Patients with SLE significantly had lower periodontal probing depths compared to healthy controls.
Wu et al. 2017 (Japan) [42]	Retrospective Case-control study	Fair	7204 SLE patients 72040 controls	Number of periodontitis-related visits History of PD	A higher risk of SLE was significantly associated with a history of PD. Prevalence of periodontitis among SLE patients was 35%.
Al Mutairi et al. 2015 (Kingdom of Saudi Arabia) [44]	Case-control study	Fair	25 SLE patients 50 controls	PI BOP CAL PD Residual teeth	Periodontal health was not different between SLE patients and controls.
Rhodus and Johnson 1990 (the USA) [45]	Case series	Poor	16 females with SLE	PD CAL	93.8% of studied patients presented periodontitis.

Note: BOP: bleeding on probing, PD: probing depth, SLE: systemic lupus erythematosus, ANUG: acute necrotizing ulcerative gingivitis, PI: plaque index, GI: gingival index, CAL: clinical attachment loss, RA: rheumatoid arthritis, ANCA: antineutrophil cytoplasmic antibodies, GBI: gingival bleeding index, GCF: gingival crevicular fluid, JSLE: juvenile systemic lupus erythematosus. The quality rating of the epidemiological studies performed according to Oxford center for evidence-based medicine 2011. OCEBM Levels of Evidence. (Electronic resource). URL: https://www.cebm.ox.ac.uk/resources/levels-of-evidence/ocebm-levels-of-evidence (accessed on 27 April 2021). "Poor" corresponds to the level 4, "fair" corresponds to levels 2 and 3, and "good" corresponds to level 1 [46].

3. Biological Basics for a Potential Relationship between PD and SLE

In addition to epidemiological data, several studies, presented in the following section, have reported that shared genetic and environmental risk factors, as well as the activation of immune pathways underlying local pathological outcomes for the two conditions have led to the relationship between SLE and PD.

3.1. Genetic Link

Several loci and genetic variants have been identified to be associated with SLE [2]; however, only three studies have addressed the link of SLE with PD. Notably, Kobayashi et al. [32,39] assessed the distribution of the FcγRIIA, FcγPIIIA and FcγPIIIb genotypes and alleles in 71 Japanese SLE patients with and without PD, and in healthy subjects with and without PD, and reported that the PD–SLE connection might be associated to the polymorphism of Fcγ receptor. Specifically, these authors reported that FcγRIIA-R131 and the combination of FcγRIIA-R131 and FcγRIIB-232T alleles are strongly in association with SLE and periodontitis. Japanese SLE patients with the combined FcγR risk alleles experienced more severe periodontal tissue destruction than other SLE patients. Further studies are needed, however, to confirm the association of FcγR with SLE in other ethnic populations. Schaefer et al. [47] sought to elucidate the shared genetic basis of either SLE or rheumatoid arthritis (RA) with aggressive periodontitis. These authors not only identified PRDM1 and IRF5 as candidate genes that play a role in IFN-signaling and have genome-wide association with SLE, but they reported that the extent of shared risk loci is limited. Further studies are required to determine the pathogenic genetic link between the two diseases and related polymorphism(s).

Besides genetics, epigenetic modifications as a result of the interaction of bacterial metabolites and epigenetic enzymatic reactions, are also involved in pathogenesis of both PD and SLE [48]. Epigenetic mechanisms, such as DNA methylation and histone modification can trigger breakdown of immunological homeostasis of periodontal environment, but further investigations are needed to a more complete understanding of cyclic inflammation/dysbiosis process.

3.2. Potential Mechanisms Linking SLE with the PD Pathogenesis

Potential mechanisms linking the SLE with the pathogenesis of PD include (i) the effects of systemic immune dysregulation on subgingival microbiota; (ii) the SLE-induced imbalance between pro-inflammatory and anti-inflammatory cytokines, which seems to be the cause of tissue damage [36]; (iii) the activation of autoreactive B cells and dysregulation of several other immune cell types, including macrophages, neutrophils, CD4+ T cells, and dendritic cells [48].

3.2.1. Effect of SLE-Associated Systemic Immune Dysregulation on Subgingival Microbiota

It has been reported that systemic inflammatory disorders such as diabetes, RA and inflammatory Bowel disease, might contribute to the destruction of periodontal tissue by disrupting the balance between host and oral microbiota [19,49]. A recent study examined the effects of SLE on the subgingival microbiota and reported that the SLE patients had a dysbiotic subgingival microbiota with higher subgingival bacterial load, and experienced major alterations in bacterial composition with a shift to greater quantities of pathogenic bacteria, including *Prevotella oulorum, P. Oris, P.nigrescens, S. noxia, Lachnospiraceae*, and *Leptotrichia*, even in periodontally healthy sites [36]. In another study, *Candida albicans* and *Lactobacilli* were observed in higher proportions in the SLE patients and *A. actinomycetemcomitans* in juvenile SLE patients as compared with controls [50]. SLE disease activity and severity has been correlated to changes of the PD-associated microbiota [51]. *Treponema denticola* and *Tannerella forsythia* were also in increased quantities in SLE-active periodontal sites in comparison to that of SLE-inactive and healthy controls [52]. SLE-associated inflammatory changes in the periodontium providing a source of nutriments by altering the subgingival microbiota may favor bacterial interactions that lead to the increased susceptibility to PD [53]. The dysbiotic microbial community may play, therefore, a central role in the mechanistic link between the two conditions, though further studies are warranted to define it.

3.2.2. SLE-Induced Imbalance Between Pro-inflammatory and Anti-Inflammatory Cytokines

In patients affected by both PD and chronic inflammation-driven disorders, changes in the oral microbiota have been linked to the increased local inflammation [19,53]. For instance, modified patterns of cytokines expression in gingival tissue and of cytokines levels in CGF and in saliva have been reported in inflammatory bowel disease [19], diabetes [53] and RA [54]. Indeed, in SLE, the salivary concentrations of IL-6 and IL-17A were significantly higher in the SLE/PD patients compared to the controls/PD subjects. Moreover, IL-6, IL-17A, and IL-33 levels were increased in the SLE/PD patients compared to the SLE patients without PD [36,55,56]. Increased levels of the same cytokines have been observed also in the saliva of RA patients [54]. Additionally, increased levels of IFN-γ, IL-10, IL-1β, and IL-4 were observed in the saliva of patients with SLE, even in the absence of PD [55]. Specifically, IL-17 involved in both PD and SLE pathogenesis was reported to play a key role in the process of inflammation/dysbiosis [57]. In CGF of SLE/PD patients' levels of visfatin, an adipokine involved in pro-inflammatory response, are increased [58]. Furthermore, the altered levels of IL-1β, IL-8, G-CSF, IFN-γ, and CMP-1 in gingival crevicular fluid (CGF) have been associated to worsened periodontal conditions in patients with juvenile SLE [50]. Some of these cytokines specifically IFN-γ, IL-10, and IL-4 were also increased in the serum samples of the SLE patients and were linked to the disease manifestation [1]. Pessoa et al. reported serum cytokine dysregulation in SLE patients to be dependent on SLE activity [51]. However, the involvement of cytokines in the periodontal tissue destruction is difficult to interpret due to the various effects of the same cytokines at different stages of SLE, as well as on the pathogenesis of PD. Furthermore, systemic use of the anti-inflammatory drugs (e.g., corticoids) affects the local production of some cytokines (e.g., IL-1β and IL-18) in the gingiva [56] and, therefore, may modify the local inflammatory response to the dysbiotic flora and the periodontium destruction.

3.3. B-Cell Hyperactivity

Destructive lesions are dominated by B-lymphocytes and plasma cells [11], and interestingly, in SLE, B-cell hyperactivity was proposed as the basic mechanism for the generation of autoantibodies [2]. The interaction between antigen presenting cells, abnormally activated T cells, and hyperactive B cells results in the production of soluble autoantibodies of the IgG isotype, as well as various cytokines. The secreted autoantibodies form immune complexes by binding autoantigens and, in turn, complement fixation, or engaging Fcγ receptors on several different cell types, leading to tissue damage [32,39]. If, and how, the increased autoantibodies in SLE contribute to the chronic tissue damage resulting from periodontitis remains to be elucidated.

4. Potential Mechanisms Underlying the Links between PD and the Pathogenesis of SLE

PD and oral dysbiosis are implicated in several autoimmune diseases, including SLE, and several pathogenic mechanisms have been proposed to explain this association [59]. In the pathogenesis of SLE, infections may play a pivotal role in addition to the genetic, hormonal, and environmental aspects [2,60]. SLE patients secrete large amounts of antibodies against various oral bacteria. Specifically, serum antibody titers against PD-associated bacteria such as *A. actinomycetemcomitans*, *P. gingivalis*, *T. denticola*, and *C. ochracea* were higher in the patients who were positive for anti-dsDNA antibodies significantly correlated with anti-dsDNA titers and reduced levels of complement [61]. Moreover, antibodies to *A. actinomycetemcomitans* were associated with higher disease activity.

Infectious agents can trigger autoimmune diseases through various mechanisms, including molecular mimicry, epitope spreading, alterations in self-antigens, and immune cell activation in genetically susceptible individuals [62]. More precisely, it has been reported that periopathogens might cause the excessive activation of immune response in the SLE by retaining a high expression of TLRs in periodontal tissues, and in turn, leading to the acceleration of the onset and progression of autoimmune reactions [55]. Indeed, the expression levels of TLR-2 TLR-4 are increased in both PD [63] and SLE [64]. These findings suggest that periopathogens (e.g., *P. gingivalis*) stimulate the expression of TLR-2 and TLR-4 in the periodontium and activate the mechanisms of local and systemic autoimmunity related to the SLE, which might be, at least partially, associated with the disease in the SLE patients.

Besides these exogenous pathogen-associated molecular patterns, TLRs can bind with damage-associated molecular patterns (DAMPs) released by damaged tissues or "endogenous" apoptotic cells [64]. DAMPs can induce inflammation and immune response in the absence of infection, promote maturation/activation of various immune cells, as well as production of pro-inflammatory cytokines, and break tolerance to self-antigens contributing to autoimmune diseases like SLE. In fact, the concentration of HMGB1 (a well-known DAMP) in gingival crevicular fluid (GCF), as well as the number of HMGB1-positive cells are higher in the inflamed gingival epithelium of patients with periodontitis than that of healthy subjects [65]. HMGB1 expression was also enhanced in the SLE patients and was correlated with the index of SLE disease activity [66].

The chronically inflamed periodontium is the site where immune tolerance to citrullinated epitopes is broken, and the production of ACPAs commences even before the clinical symptoms of RA by many years [21]. Occurrence of ANCA-positive sera in the SLE patients with periodontitis is high (83.3%) compared to that in the SLE patients without periodontitis [33]. SLE is characterized by the production of autoantibodies (e.g., antinuclear, anti-dsDNA, anti-Sm, anti-Ro, anti-CL, and anti-β2GPI antibodies) coupled with patient failure to suppress them. Some of these antibodies cause disease because of their antigen specificity. *P. gingivalis* (a keystone periodontal pathogen) is suspected to contribute to other disease-specific autoantibody responses [21]. Interestingly, patients with active SLE who harbored *P. gingivalis* alone or in combination with *T. denticola* significantly exhibited higher intraoral anti-CL and anti-β2GPI antibodies than the patients without these bacteria. Moreover, anti-CL and anti-β2GPI antibody levels were correlated with periodontal attachment loss, increased C-reactive protein level, and erythrocyte sedimentation rate [34].

5. Conclusions

Overall, to date, despite the controversial results, the available data clearly suggest a possible bidirectional association between PD and SLE that should be considered in the management of SLE patients. Prospective clinical studies that enroll large numbers of very well-defined patients (in terms of both PD and SLE) and respective control subjects, are needed to confirm the causal association and to elucidate the biochemical and immunological interaction between the two diseases.

Author Contributions: Conceptualization, B.S. and F.A.; writing—original draft preparation. B.S., C.P.N., G.M.G.L., A.Z., S.M.D., F.A.; writing—review and editing B.S., C.P.N. and F.A.; supervision, F.A.; funding acquisition F.A. All authors have read and agreed to the published version of the manuscript.

Funding: This research received no external funding.

Institutional Review Board Statement: Not applicable.

Informed Consent Statement: Not applicable.

Acknowledgments: We gratefully acknowledge the help of Rena Bizios for critically reviewing this article.

Conflicts of Interest: The authors declare no conflict of interest.

References

1. Crampton, S.P.; Morawski, P.A.; Bolland, S. Linking susceptibility genes and pathogenesis mechanisms using mouse models of systemic lupus erythematosus. *Dis. Model. Mech.* **2014**, *7*, 1033–1046. [CrossRef] [PubMed]
2. Moulton, V.R.; Suarez-Fueyo, A.; Meidan, E.; Li, H.; Mizui, M.; Tsokos, G.C. Pathogenesis of Human Systemic Lupus Erythematosus: A Cellular Perspective. *Trends Mol. Med.* **2017**, *23*, 615–635. [CrossRef] [PubMed]
3. Khatibi, M.; Shakoorpour, A.H.; Jahromi, Z.M.; Ahmadzadeh, A. The prevalence of oral mucosal lesions and related factors in 188 patients with systemic lupus erythematosus. *Lupus* **2012**, *21*, 1312–1315. [CrossRef]
4. Benli, M.; Batool, F.; Stutz, C.; Petit, C.; Jung, S.; Huck, O. Orofacial manifestations and dental management of systemic lupus erythematosus: A review. *Oral Dis.* **2021**, *27*, 151–167. [CrossRef] [PubMed]
5. Rodriguez, J.P.L.; Torres, L.J.G.; Martinez, R.E.M.; Mendoza, C.A.; Medina-Solís, C.E.; Coronel, S.R.; Cortes, J.O.G.; Pérez, R.A.D. Frequency of dental caries in active and inactive systemic lupus erythematous patients: Salivary and bacterial factors. *Lupus* **2016**, *25*, 1349–1356. [CrossRef]
6. Corrêa, J.D.; Branco, A.L.G.; Calderaro, D.C.; Mendonça, S.M.S.; Travassos, D.V.; Ferreira, A.G.; Teixeira, A.L.; Abreu, L.G.; Silva, A.T. Impact of systemic lupus erythematosus on oral health-related quality of life. *Lupus* **2017**, *27*, 283–289. [CrossRef]
7. Rutter-Locher, Z.; Smith, T.O.; Giles, I.; Sofat, N. Association between Systemic Lupus Erythematosus and Periodontitis: A Systematic Review and Meta-analysis. *Front. Immunol.* **2017**, *8*, 8. [CrossRef]
8. Murakami, S.; Mealey, B.L.; Mariotti, A.; Chapple, I.L. Dental plaque-induced gingival conditions. *J. Periodontol.* **2018**, *89*, S17–S27. [CrossRef]
9. Kassebaum, N.J.; Bernabé, E.; Dahiya, M.; Bhandari, B.; Murray, C.J.L.; Marcenes, W. Global Burden of Severe Periodontitis in 1990–2010. *J. Dent. Res.* **2014**, *93*, 1045–1053. [CrossRef]
10. Silva, N.; Abusleme, L.; Bravo, D.; Dutzan, N.; Garcia-Sesnich, J.; Vernal, R.; Hernández, M.; Gamonal, J. Host response mechanisms in periodontal diseases. *J. Appl. Oral Sci.* **2015**, *23*, 329–355. [CrossRef]
11. Pihlstrom, B.L.; Michalowicz, B.S.; Johnson, N.W. Periodontal diseases. *Lancet* **2005**, *366*, 1809–1820. [CrossRef]
12. Genco, R.J.; Sanz, M. Clinical and public health implications of periodontal and systemic diseases: An overview. *Periodontol. 2000* **2020**, *83*, 7–13. [CrossRef] [PubMed]
13. Romandini, M.; Baima, G.; Antonoglou, G.; Bueno, J.; Figuero, E.; Sanz, M. Periodontitis, Edentulism, and Risk of Mortality: A Systematic Review with Meta-analyses. *J. Dent. Res.* **2021**, *100*, 37–49. [CrossRef] [PubMed]
14. El Kholy, K.; Genco, R.J.; Van Dyke, T.E. Oral infections and cardiovascular disease. *Trends Endocrinol. Metab.* **2015**, *26*, 315–321. [CrossRef] [PubMed]
15. Casanova, L.; Hughes, F.J.; Preshaw, P.M. Diabetes and periodontal disease: A two-way relationship. *Br. Dent. J.* **2014**, *217*, 433–437. [CrossRef] [PubMed]
16. Corbella, S.; Taschieri, S.; Del Fabbro, M.; Francetti, L.; Weinstein, R.; Ferrazzi, E. Adverse pregnancy outcomes and periodontitis: A systematic review and meta-analysis exploring potential association. *Quintessence Int.* **2016**, *47*, 193–204.
17. Linden, G.J.; Herzberg, M.C. Periodontitis and systemic diseases: A record of discussions of working group 4 of the Joint EFP/AAP Workshop on Periodontitis and Systemic Diseases. *J. Clin. Periodontol.* **2013**, *40*, S20–S23. [CrossRef] [PubMed]
18. Dioguardi, M.; Crincoli, V.; Laino, L.; Alovisi, M.; Sovereto, D.; Mastrangelo, F.; Russo, L.L.; Muzio, L.L. The Role of Periodontitis and Periodontal Bacteria in the Onset and Progression of Alzheimer's Disease: A Systematic Review. *J. Clin. Med.* **2020**, *9*, 495. [CrossRef] [PubMed]
19. Baima, G.; Massano, A.; Squillace, E.; Caviglia, G.P.; Buduneli, N.; Ribaldone, D.G.; Aimetti, M. Shared microbiological and immunological patterns in periodontitis and IBD: A scoping review. *Oral Dis.* **2021**. [CrossRef]
20. Fuggle, N.R.; Smith, T.O.; Kaul, A.; Sofat, N. Hand to Mouth: A Systematic Review and Meta-Analysis of the Association between Rheumatoid Arthritis and Periodontitis. *Front. Immunol.* **2016**, *7*, 80. [CrossRef]
21. Potempa, J.; Mydel, P.; Koziel, J. The case for periodontitis in the pathogenesis of rheumatoid arthritis. *Nat. Rev. Rheumatol.* **2017**, *13*, 606–620. [CrossRef]
22. Venkataraman, A.; Almas, K. Rheumatoid Arthritis and Periodontal Disease. An Update. *N. Y. State Dent. J.* **2015**, *81*, 30–36.
23. Tsokos, G.C. Systemic Lupus Erythematosus. *N. Engl. J. Med.* **2011**, *365*, 2110–2121. [CrossRef] [PubMed]
24. Rekvig, O.P.; Van Der Vlag, J. The pathogenesis and diagnosis of systemic lupus erythematosus: Still not resolved. *Semin. Immunopathol.* **2014**, *36*, 301–311. [CrossRef]
25. Morawski, P.A.; Bolland, S. Expanding the B Cell-Centric View of Systemic Lupus Erythematosus. *Trends Immunol.* **2017**, *38*, 373–382. [CrossRef] [PubMed]
26. Vogel, R.I. Periodontal Disease Associated With Amegakaryocytic Thrombocytopenia in Systemic Lupus Erythematosus. *J. Periodontol.* **1981**, *52*, 20–23. [CrossRef] [PubMed]
27. Nagler, R.M.; Lorber, M.; Ben-Arieh, Y.; Laufer, D.; Pollack, S. Generalized periodontal involvement in a young patient with systemic lupus erythematosus. *Lupus* **1999**, *8*, 770–772. [CrossRef] [PubMed]
28. Jaworski, C.P.; Koudelka, B.M.; Roth, N.A.; Marshall, K.J. Acute necrotizing ulcerative gingivitis in a case of systemic lupus erythematosus. *J. Oral Maxillofac. Surg.* **1985**, *43*, 43–46. [CrossRef]
29. Fernandes, E.; Savioli, C.; Siqueira, J.; Silva, C. Oral health and the masticatory system in juvenile systemic lupus erythematosus. *Lupus* **2007**, *16*, 713–719. [CrossRef]

30. Calderaro, D.C.; Ferreira, G.A.; De Mendonça, S.M.S.; Corrêa, J.D.; Santos, F.X.; Sanção, J.G.C.; Da Silva, T.A.; Teixeira, A.L. Is there an association between systemic lupus erythematosus and periodontal disease? *Rev. Bras. Reum.* **2016**, *56*, 280–284. [CrossRef]
31. Fabbri, C.; Fuller, R.; Bonfá, E.; Guedes, L.K.N.; D'Alleva, P.S.R.; Borba, E.F. Periodontitis treatment improves systemic lupus erythematosus response to immunosuppressive therapy. *Clin. Rheumatol.* **2014**, *33*, 505–509. [CrossRef] [PubMed]
32. Kobayashi, T.; Ito, S.; Yasuda, K.; Kuroda, T.; Yamamoto, K.; Sugita, N.; Tai, H.; Narita, I.; Gejyo, F.; Yoshie, H. The Combined Genotypes of Stimulatory and Inhibitory Fcγ Receptors Associated With Systemic Lupus Erythematosus and Periodontitis in Japanese Adults. *J. Periodontol.* **2007**, *78*, 467–474. [CrossRef]
33. Novo, E.; Garcia-MacGregor, E.; Viera, N.; Chaparro, N.; Crozzoli, Y. Periodontitis and Anti-Neutrophil Cytoplasmic Antibodies in Systemic Lupus Erythematosus and Rheumatoid Arthritis: A Comparative Study. *J. Periodontol.* **1999**, *70*, 185–188. [CrossRef] [PubMed]
34. Wang, C.-Y.; Chyuan, I.-T.; Wang, Y.-L.; Kuo, M.Y.-P.; Chang, C.-W.; Wu, K.-J.; Hsu, P.-N.; Nagasawa, T.; Wara-Aswapati, N.; Chen, Y.-W. β2-Glycoprotein I-Dependent Anti-Cardiolipin Antibodies Associated with Periodontitis in Patients with Systemic Lupus Erythematosus. *J. Periodontol.* **2015**, *86*, 995–1004. [CrossRef] [PubMed]
35. De Pablo, P.; Dewan, K.; Dietrich, T.; Chapple, I.; Gordon, C. AB0603 Periodontal Disease is Common in Patients with Systemic Lupus Erythematosus. *Ann. Rheum. Dis.* **2015**, *74* (Suppl. 2), 1101. [CrossRef]
36. Corrêa, J.D.; Calderaro, D.C.; Ferreira, G.A.; Mendonça, S.M.S.; Fernandes, G.R.; Xiao, E.; Teixeira, A.L.; Leys, E.J.; Graves, D.T.; Silva, T.A. Subgingival microbiota dysbiosis in systemic lupus erythematosus: Association with periodontal status. *Microbiome* **2017**, *5*, 1–13. [CrossRef] [PubMed]
37. Zhang, Q.; Feng, G.; Fu, T.; Yin, R.; Li, L.; Gu, Z. Periodontal disease in Chinese patients with systemic lupus erythematosus. *Rheumatol. Int.* **2017**, *37*, 1373–1379. [CrossRef]
38. Figueredo, C.M.S.; Areas, A.; Sztajnbok, F.R.; Miceli, V.; Miranda, A.L.; Fischer, R.G.; Gustafsson, A. Higher elastase activity associated with lower IL-18 in GCF from juvenile systemic lupus patients. *Oral Health Prev. Dent.* **2008**, *6*, 9.
39. Kobayashi, T.; Ito, S.; Yamamoto, K.; Hasegawa, H.; Sugita, N.; Kuroda, T.; Kaneko, S.; Narita, I.; Yasuda, K.; Nakano, M.; et al. Risk of Periodontitis in Systemic Lupus Erythematosus Is Associated with Fcγ Receptor Polymorphisms. *J. Periodontol.* **2003**, *74*, 378–384. [CrossRef]
40. Mutlu, S.; Richards, A.; Maddison, P.; Scully, C. Gingival and periodontal health in systemic lupus erythematosus. *Community Dent. Oral Epidemiol.* **1993**, *21*, 158–161. [CrossRef]
41. Zhong, H.-J.; Xie, H.-X.; Luo, X.-M.; Zhang, E.-H. Association between periodontitis and systemic lupus erythematosus: A meta-analysis. *Lupus* **2020**, *29*, 1189–1197. [CrossRef]
42. Wu, Y.-D.; Lin, C.-H.; Chao, W.-C.; Liao, T.-L.; Chen, D.-Y.; Chen, H.-H. Association between a history of periodontitis and the risk of systemic lupus erythematosus in Taiwan: A nationwide, population-based, case-control study. *PLoS ONE* **2017**, *12*, e0187075. [CrossRef] [PubMed]
43. Bae, S.-C.; Lee, Y.H. Causal association between periodontitis and risk of rheumatoid arthritis and systemic lupus erythematosus: A Mendelian randomization. *Z. Rheumatol.* **2020**, *79*, 929–936. [CrossRef] [PubMed]
44. Al-Mutairi, K.D.; Al-Zahrani, M.S.; Bahlas, S.M.; Kayal, R.A.; Zawawi, K.H. Periodontal findings in systemic lupus erythematosus patients and healthy controls. *Saudi Med. J.* **2015**, *36*, 463–468. [CrossRef]
45. Rhodus, N.L.; Johnson, D.K. The prevalence of oral manifestations of systemic lupus erythematosus. *Quintessence Int.* **1990**, *21*, 461–465.
46. OCEBM Levels of Evidence-Centre for Evidence-Based Medicine (CEBM), University of Oxford. Available online: https://www.cebm.ox.ac.uk/resources/levels-of-evidence/ocebm-levels-of-evidence (accessed on 27 April 2021).
47. Schaefer, A.S.; Jochens, A.; Dommisch, H.; Graetz, C.; Jockel-Schneider, Y.; Harks, I.; Staufenbiel, I., Meyle, J.; Eickholz, P.; Folwaczny, M.; et al. A large candidate-gene association study suggests genetic variants at IRF5 and PRDM1 to be associated with aggressive periodontitis. *J. Clin. Periodontol.* **2014**, *41*, 1122–1131. [CrossRef] [PubMed]
48. Suárez, L.J.; Garzón, H.; Arboleda, S.; Rodríguez, A. Oral Dysbiosis and Autoimmunity: From Local Periodontal Responses to an Imbalanced Systemic Immunity. A Review. *Front. Immunol.* **2020**, *11*, 591255. [CrossRef] [PubMed]
49. Hajishengallis, G.; Lamont, R.J. Dancing with the Stars: How Choreographed Bacterial Interactions Dictate Nososymbiocity and Give Rise to Keystone Pathogens, Accessory Pathogens, and Pathobionts. *Trends Microbiol.* **2016**, *24*, 477–489. [CrossRef]
50. Sete, M.; Carlos, J.; Lira-Junior, R.; Boström, E.; Sztajnbok, F.; Figueredo, C. Clinical, immunological and microbial gingival profile of juvenile systemic lupus erythematosus patients. *Lupus* **2018**, *28*, 189–198. [CrossRef]
51. Pessoa, L.; Aleti, G.; Choudhury, S.; Nguyen, D.; Yaskell, T.; Zhang, Y.; Li, W.; Nelson, K.E.; Neto, L.L.S.; Sant'Ana, A.C.P.; et al. Host-Microbial Interactions in Systemic Lupus Erythematosus and Periodontitis. *Front. Immunol.* **2019**, *10*, 2602. [CrossRef]
52. Jensen, J.L.; Bergem, H.O.; Gilboe, I.-M.; Husby, G.; Axéll, T. Oral and ocular sicca symptoms and findings are prevalent in systemic lupus erythematosus. *J. Oral Pathol. Med.* **2007**, *28*, 317–322. [CrossRef]
53. Graves, D.; Corrêa, J.; Silva, T. The Oral Microbiota Is Modified by Systemic Diseases. *J. Dent. Res.* **2018**, *98*, 148–156. [CrossRef] [PubMed]
54. Corrêa, J.D.; Fernandes, G.R.; Calderaro, D.C.; Mendonça, S.M.S.; Silva, J.M.; Albiero, M.L.; Cunha, F.Q.; Xiao, E.; Ferreira, G.A.; Teixeira, A.L.; et al. Oral microbial dysbiosis linked to worsened periodontal condition in rheumatoid arthritis patients. *Sci. Rep.* **2019**, *9*, 1–10. [CrossRef] [PubMed]

55. Marques, C.P.C.; Victor, E.C.; Franco, M.M.; Fernandes, J.M.C.; Maor, Y.; de Andrade, M.S.; Rodrigues, V.P.; Benatti, B.B. Salivary levels of inflammatory cytokines and their association to periodontal disease in systemic lupus erythematosus patients. A case-control study. *Cytokine* **2016**, *85*, 165–170. [CrossRef]
56. Mendonça, S.M.S.; Corrêa, J.D.; Souza, A.F.; Travassos, D.V.; Calderaro, D.C.; Rocha, N.P.; Vieira, É.L.M.; Teixeira, A.L.; Ferreira, A.G.; Silva, A.T. Immunological signatures in saliva of systemic lupus erythematosus patients: Influence of periodontal condition. *Clin. Exp. Rheumatol.* **2018**, *37*, 208–214. [PubMed]
57. Bunte, K.; Beikler, T. Th17 Cells and the IL-23/IL-17 Axis in the Pathogenesis of Periodontitis and Immune-Mediated Inflammatory Diseases. *Int. J. Mol. Sci.* **2019**, *20*, 3394. [CrossRef]
58. Rezaei, M.; Bayani, M.; Tasorian, B.; Mahdian, S. The comparison of visfatin levels of gingival crevicular fluid in systemic lupus erythematosus and chronic periodontitis patients with healthy subjects. *Clin. Rheumatol.* **2019**, *38*, 3139–3143. [CrossRef]
59. Nair, S.; Faizuddin, M.; Dharmapalan, J. Role of Autoimmune Responses in Periodontal Disease. *Autoim. Dis.* **2014**, *2014*, 1–7. [CrossRef]
60. Sete, M.R.C.; Figueredo, C.M.D.S.; Sztajnbok, F. Periodontitis and systemic lupus erythematosus. *Rev. Bras. Reum.* **2016**, *56*, 165–170. [CrossRef]
61. Bagavant, H.; Dunkleberger, M.L.; Wolska, N.; Sroka, M.; Rasmussen, A.; Adrianto, I.; Montgomery, C.; Sivils, K.; Guthridge, J.M.; James, J.A.; et al. Antibodies to periodontogenic bacteria are associated with higher disease activity in lupus patients. *Clin. Exp. Rheumatol.* **2018**, *37*, 106–111.
62. Getts, D.R.; Spiteri, A.; King, N.J.; Miller, S.D. Microbial Infection as a Trigger of T-Cell Autoimmunity. *Autoimmune Dis.* **2020**, 363–374. [CrossRef]
63. Ilango, P.; Mahalingam, A.; Parthasarathy, H.; Katamreddy, V.; Subbareddy, V. Evaluation of TLR2 and 4 in Chronic Periodontitis. *J. Clin. Diagn. Res.* **2016**, *10*, ZC86–ZC89. [CrossRef]
64. Liu, Y.; Yin, H.; Zhao, M.; Lu, Q. TLR2 and TLR4 in Autoimmune Diseases: A Comprehensive Review. *Clin. Rev. Allergy Immunol.* **2014**, *47*, 136–147. [CrossRef] [PubMed]
65. Luo, L.; Xie, P.; Gong, P.; Tang, X.-H.; Ding, Y.; Deng, L.-X. Expression of HMGB1 and HMGN2 in gingival tissues, GCF and PICF of periodontitis patients and peri-implantitis. *Arch. Oral Biol.* **2011**, *56*, 1106–1111. [CrossRef] [PubMed]
66. Abdulahad, A.D.; Westra, J.; Bijzet, J.; Limburg, P.C.; Kallenberg, C.G.; Bijl, M. High mobility group box 1 (HMGB1) and anti-HMGB1 antibodies and their relation to disease characteristics in systemic lupus erythematosus. *Arthritis Res. Ther.* **2011**, *13*, R71–R79. [CrossRef] [PubMed]

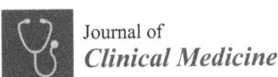

Journal of Clinical Medicine

Article

The Correlation between Periodontal Parameters and Cell-Free DNA in the Gingival Crevicular Fluid, Saliva, and Plasma in Chinese Patients: A Cross-Sectional Study

Xuanzhi Zhu [1,2], Chao-Jung Chu [1,2], Weiyi Pan [1,3], Yan Li [1], Hanyao Huang [1,4,*] and Lei Zhao [1,2,*]

1 State Key Laboratory of Oral Diseases, National Clinical Research Center for Oral Diseases, West China Hospital of Stomatology, Sichuan University, Chengdu 610041, China
2 Department of Periodontics, West China Hospital of Stomatology, Sichuan University, Chengdu 610041, China
3 Department of Oral Medicine, West China Hospital of Stomatology, Sichuan University, Chengdu 610041, China
4 Department of Oral and Maxillofacial Surgery, West China Hospital of Stomatology, Sichuan University, Chengdu 610041, China
* Correspondence: huanghanyao_cn@scu.edu.cn (H.H.); zhaolei@scu.edu.cn (L.Z.)

Abstract: Purpose: To investigate the correlation between periodontal parameters and cell-free DNA (cfDNA) concentrations in gingival crevicular fluid (GCF), saliva, and plasma. Methods: Full mouth periodontal parameters, including probing depth (PD), bleeding on probing (BOP), and plaque index (PI) were recorded from 25 healthy volunteers, 31 patients with untreated gingivitis, and 25 patients with untreated periodontitis. GCF, saliva, and plasma samples were collected from all subjects. Extraction and quantification assays were undertaken to determine cfDNA concentrations of each sample. Results: GCF and salivary cfDNA levels were increased with aggravation of periodontal inflammation (GCF $p < 0.0001$; saliva $p < 0.001$). Plasma cfDNA concentrations in patients with periodontitis were significantly higher than those in healthy volunteers and patients with gingivitis. GCF and salivary cfDNA were positively correlated with mean PD, max PD, BOP, and mean PI ($p < 0.0001$), whereas plasma cfDNA was not correlated with BOP ($p = 0.099$). Conclusion: GCF, saliva, and plasma concentrations of cfDNA were significantly elevated in patients with periodontal disease. There were also positive correlations between cfDNA levels in GCF and saliva and periodontal parameters.

Keywords: cell-free DNA; periodontal disease; gingival crevicular fluid; innate immunity

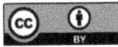

1. Introduction

Periodontitis is a chronic and inflammatory disease that leads to the destruction of periodontal tissue [1]. During the development of periodontitis, innate immunity plays an important role; an inappropriate immune response that happens after the infection of biofilm microorganisms is regarded as one of the main reasons for this hard-to-control inflammation [2]. The initiation of innate immunity depends on the recognition between molecular patterns and toll-like receptors (TLRs) or other pattern-recognition receptors (PRRs) of host cells, activating a series of signaling pathways [3]. Molecular patterns include pathogen-associated molecular patterns (PAMPs) and damage-associated molecular patterns (DAMPs) [4]. Cell-free deoxyribonucleic acid (cfDNA) is a general term for extracellular molecular patterns present in body fluids, also called circulating DNA in plasma or serum, which is mainly recognized by TLR9. The level of cfDNA is directly associated with cancer, diabetes, stroke, systemic lupus erythematosus, trauma, rheumatoid arthritis, infection, and coronary heart disease [5]. cfDNA mainly comes from endogenous nuclear and mitochondrial DNA released from damaged host cells [6], as well as exogenous bacterial or viral DNA [7].

The sources of cfDNA in the periodontal microenvironment are bacterial DNA (bDNA) [8,9], DNA released by the death and lysis of periodontal tissue cells [10], and neutrophil extracellular traps (NETs) [11]. Nucleic acid sensors and their downstream signaling pathways are keys to the regulation of periodontal immunity by periodontal cfDNA. The cfDNA sensors are either in the cytoplasm or in the endolysosomal region. The endosomal nucleic acid sensor, represented by TLR9, recognizes unmethylated CpG DNA from bDNA and generates pro-inflammatory responses via MyD88, activating nuclear factor κ light-chain enhancer of activated B cells (NF-κB), activator protein 1 (AP-1), and mitogen-activated protein kinase signaling pathways [12]. Cytoplasmic nucleic acid sensors, represented by absent in melanoma 2 (AIM2), DNA-dependent activator of interferon regulatory factor (DAI), and cyclic GMP-AMP synthase (cGAS), act through mediators such as caspase-1, TBK1, and IRF3, catalyzing interleukin-1β (IL-1β) activation and amplifying NF-κB pathway activation [13]. In addition, periodontal cfDNA is detectable in peripheral blood [14], synovial fluid [15], and atherosclerotic plaque [16], suggesting that cfDNA may bridge periodontitis and systemic inflammatory disease. Thus, we hypothesized that cfDNA could possibly be a biomarker for periodontitis and the level of cfDNA might correlate with the level of periodontal inflammation.

This study intends to detect the correlation between the levels of cfDNA in GCF, saliva, and plasma, and provide comprehensive clinical evidence for later research on the role of cfDNA and its representative innate immune response in periodontitis and periodontitis-related systemic diseases.

2. Materials and Methods

2.1. Patient Selection

Patients who visited the Department of Periodontics in West China Hospital of Stomatology, Sichuan University, from February 2022 to May 2022, and periodontal health volunteers were assessed for eligibility. We recruited 25 healthy volunteers and 56 patients with untreated gingivitis or periodontitis. Inclusion criteria included being between 18 and 60 years of age, with at least 14 permanent teeth and ≥4 molars. Participants were classified into three groups based on the consensus report on the classification of periodontal and peri-implant diseases and conditions in 2018, as shown in [17]. Periodontal health with intact periodontium (healthy) had no probing attachment loss, probing pocket depth ≤ 3 mm, bleeding on probing < 10%, and no radiological bone loss. Gingivitis with intact periodontium (gingivitis) had no probing attachment loss, bleeding on probing ≥ 10%, and no radiological bone loss. Stage II-IV periodontitis (periodontitis) had more than two non-adjacent sites with interdental probing attachment loss ≥ 3 mm, more than two non-adjacent sites with probing pocket depth ≥ 5 mm, and radiological bone loss ≥ 15%.

Exclusion criteria included having a history of smoking or long-term alcohol abuse, women who were pregnant or breastfeeding, having received antibiotic therapy or periodontal treatment in the last 6 months, having systemic disease (such as hypertension, diabetes, hyperlipidemia, respiratory diseases, malignant tumors, liver or renal insufficiency, etc.), undergoing orthodontic treatment, having received head and neck radiotherapy or chemotherapy, or inability to sign informed consent.

Each subject was examined and evaluated by the same calibrated periodontist (C.C.). Baseline full mouth probing depth (PD), bleeding on probing (BOP) [18], and plaque index (PI) [19] were recorded. Five patients were chosen from among the study participants for calibration. PD, BOP, and PI were measured twice, with 2 days between the examinations. For PD, the percentage of agreement within ±1 mm between repeated measurements was 97.5%. For BOP, the percentage of agreement within ±2% between repeated measurements was 96%. For PI, the percentage of agreement within ±1 between repeated measurements was 97.5%.

2.2. Sample Collection

Statistical power calculations for this study was conducted using G*Power 3.1.9.7 software (Heinrich-Heine-Universität Düsseldorf, Germany), based on data collected in a previous pilot study [20]. The sample size analysis was determined by considering three groups of participants, with an expected standard deviation of 0.5, two-tailed significance of 0.05, and a power level of 80%. It was established that a minimum sample of 25 per group was required for a good power. Sites with PD $\leq$ 3 mm and negative BOP in the healthy group and sites with the deepest PD for the gingivitis and periodontitis groups were selected for GCF sampling. Sites with periodontal abscess, endo-periodontal lesion, caries, and prosthesis were excluded. GCF sampling were conducted at another appointment after periodontal parameter measurements. GCF samples were collected using Whatman 3 mm chromatography paper (Whatman Inc., Clifton, NJ, USA). All papers were cut into 2 × 10 mm strips with sterile tissue scissors. After isolation of the selected tooth with a cotton pellet and being gently air-dried, one paper strip was slowly inserted 1–2 mm into the periodontal pocket or gingival sulcus and left for 30 s [21]. Paper strips were transferred into a 1.5 ml centrifuge tube. Blood or saliva-contaminated samples were discarded. GCF samples from each site were eluted by adding 220 μL of phosphate-buffered saline (PBS) and gently shaking for 1 h at room temperature, followed by centrifugation at 5500 rpm at 4 °C for 20 min. Supernatants were then stored at −80 °C.

Unstimulated whole saliva was collected from each subject between 8 and 10 a.m., as previously described [22]. All participants were asked to refrain from eating, drinking, and brushing their teeth for at least 1 h before saliva collection. Saliva samples were centrifuged at 3000 rpm for 10 min at 4 °C. Supernatants were collected and stored at −80 °C.

Venous blood was collected using an EDTAK2 vacuum blood collection tube and left to stand at room temperature for 30 min. Samples were then centrifuged at 3000 rpm for 10 min at 4 °C. The plasma of each sample was pipetted into a 1.5 mL centrifuge tube and centrifuged at 20,000 rpm for 10 min at 4 °C. Supernatants were collected and stored at −80 °C.

2.3. Extraction and Quantification of cfDNA

Extraction and quantification of cfDNA from samples was performed with a DNeasy Blood & Tissue Kit (QIAGEN, Hilden, Germany) and Quant-iT PicoGreen double-stranded DNA Assay Kit (Thermo Fisher Scientific, Waltham, MA, USA) by one trained laboratory analysis researcher (X.Z.), according to the manufacturers' instructions. To avoid subjective bias, we adopted blinding. The laboratory analysis researcher was not aware of specific sample groupings. In detail, the following steps were followed: we mixed 100 μL sample, 20 μL proteinase K, 150 μL PBS buffer, and 200 μL AL buffer by vortexing, incubated the mixture for 10 min at 56 °C, mixed in 200 μL ethanol (96–100%), then placed the DNeasy Mini spin column into a 2 mL EP tube, added the above mixture, and centrifuged at 6000× g for 1 min, discarding the filtrate and the collection tube. Then, we transferred the DNeasy Mini spin column to a new 2 mL EP tube, added 500 μL AW1 buffer, and centrifuged at 6000× g for 1 min, discarding the filtrate and collection tube. Then, we transferred the DNeasy Mini spin column to a new 2 mL EP tube, added 500 μL AW2 buffer, centrifuged at 20,000× g for 3 min, discarded the filtrate and collection tube, transferred the DNeasy Mini spin column to a new EP tube, added 100 μL of AE buffer, incubated at room temperature for 1 min, centrifuged at 6000× g for 1 min, and collected the eluate for further use. We added 50 μL of PicoGreen and 50 μL of the cfDNA eluate to a 96-well plate and incubated it in the dark for 2 to 5 min at room temperature. The cfDNA content was calculated by measuring the fluorescence intensity (excitation 490 nm, emission 520 nm). Note that in the methods, the original GCF paper strip samples were eluted in 220 μL of PBS, and the GCF cfDNA concentration data were reported in ng/μL per 30-s sample, as previously described [21].

2.4. Statistical Analysis

Statistical analysis was performed using GraphPad Prism 9 (La Jolla, CA, USA). Data distributions were evaluated for the violation of normality. Parametric data were assessed using a one-way analysis of variance (ANOVA) with Tukey's post hoc tests (for multiple comparisons), Pearson's correlation, and simple linear regression analysis. Non-parametric data were assessed by Mann–Whitney test and Spearman's correlation. A stepwise multivariable linear regression model was used to analyze the dependence of every single cfDNA concentration by explicable variables such as sex, age, and periodontal parameters.

3. Results

3.1. Demographics and Clinical Parameters

A total of 114 candidate subjects were included and evaluated in this study. Based on exclusion criteria, 33 subjects were excluded, and 81 subjects completed the trial. Trial participants included 25 healthy volunteers, 31 patients with gingivitis, and 25 patients with periodontitis. Demographic and clinical parameters are shown in Table 1.

Table 1. Patient demographics and clinical parameters.

Characteristics	Groups		
	Healthy	Gingivitis	Periodontitis
Number of subjects (n)	25	31	25
Male/female	16/9	13/18	11/24
Cigarette (Y/N)	0/25	0/31	0/25
			Mean ± SD
Age range (years)	25.08 ± 1.96 (range 23–32)	26.16 ± 4.12 (range 21–33)	33.52 ± 11.31 (range 22–60)
	Clinical parameters		
Mean PD (mm)	1.87 ± 0.31	2.55 ± 0.43	3.44 ± 0.61
Max PD (mm)	2.92 ± 0.28	4.03 ± 0.66	7.16 ± 1.84
BOP (%)	6.56 ± 2.04	46.35 ± 13.51	74.24 ± 19.06
Mean PI	0.57 ± 0.29	1.15 ± 0.31	1.83 ± 0.43

Abbreviations: PD, probing depth; BOP, bleeding on probing; PI, plaque index.

3.2. Comparison of GCF cfDNA Concentration in Relation to Periodontal Parameters

The cfDNA concentration in GCF (ng/µL per 30-s sample) increased with the degree of periodontal inflammation (healthy 31.62 ± 28.20, gingivitis 236.29 ± 182.41, periodontitis 521.56 ± 217.95, $p < 0.0001$, Figure 1A). Significant positive correlations were found between cfDNA concentrations in GCF and mean PD ($r = 0.644$, $p < 0.0001$), max PD ($r = 0.680$, $p < 0.0001$), BOP ($r = 0.670$, $p < 0.0001$), and mean PI ($r = 0.576$, $p < 0.0001$). Linear regression analysis showed that the cfDNA concentration in GCF had good predictability for mean PD ($R^2 = 0.415$, $p < 0.0001$), max PD ($R^2 = 0.463$, $p < 0.0001$), BOP ($R^2 = 0.449$, $p < 0.0001$), and mean PI ($R^2 = 0.331$, $p < 0.0001$) (Table 2). The relationship between GCF cfDNA concentration and periodontal parameters are presented in Figure 2A–D.

3.3. Comparison of Saliva cfDNA Concentration in Relation to Periodontal Parameters

Similar to the results in GCF, the cfDNA concentrations in saliva were also positively correlated with periodontal parameters (Table 3). Saliva levels of cfDNA progressively increased between healthy, gingivitis, and periodontitis groups. There were statistical differences among the three groups (healthy 131.99 ± 70.79 ng/mL, gingivitis 260.25 ± 93.93 ng/mL, periodontitis 403.92 ± 154.74 ng/mL, $p < 0.001$, Figure 1B). Linear regression analysis showed that the predictive power of salivary cfDNA for periodontal indicators was also statistically significant (Table 3, Figure 2E–H).

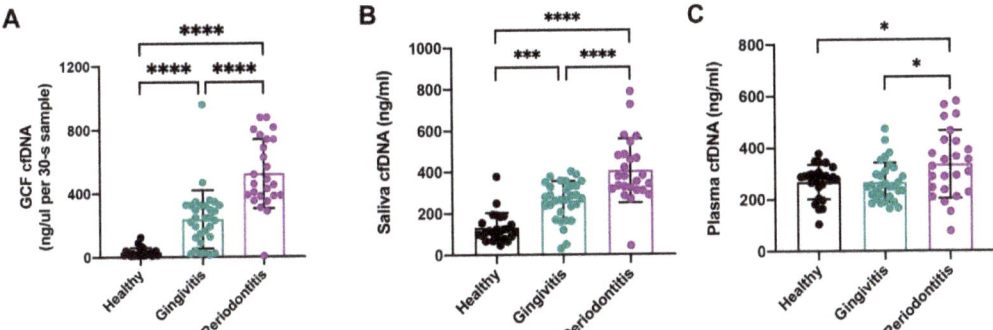

Figure 1. Comparison of cfDNA concentrations in GCF (ng/μl per 30-s sample), saliva (ng/mL), and plasma (ng/mL) in different states of periodontal inflammation. (**A**) Comparison of GCF cfDNA in different periodontal states. (**B**) Comparison of saliva cfDNA in different periodontal states. (**C**) Comparison of plasma cfDNA in different periodontal states. (Abbreviation: cfDNA, cell-free DNA; GCF, gingival crevicular fluid. n = 25 (healthy), 31 (gingivitis) and 25 (periodontitis). Differences were assessed via one-way ANOVA with Tukey's multiple comparison tests. * $p < 0.05$; *** $p < 0.001$; and **** $p < 0.0001$).

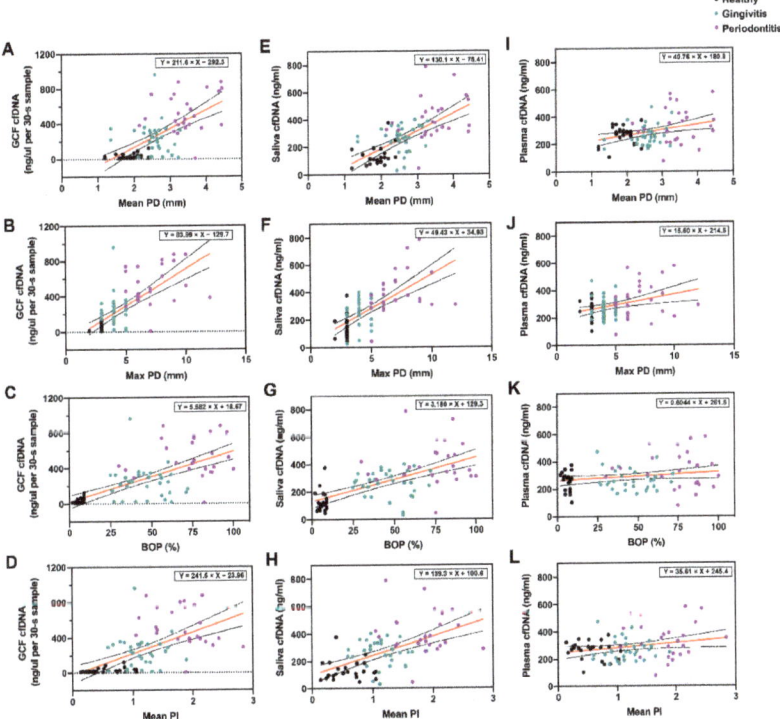

Figure 2. The relationships between cfDNA levels and periodontal parameters. (**A–D**) Correlations between GCF cfDNA (ng/uL per 30-s sample) and periodontal parameters. (**E–H**) Correlations between saliva cfDNA (ng/mL) and periodontal parameters. (**I–L**) Correlations between plasma cfDNA (ng/mL) and periodontal parameters. Lines represent mean and 95% confidence interval. Pearson correlation analysis and linear regression analysis were conducted. n = 81.

Table 2. Correlations between GCF cfDNA concentration and clinical parameters.

		Correlation Coefficient (r Value) [a]		
		Clinical Parameters		
Mean PD (mm)	Max PD (mm)		BOP (%)	Mean PI
0.644 ($p < 0.0001$)	0.680 ($p < 0.0001$)		0.670 ($p < 0.0001$)	0.576 ($p < 0.0001$)
		Regression analyses (R^2 value) [b]		
		Mean PD (mm)	Max PD (mm)	BOP (%)	Mean PI
Mean GCF cfDNA conc.	Model	$R^2 = 0.415$	$R^2 = 0.463$	$R^2 = 0.449$	$R^2 = 0.331$
	SE	196,025.625	187,864.649	190,166.355	209,571.977
	p value	<0.0001	<0.0001	<0.0001	<0.0001

Abbreviations: GCF, gingival crevicular fluid; cfDNA, cell-free DNA; PD, probing depth; BOP, bleeding on probing; PI, plaque index. [a] Pearson correlation for parametric data (Mean PD, max PD, BOP, and PI); $n = 81$. [b] Linear regression analysis; $n = 81$.

Table 3. Correlations between saliva cfDNA concentration and clinical parameters.

		Correlation Coefficient (r Value) [a]		
		Clinical Parameters		
Mean PD (mm)	Max PD (mm)		BOP (%)	Mean PI
0.657 ($p < 0.0001$)	0.664 ($p < 0.0001$)		0.622 ($p < 0.0001$)	0.550 ($p < 0.0001$)
		Regression analyses (R^2 value) [b]		
		Mean PD (mm)	Max PD (mm)	BOP (%)	Mean PI
Mean saliva cfDNA conc.	Model	$R^2 = 0.432$	$R^2 = 0.441$	$R^2 = 0.387$	$R^2 = 0.303$
	SE	116.411	115.485	120.905	128.942
	p value	<0.0001	<0.0001	<0.0001	<0.0001

Abbreviations: cfDNA, cell-free DNA; PD, probing depth; BOP, bleeding on probing; PI, plaque index. [a] Pearson correlation for parametric data (Mean PD, max PD, BOP, and PI); $n = 81$. [b] Linear regression analysis; $n = 81$.

3.4. Comparison of Plasma cfDNA Concentration in Relation to Periodontal Parameters

Plasma levels of cfDNA in patients with periodontitis (334.78 ± 131.55 ng/mL) were significantly higher than in healthy volunteers (267.49 ± 65.9 ng/mL, $p = 0.036$) and patients with gingivitis (265.29 ± 75.93 ng/mL, $p = 0.020$, Figure 1C). Pearson correlation analysis showed that plasma cfDNA levels were only significantly positively correlated with mean PD ($r = 0.321$, $p = 0.003$), max PD ($r = 0.327$, $p = 0.003$), mean PI ($r = 0.220$, $p = 0.049$), and weakly correlated with BOP ($r = 0.185$, $p = 0.099$, Table 4). Linear regression analysis also showed that plasma cfDNA was a strong predictor for mean PD ($R^2 = 0.103$, $p = 0.003$), max PD ($R^2 = 0.107$, $p = 0.003$), and mean PI ($R^2 = 0.103$, $p = 0.049$), but was not significant in predicting BOP ($R^2 = 0.034$, $p = 0.099$, Table 4). The relationships between plasma cfDNA and periodontal parameters are shown in Figure 2I–L.

3.5. Multivariate Analysis of Age, Sex, and Clinical Parameters on cfDNA Concentrations

The stepwise analysis performed on all enrolled subjects indicated that GCF and salivary cfDNA concentrations were significantly correlated to mean PD, max PD, BOP, and mean PI ($p < 0.001$ for all outcomes) (Table S1). More specifically, the GCF cfDNA levels were significantly dependent on age, co-analyzed with mean PD ($p = 0.044$), BOP ($p = 0.003$), and mean PI ($p = 0.015$). Salivary cfDNA levels were significantly dependent on age, co-analyzed with BOP ($p = 0.006$) and mean PI ($p = 0.014$). Salivary cfDNA levels were also significantly dependent on sex, co-analyzed with mean PD ($p = 0.019$), max PD ($p = 0.011$), BOP ($p = 0.022$), and mean PI ($p = 0.014$) (Table S1).

Table 4. Correlations between plasma cfDNA concentration and clinical parameters.

		Correlation Coefficient (r Value) [a]		
		Clinical Parameters		
Mean PD (mm)		Max PD (mm)	BOP (%)	Mean PI
0.321 ($p = 0.003$)		0.327 ($p = 0.003$)	0.185 ($p = 0.099$)	0.220 ($p = 0.049$)
		Regression analyses (R^2 value) [b]		
		Mean PD (mm) / Max PD (mm)	BOP (%)	Mean PI
Mean plasma cfDNA conc.	Model	$R^2 = 0.103$ / $R^2 = 0.107$	$R^2 = 0.034$	$R^2 = 0.048$
	SE	93.723 / 93.526	97.270	96.552
	p value	0.003 / 0.003	0.099	0.049

Abbreviations: cfDNA, cell-free DNA; PD, probing depth; BOP, bleeding on probing; PI, plaque index. [a] Pearson correlation for parametric data (Mean PD, max PD, BOP, and PI); $n = 81$. [b] Linear regression analysis; $n = 81$.

4. Discussion

The use of cfDNA as a tool for disease diagnosis and research has already been widely used in fields such as oncology [23,24], prenatal genetic testing [25], myocardial infarction [26], and autoimmune disorders [27]. Hajishengallis et al. [28] found that TLR9 specifically recognizes bacterial-derived CpG DNA, and the downstream NF-κB pathway plays an essential role in periodontitis by stimulating macrophages to produce pro-inflammatory factors. In addition, cytoplasmic nucleic acid sensors such as DAI, AIM2 [29], and cGAS [30] were also highly expressed in periodontal and pulpal inflammation. Thus, DNA-sensing could play a key role in the immune response elicited by periodontal cfDNA, and we hypothesized that the level of cfDNA might correlate with the pathogenesis of periodontitis. After strict inclusion and exclusion criteria and diagnostic grouping, our study found that cfDNA levels were significantly elevated in patients with periodontal disease, and GCF and salivary cfDNA were positively correlated with periodontal parameters. Interestingly, circulating cfDNA levels were significantly elevated only in patients with periodontitis, whereas patients with gingivitis were not significantly different from healthy individuals.

GCF refers to the fluid infiltrating from the gingival connective tissue into the gingival crevice through the epithelium of the gingival sulcus and the junctional epithelium, and its main component is derived from serum. The outflow of GCF was positively correlated with the degree of inflammation [31]. Changes in the levels of inflammatory factors in GCF were the most reflective of periodontal inflammatory destruction [31]. Suwannagindra et al. [20] measured GCF cfDNA concentration in patients with periodontitis and found no correlation between GCF cfDNA and periodontal parameters, which appears to be contradictory to studies in other systemic diseases [27,32]. In their study, only 20 patients with mild to severe periodontitis were included, patient GCF collection methods were not consistent, and saliva and peripheral blood cfDNA levels were not measured. Thus, we designed a cross-sectional study with strict inclusion and exclusion criteria for healthy, gingivitis, and periodontitis groups, as well as saliva and plasma collection. The cfDNA extraction and quantification methods we used were consistent with previous studies, which allowed us to compare our results with other systemic diseases. Our results showed a significant difference between healthy, gingivitis, and periodontitis groups with sequentially higher GCF cfDNA concentrations. This suggests that cfDNA concentration in GCF is closely related to the level of periodontal inflammation in individuals. Interestingly, the concentration of cfDNA in GCF was much higher than in saliva and plasma, with a difference of three orders of magnitude. Similar results have been reported for other types of inflammatory markers in previous studies, such as significantly higher levels of interleukin (IL) -1β in the GCF of patients with gingivitis than in serum [33]. In addition, GCF cfDNA concentrations had strong positive correlations with mean PD, max PD, BOP, and mean PI. GCF cfDNA levels also had statistically significant predictive effects on the above periodontal parameters. Once again, this shows that GCF is objectively representative of the specimen concerned in periodontal research.

Microorganisms and inflammatory factors in saliva have also been shown to reflect the process of periodontal disease [34]. Compared with GCF, saliva is more convenient to collect in clinical and animal models. The molecular substances in saliva can reflect changes in human metabolism, which is of great significance for the detection of disease molecular markers [35]. Salivary cfDNA in this study showed similar results to GCF, with positive correlations with all four periodontal parameters and predictive power. Therefore, it is feasible to use saliva as a surrogate specimen for GCF for the clinical detection of cfDNA and subsequent mechanism exploration.

Periodontal inflammation could be linked to systemic disease through blood circulation [36]. The levels of inflammatory factors in the plasma of patients with periodontitis are higher than those of healthy people [37]. In this study, the plasma cfDNA level of periodontitis patients was significantly higher than in both the healthy and gingivitis groups, whereas the plasma cfDNA level of the gingivitis group was not significantly higher than in healthy individuals. This suggests that changes in cfDNA in the blood circulation are associated with moderate to severe periodontal inflammation and that the more severe the inflammation, the more significant the elevation of cfDNA in the blood circulation. In moderate to severe periodontitis, a large number of microorganisms die and cleave to release bDNA, and host cells (e.g., gingival epithelial cells, periodontal ligament cells, osteocytes, etc.) undergo different forms of cell death, such as apoptosis [38] and pyroptosis [39], releasing mitochondrial DNA and nuclear DNA. Meanwhile, neutrophils are massively activated to release NETs. The released cfDNA may enter the blood circulation. In addition, other inflammatory mediators in periodontitis, such as IL-1β, IL-6, tumor necrosis factor-α, etc., can be secreted into the blood to activate the systemic immune response [40,41], which may lead to tissue destruction in other organs to release DAMPs-derived cfDNA. Moreover, periodontal pathogens, such as *Porphyromonas gingivalis* (*P. gingivalis*.), could also colonize arterial tissues by adhering to erythrocytes through blood circulation, causing vascular damage and releasing DAMPs through other innate immune pathways such as TLR2/TLR4, whereas the self-death lysis of systemic colonized periodontal pathogens could also release a large amount of exogenous bDNA. Studies have found that elevated cfDNA levels were closely related to periodontitis-related systemic inflammation (e.g., diabetes [42], rheumatoid arthritis [27], and atherosclerosis [43]). Therefore, cfDNA could be the bridging molecule between periodontitis and systemic diseases.

In this study, we found that patients with periodontitis had higher cfDNA concentrations in GCF, saliva, and plasma than healthy volunteers or gingivitis patients, and were significantly positively correlated with severe clinical parameters. This shows that cfDNA as a whole collection has the same potential as a diagnostic biomarker of periodontitis as a specific protein or small molecule mediator. The results of this trial are consistent with previous studies of systemic disease. Shi C et al. [44] in a cross-sectional study, showed that serum cfDNA in patients with inflammatory bowel disease was significantly higher than in healthy subjects, and cfDNA concentration was positively correlated with disease grade, TLR9, TNF-α, iNOS, and F4/80 expressions. Using the same extraction and quantification method as our study, Dawulieti J et al. [45] also demonstrated that serum cfDNA levels in sepsis patients were higher than in healthy volunteers. Fast diagnosis of periodontitis by detecting biomarkers in saliva, such as haemoglobin [46], holds promise for research in community disease screening. Our results showed that the correlation between cfDNA levels in saliva and periodontal parameters was similar to that of GCF. The cfDNA detection method was nonspecific compared with other biomarkers. Saliva cfDNA detection kits may be used in community screening for periodontal disease or in extensive oral epidemiological surveys.

These findings suggest that cfDNA could be used as a potential therapeutic target. Intraperitoneal injection of DNase I to neutralize NETs significantly reduced bone resorption in mice with plasminogen deficiency [11]. The intervention of the nucleic acid-sensing pathway was also shown to inhibit periodontal inflammation. It was reported that, compared with wild-type mice, TLR9 knockout mice had less bone resorption and pro-inflammatory factor release in *Porphyromonas gingivalis*-induced experimental periodontitis [47]. Unlike other biological macromolecules, cfDNA is negatively charged in its natural state, and a strategy of targeted clearance by cationic polymers for traditional gene presentation has been demonstrated to be feasible. Studies have shown that cationic nanoparticles effectively alleviate joint swelling, synovial hyperplasia, and bone destruction by scavenging cfDNA in collagen-induced arthritis rat models [48,49]. In addition, the experiments of Pan W et al. [50] showed that the promotion of periodontitis in rheumatoid arthritis could be inhibited by downregulating the TLR9 pathway. Therefore, topical or systemic applications of cfDNA scavengers may have potential therapeutic effects in periodontitis and periodontitis-related systemic inflammatory diseases.

However, this cross-sectional study faces some limitations. First, we did not include clinical attachment loss (CAL) and tooth mobility in periodontitis patients to quickly and accurately record periodontal parameters. Although CAL changes and original tooth mobility are reliable in terms of disease prediction [51,52], given that there was neither probing attachment loss nor pathological mobility in the healthy and gingivitis groups, the sample size included in the statistical analysis using PD, BOP, and PI was more significant than an analysis using CAL or mobility within the periodontitis group, providing a more objective picture of the association with cfDNA in the current inflammatory state. This was also consistent with our cross-sectional study design. In the future, more prospective cohort studies are needed to reveal the role of cfDNA in the pathogenesis and prognosis of periodontitis. Second, the prevalence of periodontitis in Chinese adults was 69.3% according to the 4th National Oral Health Survey in the Mainland of China [53], which made including healthy volunteers in this study very difficult. These resulted in the inability to perform more objective age- and sex-matched analyses between the three groups. This may also be the reason why our multivariate analysis including sex and age contradicted results from a prospective study with a larger sample size [54]. In addition, gene polymorphisms determine the differences in susceptibility to periodontitis among individuals [55], and the subjects included in this study were all Chinese adults. Hence, differences in cfDNA in more diverse populations need further research.

5. Conclusions

The cfDNA concentrations in GCF, saliva, and plasma increased with aggravation of periodontal inflammation, suggesting that cfDNA may be associated with periodontal disease. cfDNA was positively correlated with mean PD, max PD, BOP, and mean PI and had statistically significant predictive effects on the above periodontal parameters. Compared with plasma, cfDNA levels in GCF and saliva were more strongly associated with periodontal parameters. More research is needed to explore the role of cfDNA in periodontal and periodontitis-related systemic inflammation.

Supplementary Materials: The following supporting information can be downloaded at: https://www.mdpi.com/article/10.3390/jcm11236902/s1, Table S1: Multivariate analysis of age, sex, and clinical parameters on cfDNA concentrations.

Author Contributions: Conceptualization, H.H. and L.Z.; methodology, C.-J.C., W.P. and Y.L.; formal analysis, X.Z.; investigation, X.Z. and C.-J.C.; writing—original draft preparation, X.Z.; writing—review and editing, H.H. and L.Z.; visualization, X.Z.; supervision, H.H. and L.Z.; funding acquisition, Y.L., H.H. and L.Z. All authors have read and agreed to the published version of the manuscript.

Funding: This research was funded by National Natural Science Foundation of China, grant numbers 81970944 and 81991502; Research and Develop Program, West China Hospital of Stomatology Sichuan University, grant number RD-02-202107; Sichuan Province Science and Technology Support Program, grant number 2022NSFSC0743; Sichuan Postdoctoral Science Foundation, grant number TB2022005; and Key Projects of Sichuan Provincial Department of Science and Technology, grant number 2020YFSY0008.

Institutional Review Board Statement: This study was approved by the West China Hospital of Stomatology Institutional Review Board (WCSHIRB-CT-2022-173). Clinical trial registration number ChiCTR2200059510.

Informed Consent Statement: Informed consent was obtained from all subjects involved in the study.

Data Availability Statement: The authors declare that all data supporting the findings of this study are available upon request to the corresponding author.

Conflicts of Interest: The authors declare no conflict of interest.

References

1. Hajishengallis, G. Periodontitis: From microbial immune subversion to systemic inflammation. *Nat. Rev. Immunol.* **2015**, *15*, 30–44. [CrossRef]
2. Thaiss, C.A.; Zmora, N.; Levy, M.; Elinav, E. The microbiome and innate immunity. *Nature* **2016**, *535*, 65–74. [CrossRef]
3. Olive, C. Pattern recognition receptors: Sentinels in innate immunity and targets of new vaccine adjuvants. *Expert Rev. Vaccines* **2012**, *11*, 237–256. [CrossRef] [PubMed]
4. Takeuchi, O.; Akira, S. Pattern recognition receptors and inflammation. *Cell* **2010**, *140*, 805–820. [CrossRef] [PubMed]
5. Swarup, V.; Rajeswari, M.R. Circulating (cell-free) nucleic acids–a promising, non-invasive tool for early detection of several human diseases. *FEBS Lett.* **2007**, *581*, 795–799. [CrossRef] [PubMed]
6. Jahr, S.; Hentze, H.; Englisch, S.; Hardt, D.; Fackelmayer, F.O.; Hesch, R.D.; Knippers, R. DNA fragments in the blood plasma of cancer patients: Quantitations and evidence for their origin from apoptotic and necrotic cells. *Cancer Res.* **2001**, *61*, 1659–1665.
7. Mortaz, E.; Adcock, I.M.; Abedini, A.; Kiani, A.; Kazempour-Dizaji, M.; Movassaghi, M.; Garssen, J. The role of pattern recognition receptors in lung sarcoidosis. *Eur. J. Pharmacol.* **2017**, *808*, 44–48. [CrossRef]
8. Kim, Y.; Jo, A.R.; Jang, D.H.; Cho, Y.J.; Chun, J.; Min, B.M.; Choi, Y. Toll-like receptor 9 mediates oral bacteria-induced IL-8 expression in gingival epithelial cells. *Immunol. Cell Biol.* **2012**, *90*, 655–663. [CrossRef] [PubMed]
9. Sahingur, S.E.; Xia, X.J.; Schifferle, R.E. Oral bacterial DNA differ in their ability to induce inflammatory responses in human monocytic cell lines. *J. Periodontol.* **2012**, *83*, 1069–1077. [CrossRef] [PubMed]
10. Govindarajan, S.; Veeraraghavan, V.P.; Dillibabu, T.; Patil, S. Oral Cavity-A Resilient Source for DNA Sampling. *J. Contemp. Dent. Pract.* **2022**, *23*, 1–2. [PubMed]
11. Silva, L.M.; Doyle, A.D.; Greenwell-Wild, T.; Dutzan, N.; Tran, C.L.; Abusleme, L.; Juang, L.J.; Leung, J.; Chun, E.M.; Lum, A.G.; et al. Fibrin is a critical regulator of neutrophil effector function at the oral mucosal barrier. *Science* **2021**, *374*, eabl5450. [CrossRef] [PubMed]
12. Pandey, S.; Kawai, T.; Akira, S. Microbial sensing by Toll-like receptors and intracellular nucleic acid sensors. *Cold Spring Harb. Perspect. Biol.* **2014**, *7*, a016246. [CrossRef] [PubMed]
13. Wu, J.; Chen, Z.J. Innate immune sensing and signaling of cytosolic nucleic acids. *Annu. Rev. Immunol.* **2014**, *32*, 461–488. [CrossRef]
14. Kaneko, C.; Kobayashi, T.; Ito, S.; Sugita, N.; Murasawa, A.; Nakazono, K.; Yoshie, H. Circulating levels of carbamylated protein and neutrophil extracellular traps are associated with periodontitis severity in patients with rheumatoid arthritis: A pilot case-control study. *PLoS ONE* **2018**, *13*, e0192365. [CrossRef]
15. Martinez-Martinez, R.E.; Abud-Mendoza, C.; Patino-Marin, N.; Rizo-Rodriguez, J.C.; Little, J.W.; Loyola-Rodriguez, J.P. Detection of periodontal bacterial DNA in serum and synovial fluid in refractory rheumatoid arthritis patients. *J. Clin. Periodontol.* **2009**, *36*, 1004–1010. [CrossRef]
16. Rao, A.; D'Souza, C.; Subramanyam, K.; Rai, P.; Thomas, B.; Gopalakrishnan, M.; Karunasagar, I.; Kumar, B.K. Molecular analysis shows the presence of periodontal bacterial DNA in atherosclerotic plaques from patients with coronary artery disease. *Indian Heart J.* **2021**, *73*, 218–220. [CrossRef]
17. Papapanou, P.N.; Sanz, M.; Buduneli, N.; Dietrich, T.; Feres, M.; Fine, D.H.; Flemmig, T.F.; Garcia, R.; Giannobile, W.V.; Graziani, F.; et al. Periodontitis: Consensus report of workgroup 2 of the 2017 World Workshop on the Classification of Periodontal and Peri-Implant Diseases and Conditions. *J. Periodontol.* **2018**, *89* (Suppl. S1), S173–S182. [CrossRef]
18. Joss, A.; Adler, R.; Lang, N.P. Bleeding on probing. A parameter for monitoring periodontal conditions in clinical practice. *J. Clin. Periodontol.* **1994**, *21*, 402–408. [CrossRef]
19. Fischman, S.L. Clinical index systems used to assess the efficacy of mouthrinses on plaque and gingivitis. *J. Clin. Periodontol.* **1988**, *15*, 506–510. [CrossRef]

20. Suwannagindra, S.; Thaweboo, B.; Kerdvongbundit, V. Correlation between cell free DNA in gingival crevicular fluid and clinical periodontal parameters by using two collection techniques. *M. Dent. J.* **2020**, *40*, 165–174.
21. Wassall, R.R.; Preshaw, P.M. Clinical and technical considerations in the analysis of gingival crevicular fluid. *Periodontol* **2016**, *70*, 65–79. [CrossRef]
22. Henson, B.S.; Wong, D.T. Collection, storage, and processing of saliva samples for downstream molecular applications. *Methods Mol. Biol.* **2010**, *666*, 21–30. [CrossRef] [PubMed]
23. Green, E.A.; Li, R.; Albiges, L.; Choueiri, T.K.; Freedman, M.; Pal, S.; Dyrskjot, L.; Kamat, A.M. Clinical Utility of Cell-free and Circulating Tumor DNA in Kidney and Bladder Cancer: A Critical Review of Current Literature. *Eur. Urol. Oncol.* **2021**, *4*, 893–903. [CrossRef]
24. Corcoran, R.B.; Chabner, B.A. Application of Cell-free DNA Analysis to Cancer Treatment. *N. Engl. J. Med.* **2018**, *379*, 1754–1765. [CrossRef] [PubMed]
25. Zhang, S.; Han, S.; Zhang, M.; Wang, Y. Non-invasive prenatal paternity testing using cell-free fetal DNA from maternal plasma: DNA isolation and genetic marker studies. *Leg. Med.* **2018**, *32*, 98–103. [CrossRef]
26. Shimony, A.; Zahger, D.; Gilutz, H.; Goldstein, M.; Orlov, G.; Merkin, M.; Shalev, A.; Ilia, R.; Douvdevani, A. Cell free DNA detected by a novel method in acute ST-elevation myocardial infarction patients. *Acute Card. Care* **2010**, *12*, 109–111. [CrossRef]
27. Duvvuri, B.; Lood, C. Cell-Free DNA as a Biomarker in Autoimmune Rheumatic Diseases. *Front. Immunol.* **2019**, *10*, 502. [CrossRef] [PubMed]
28. Hajishengallis, G.; Sahingur, S.E. Novel inflammatory pathways in periodontitis. *Adv. Dent. Res.* **2014**, *26*, 23–29. [CrossRef]
29. Sahingur, S.E.; Xia, X.J.; Voth, S.C.; Yeudall, W.A.; Gunsolley, J.C. Increased nucleic Acid receptor expression in chronic periodontitis. *J. Periodontol.* **2013**, *84*, e48–e57. [CrossRef] [PubMed]
30. Tian, X.; Liu, C.; Wang, Z. The induction of inflammation by the cGAS-STING pathway in human dental pulp cells: A laboratory investigation. *Int. Endod. J.* **2022**, *55*, 54–63. [CrossRef]
31. Barros, S.P.; Williams, R.; Offenbacher, S.; Morelli, T. Gingival crevicular fluid as a source of biomarkers for periodontitis. *Periodontol* **2016**, *70*, 53–64. [CrossRef] [PubMed]
32. Sandquist, M.; Wong, H.R. Biomarkers of sepsis and their potential value in diagnosis, prognosis and treatment. *Expert Rev. Clin. Immunol.* **2014**, *10*, 1349–1356. [CrossRef] [PubMed]
33. Trombelli, L.; Scapoli, C.; Carrieri, A.; Giovannini, G.; Calura, G.; Farina, R. Interleukin-1 beta levels in gingival crevicular fluid and serum under naturally occurring and experimentally induced gingivitis. *J. Clin. Periodontol.* **2010**, *37*, 697–704. [CrossRef] [PubMed]
34. Kim, E.H.; Joo, J.Y.; Lee, Y.J.; Koh, J.K.; Choi, J.H.; Shin, Y.; Cho, J.; Park, E.; Kang, J.; Lee, K.; et al. Grading system for periodontitis by analyzing levels of periodontal pathogens in saliva. *PLoS ONE* **2018**, *13*, e0200900. [CrossRef]
35. Shakeeb, N.; Varkey, P.; Ajit, A. Human Saliva as a Diagnostic Specimen for Early Detection of Inflammatory Biomarkers by Real-Time RT-PCR. *Inflammation* **2021**, *44*, 1713–1723. [CrossRef]
36. Zhu, X.; Huang, H.; Zhao, L. PAMPs and DAMPs as the Bridge Between Periodontitis and Atherosclerosis: The Potential Therapeutic Targets. *Front. Cell Dev. Biol.* **2022**, *10*, 856118. [CrossRef]
37. Hegde, R.; Awan, K.H. Effects of periodontal disease on systemic health. *Dis. Mon.* **2019**, *65*, 185–192. [CrossRef]
38. Listyarifah, D.; Al-Samadi, A.; Salem, A.; Syaify, A.; Salo, T.; Tervahartiala, T.; Grenier, D.; Nordstrom, D.C.; Sorsa, T.; Ainola, M. Infection and apoptosis associated with inflammation in periodontitis: An immunohistologic study. *Oral Dis.* **2017**, *23*, 1144–1154. [CrossRef]
39. Sordi, M.B.; Magini, R.S.; Panahipour, L.; Gruber, R. Pyroptosis-Mediated Periodontal Disease. *Int. J. Mol. Sci.* **2021**, *23*, 372. [CrossRef]
40. Ribeiro, C.C.C.; Carmo, C.D.S.; Benatti, B.B.; Casarin, R.V.C.; Alves, C.M.C.; Nascimento, G.G.; Moreira, A.R.O. Systemic circulating inflammatory burden and periodontitis in adolescents. *Clin. Oral Investig.* **2021**, *25*, 5855–5865. [CrossRef]
41. Furutama, D.; Matsuda, S.; Yamawaki, Y.; Hatano, S.; Okanobu, A.; Memida, T.; Oue, H.; Fujita, T.; Ouhara, K.; Kajiya, M.; et al. IL-6 Induced by Periodontal Inflammation Causes Neuroinflammation and Disrupts the Blood-Brain Barrier. *Brain Sci.* **2020**, *10*, 679. [CrossRef] [PubMed]
42. Padilla-Martinez, F.; Wojciechowska, G.; Szczerbinski, L.; Kretowski, A. Circulating Nucleic Acid-Based Biomarkers of Type 2 Diabetes. *Int. J. Mol. Sci.* **2021**, *23*, 295. [CrossRef] [PubMed]
43. Cerne, D.; Bajalo, J.L. Cell-free nucleic acids as a non-invasive route for investigating atherosclerosis. *Curr. Pharm. Des.* **2014**, *20*, 5004–5009. [CrossRef]
44. Shi, C.; Dawulieti, J.; Shi, F.; Yang, C.; Qin, Q.; Shi, T.; Wang, L.; Hu, H.; Sun, M.; Ren, L.; et al. A nanoparticulate dual scavenger for targeted therapy of inflammatory bowel disease. *Sci. Adv.* **2022**, *8*, eabj2372. [CrossRef] [PubMed]
45. Dawulieti, J.; Sun, M.; Zhao, Y.; Shao, D.; Yan, H.; Lao, Y.H.; Hu, H.; Cui, L.; Lv, X.; Liu, F.; et al. Treatment of severe sepsis with nanoparticulate cell-free DNA scavengers. *Sci. Adv.* **2020**, *6*, eaay7148. [CrossRef]
46. Deng, K.; Pelekos, G.; Jin, L.; Tonetti, M.S. Gingival bleeding on brushing as a sentinel sign of gingival inflammation: A diagnostic accuracy trial for the discrimination of periodontal health and disease. *J. Clin. Periodontol.* **2021**, *48*, 1537–1548. [CrossRef]
47. Kim, P.D.; Xia-Juan, X.; Crump, K.E.; Abe, T.; Hajishengallis, G.; Sahingur, S.E. Toll-Like Receptor 9-Mediated Inflammation Triggers Alveolar Bone Loss in Experimental Murine Periodontitis. *Infect. Immun.* **2015**, *83*, 2992–3002. [CrossRef]

48. Liang, H.; Peng, B.; Dong, C.; Liu, L.; Mao, J.; Wei, S.; Wang, X.; Xu, H.; Shen, J.; Mao, H.Q.; et al. Cationic nanoparticle as an inhibitor of cell-free DNA-induced inflammation. *Nat. Commun.* **2018**, *9*, 4291. [CrossRef]
49. Peng, B.; Liang, H.; Li, Y.; Dong, C.; Shen, J.; Mao, H.Q.; Leong, K.W.; Chen, Y.; Liu, L. Tuned Cationic Dendronized Polymer: Molecular Scavenger for Rheumatoid Arthritis Treatment. *Angew. Chem. Int. Ed. Engl.* **2019**, *58*, 4254–4258. [CrossRef]
50. Pan, W.; Yin, W.; Yang, L.; Xue, L.; Ren, J.; Wei, W.; Lu, Q.; Ding, H.; Liu, Z.; Nabar, N.R.; et al. Inhibition of Ctsk alleviates periodontitis and comorbid rheumatoid arthritis via downregulation of the TLR9 signalling pathway. *J. Clin. Periodontol.* **2019**, *46*, 286–296. [CrossRef]
51. Michalowicz, B.S.; Hodges, J.S.; Pihlstrom, B.L. Is change in probing depth a reliable predictor of change in clinical attachment loss? *J. Am. Dent. Assoc.* **2013**, *144*, 171–178. [CrossRef] [PubMed]
52. Fleszar, T.J.; Knowles, J.W.; Morrison, E.C.; Burgett, F.G.; Nissle, R.R.; Ramfjord, S.P. Tooth mobility and periodontal therapy. *J. Clin. Periodontol.* **1980**, *7*, 495–505. [CrossRef] [PubMed]
53. Jiao, J.; Jing, W.; Si, Y.; Feng, X.; Tai, B.; Hu, D.; Lin, H.; Wang, B.; Wang, C.; Zheng, S.; et al. The prevalence and severity of periodontal disease in Mainland China: Data from the Fourth National Oral Health Survey (2015–2016). *J. Clin. Periodontol.* **2021**, *48*, 168–179. [CrossRef] [PubMed]
54. Meddeb, R.; Dache, Z.A.A.; Thezenas, S.; Otandault, A.; Tanos, R.; Pastor, B.; Sanchez, C.; Azzi, J.; Tousch, G.; Azan, S.; et al. Quantifying circulating cell-free DNA in humans. *Sci. Rep.* **2019**, *9*, 5220. [CrossRef]
55. Laine, M.L.; Crielaard, W.; Loos, B.G. Genetic susceptibility to periodontitis. *Periodontol* **2012**, *58*, 37–68. [CrossRef]

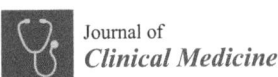

Article

Periodontitis-Related Knowledge and Its Relationship with Oral Health Behavior among Adult Patients Seeking Professional Periodontal Care

Ewa Dolińska [1,*], Robert Milewski [2], Maria Julia Pietruska [3], Katarzyna Gumińska [3], Natalia Prysak [3], Tomasz Tarasewicz [3], Maciej Janica [4] and Małgorzata Pietruska [1]

[1] Department of Periodontal and Oral Mucosa Diseases, Medical University of Bialystok, ul. Waszyngtona 13, 15-269 Bialystok, Poland; mpietruska@wp.pl
[2] Department of Statistics and Medical Informatics, Medical University of Bialystok, ul. Szpitalna 37, 15-295 Bialystok, Poland; robert.milewski@umb.edu.pl
[3] Student's Research Group, Department of Periodontal and Oral Mucosa Diseases, Medical University of Bialystok, ul. Waszyngtona 13, 15-269 Bialystok, Poland; maria.pietruska@gmail.com (M.J.P.); k.guminska@wp.pl (K.G.); natalia.prysak@gmail.com (N.P.); tarasewiczt@gmail.com (T.T.)
[4] Student's Research Group, Department of Statistics and Medical Informatics, Medical University of Bialystok, ul. Szpitalna 37, 15-295 Bialystok, Poland; janmac1e@gmail.com
* Correspondence: ewa.dolinska@umb.edu.pl; Tel.: +48-85-748-59-05

Abstract: Background: Periodontitis is a chronic inflammatory disease that not only damages the stomatognathic system, but may also adversely influence other systems and organs. Patients with low oral health literacy levels are more prone to gingivitis/periodontitis and have a more severe disease course. Methods: A written questionnaire was carried out to assess the knowledge of patients of the Outpatient Clinic of Department of Periodontal and Oral Mucosa Diseases, Medical University of Bialystok, Poland. The questions concerned knowledge regarding the causes of periodontal disease, its risk factors, and the connection between periodontal disease and general health status. To analyze the population, patients were divided according to gender, age and if they were first-time or regular outpatients. Results: Written questionnaires were completed by a total of 302 patients. In the studied population, we noted knowledge deficits, particularly related to weaker periodontal disease risk factors (stress, diabetes, osteoporosis, obesity) and the genetic factor, which is the determinant of periodontitis. The patients' awareness of the role of plaque bacteria and the effect of smoking on the periodontium was at a relatively high level. The respondents were also aware of the impact of periodontal disease on general health as well as the role of oral hygiene in preventing the disease. At the same time, few of them (26%) used interdental brushes or an irrigator (8%). Conclusions: We demonstrated that patients have an insufficient level of knowledge related to risk factors as well as the prevention of periodontal disease. Awareness of the extent of oral health literacy among patients will help to identify key issues connected with health education interventions

Keywords: periodontitis; global health; current pathophysiological understanding of periodontitis; risk factors; modulators linking periodontitis and systemic diseases; oral hygiene; questionnaire study

1. Introduction

Periodontitis is a chronic inflammatory disease leading to bone and soft tissue destruction and, consequently, tooth loss. After dental caries, it is the major cause of tooth loss in adults [1]. Moreover, it is also the 11th most common disease in the world, and is more prevalent than cardiovascular diseases [2,3]. Severe forms of periodontitis may affect 10% of the adult population worldwide. The incidence of periodontal disease increases with age and rises rapidly in people aged 50–60 years. The proportion of people with periodontitis is expected to increase further as the population ages [4]. Despite efforts to improve oral health in recent years, periodontitis remains widespread and is a significant public health

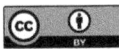

issue [5]. The World Health Organization (WHO) highlights that oral diseases (including periodontitis) are an important population problem due to their connections with other chronic diseases such as cardiovascular disease, diabetes and cancer, as well as their strong impact on people's well-being and the high economic costs generated by treating these conditions [6]. Therefore, periodontal disease prevention should be approached from a new socio-economic perspective.

The prevention of diseases significantly determines an individual's health and enables a considerable reduction in treatment-related costs. The patient's engagement in oral health care correlates with their level of knowledge and health literacy (HL), defined as the ability to obtain, process, and use information to make appropriate decisions with an impact on one's health. Patients with a low level of health literacy are less likely to adhere to the prescribed treatment, skip follow-up appointments, and apply a limited range of prophylaxis, and are more likely to suffer from general illnesses [7–9]. The same mechanism is crucial in terms of oral health literacy (OHL). Unfortunately, a limited ability to understand basic health information is common among adults and might have a significantly negative effect on the achievement of better results in maintaining sufficient oral hygiene [10]. Patients with low OHL levels are more prone to gingivitis/periodontitis and experience a more severe disease course. An increase in OHL level is correlated with undertaking preventive measures, following medical advice and an improvement in patients' quality of life [7,8].

Periodontitis is a multifactorial disease affected by genetic and environmental risk factors, which may be divided into determinants (age, gender, ethnicity, gene polymorphisms) and acquired factors: environmental and behavioral (specific bacterial flora, smoking, stress, diabetes, obesity, osteoporosis, or socio-economic status) [11–13]. The development of periodontal disease is generally determined by biofilm accumulation, but the presence of other factors is individually responsible for one's susceptibility or resistance to the disease. Reducing the influence of modifiable risk factors may alter the effectiveness of the prevention and treatment of periodontal disease.

Periodontitis not only damages the stomatognathic system, but also affects the chewing function and phonetics, and may adversely influence other systems and organs. Correlations between periodontitis and general diseases have been well documented and described since the 1990s. At present, there is a separate field of knowledge called "periodontal medicine" that evaluates the above-mentioned mechanisms [14–16]. Evidence supporting the link between periodontal disease and systemic diseases was discussed at the Joint EFP/AAP Workshop on Periodontitis and Systemic Diseases in 2012. Researchers from Europe and the USA mainly focused on the most thoroughly described associations of periodontal disease with diabetes, pregnancy complications and cardiovascular diseases. It was concluded that periodontal disease leads to a bacterial load, which results in a significant overall immune system response. This is likely to directly and indirectly affect the pathophysiology of general diseases [17–19]. As an example, both periodontitis and diabetes have an inflammatory basis and are linked together by different biochemical and metabolic interactions. Poorly controlled diabetes can increase the risk of periodontal disease, and periodontitis can adversely affect glycemic control mechanisms and increase the risk of diabetes complications [20]. It has been suggested that periodontal therapy may improve insulin sensitivity by reducing peripheral inflammatory cytokine levels. An improvement in glycemic status, defined as a reduction in glycated hemoglobin (HbA1c) was demonstrated in diabetic patients suffering from periodontitis [21,22]. There is also more evidence that periodontal therapy decreases plasma reactive oxygen species (ROMs), which are indicators of systemic oxidative stress [23].

The most widely reported associations in the literature on the subject are links between periodontitis and diabetes [20], cardiovascular disease [24], pregnancy and perinatal complications [25], obesity and metabolic syndrome [26], as well as rheumatoid arthritis [27], cancer [28], respiratory diseases [29], Alzheimer's disease [30] and other cognitive disorders [16]. This knowledge is available to professionals but is not always available to a wider audience, including patients.

The aim of our study was to assess the level of patient knowledge regarding the causes of periodontal disease, its risk factors and the connection between periodontal disease and general health status in different age groups. We also evaluated patients' health-promoting behaviors concerning oral hygiene.

2. Materials and Methods

2.1. General Methodology and a Questionnaire

We assessed the knowledge of periodontal disease in the patient population at the Outpatient Clinic of Department of Periodontal and Oral Mucosa Diseases at the Medical University of Bialystok, Poland, in the period from April 2016 to November 2017.

Patients specified their age, gender and whether it was their first visit to the Outpatient Clinic. The main questions included in the questionnaire were connected to the following:

- Causes of periodontal disease;
- Risk factors of periodontal disease;
- Impact of periodontal disease on general health;
- Pro-health behaviors of patients, aimed at prevention of periodontal disease.

Furthermore, the patients were asked which dental hygiene devices they used. We assumed that the use of interdental hygiene utensils (interdental brushes, dental floss) was a positive, health-promoting behavior resulting from awareness of periodontal disease prevention.

Additional questions pertained to:

- The frequency of tooth brushing;
- The use of a manual or mechanical toothbrush;
- The use of dental floss, interdental brushes, single-tuft brushes toothpicks or irrigators;
- The use of additional pharmacological agents such as mouthwashes, ointments, gels, breath fresheners and herbal remedies.

The questionnaire administered to participants is reported in Table 1.

Table 1. Questionnaire administered to participants.

1.	Gender					Male	Female
2.	Age	21–30	31–40	41–50	51–60	61–70	71–80
3.	Is it your first visit in the Outpatient Clinic of Department of Periodontal and Oral Mucosa Diseases?					Yes	No
4.	Do you think that oral bacteria contribute to the presence of periodontal disease?					Yes	No
5.	Do you think hereditary factors contribute to the presence of periodontal disease?					Yes	No
6.	Do you think that smoking contributes to the presence of periodontal disease?					Yes	No
7.	Are you a smoker?					Yes	No
8.	Do you think that stress affects the presence of periodontal disease?					Yes	No
9.	Do you think that diabetes contributes to the presence of periodontal disease?					Yes	No
10.	Do you think that osteoporosis contributes to the presence of periodontal disease?					Yes	No
11.	Do you think that obesity contributes to the presence of periodontal disease?					Yes	No
12.	Do you think that periodontal disease affects your overall health?					Yes	No
13.	Do you think that inadequate oral hygiene affects the presence of periodontal disease?					Yes	No
14.	How many times a day do you brush your teeth?					0	
						1	
						2	
						More than 2	

Table 1. *Cont.*

15.	What kind of brush do you use?	Manual toothbrush
		Mechanical toothbrush
16.	Do you regularly use any additional dental devices?	No
		Dental floss
		Interdental brushes
		Single-tuft brushes
		Toothpicks
		Irrigator
17.	Do you use any additional pharmacological agents?	No
		Mouthwashes
		Oral gels
		Oral ointments
		Breath fresheners
		Herbal remedies

The research was conducted in accordance with the Declaration of Helsinki, and approval was obtained from the local bioethics committee (R-I-002/80/2016). Subjects filled in the anonymous questionnaire form voluntarily, which was considered equivalent to consenting to participate in the study.

2.2. Statistical Analysis

For descriptive purposes, we first analyzed the number of correct answers to each question. If the number of the respondents who answered a question correctly did not exceed 80%, we concluded that the given group had insufficient knowledge about the topic included in the given question. We analyzed answers to each question according to the gender and age of the participants. The patients were also divided into two groups based on whether they were first-time patients or on a subsequent visit to the Clinic.

In the statistical analysis, the Chi-square test of independence was used to check the relationship between qualitative characteristics. Statistical significance was established at $p < 0.05$. Calculations were made by means of a Statistica 13.3 package from TIBCO Software Inc. (Palo Alto, CA, USA).

3. Results

3.1. Description of the Studied Group

Written questionnaires were completed by a total of 302 patients, including 180 women and 105 men (gender of 17 participants was not documented). The majority of patients completing the questionnaire were former outpatients ($n = 189$), and 36% were first-time patients. Smokers constituted 15% of the surveyed group. The patients were divided into the following age groups: 21–30 years (10% of the respondents), 31–40 years (15%), 41–50 years (22%), 51–60 (26.5%), 61–70 (17%) and 71–80 (7%) (the age of the remaining percentage of patients was not documented). The characteristics of the study group according to age, gender and status in the outpatient clinic are presented in Table 2. As some questionnaire variables were incomplete, the total numbers for some of the data collected in the questionnaire differ.

Table 2. Sample characteristics: number of patients in the respective groups. As some questionnaires variables were incomplete, the total numbers for some of the collected in the questionnaire data differs.

	Total	Man	Women	First Time Patient	Regular Patient
Total	302	105	180	110	189
21–30	31	10	19	15	16
31–40	45	18	25	25	20
41–50	67	27	39	24	43
51–60	80	23	53	25	53
61–70	52	16	31	11	41
71–80	22	10	11	8	14

The response rate to the questionnaire was 15.2% (out of 1988 patients who attended an appointment at the Outpatient Clinic in the period from April 2016 to November 2017, 302 people completed the questionnaire).

3.2. Knowledge Regarding the Causes of Periodontal Disease

Participants in our study answered seven questions about the risk factors for periodontal disease. The questions concerned bacteria forming the dental plaque, genetic factors, smoking, stress, diabetes, osteoporosis, and obesity. The involvement of bacteria in the etiology of periodontal disease was confirmed by 81% of the survey respondents. Insufficient knowledge on the subject (<80% of correct answers) was mostly demonstrated by men (77% correct answers), and those in the 41–50 age group (70%). The link between genetic factors and the occurrence of periodontal disease was reported by 61% of the patients. Lack of knowledge about this determinant of periodontal disease was evident in all age and gender groups, regardless of whether the patient was an outpatient or in the clinic for the first time. Tobacco smoking was associated with periodontal disease by 85% of respondents. Only patients aged 71–80 years showed insufficient knowledge (77% of correct answers) in this field. Significant knowledge deficiencies were noted for weaker risk factors. Stress was confirmed to be related to periodontal disease by 61% of respondents, diabetes by 64%, osteoporosis by 62% and obesity by only 39% of the surveyed patients. Stress and osteoporosis were statistically significantly more often reported as risk factors leading to periodontal disease by women. A detailed analysis of the respondents' knowledge of periodontal disease risk factors is presented in Table 3.

Table 3. Patient's knowledge about the influence of risk factors on the occurrence of periodontal disease.

	Age Group						Chi-Square	p
	21–30 (n = 26) 84%	31–40 (n = 43) 96%	41–50 (n = 46) 70%	51–60 (n = 67) 84%	61–70 (n = 43) 83%	71–80 (n = 18) 82%	12.7	p = 0.03
Bacteria	Male (n = 81) 77%			Female (n = 152) 85%			2.7	NS
	First time patients (n = 91) 83%			Regular patients (n = 152) 81%			0.2	NS
	Age group							
	21–30 (n = 23) 74%	31–40 (n = 32) 73%	41–50 (n = 44) 68%	51–60 (n = 49) 63%	61–70 (n = 22) 42%	71–80 (n = 11) 50%	14.9	p = 0.01
Genetics	Male (n = 61) 59%			Female (n = 112) 63%			0.4	NS
	First time patients (n = 70) 64%			Regular patients (n = 114) 62%			0.2	NS

Table 3. Cont.

	Age Group						Chi-Square	p
Smoking	Age group							
	21–30 (n = 26) 84%	31–40 (n = 41) 91%	41–50 (n = 63) 94%	51–60 (n = 64) 81%	61–70 (n = 43) 84%	71–80 (n = 17) 77%	7.9	NS
	Male (n = 90) 87%			Female (n = 154) 86%			0.01	NS
	First time patients (n = 96) 88%			Regular patients (n = 160) 85%			0.5	NS
Stress	Age group							
	21–30 (n = 19) 61%	31–40 (n = 27) 60%	41–50 (n = 46) 69%	51–60 (n = 42) 54%	61–70 (n = 37) 73%	71–80 (n = 10) 48%	7.8	NS
	Male (n = 54) 51%			Female (n = 121) 68%			7.7	p = 0.006
	First time patients (n = 65) 60%			Regular patients (n = 118) 63%			0.3	NS
Diabetes	Age group							
	21–30 (n = 23) 74%	31–40 (n = 33) 73%	41–50 (n = 44) 66%	51–60 (n = 48) 65%	61–70 (n = 29) 56%	71–80 (n = 10) 45%	8.0	NS
	Male (n = 66) 64%			Female (n = 112) 64%			0.005	NS
	First time patients (n = 75) 69%			Regular patients (n = 114) 62%			1.1	NS
Osteoporosis	Age group							
	21–30 (n = 18) 60%	31–40 (n = 31) 69%	41–50 (n = 43) 64%	51–60 (n = 49) 64%	61–70 (n = 34) 65%	71–80 (n = 9) 41%	5.6	NS
	Male (n = 54) 51%			Female (n = 120) 68%			7.8	p = 0.005
	First time patients (n = 73) 68%			Regular patients (n = 112) 60%			2.0	NS
Obesity	Age group							
	21–30 (n = 15) 48%	31–40 (n = 14) 32%	41–50 (n = 27) 41%	51–60 (n = 27) 36%	61–70 (n = 25) 50%	71–80 (n = 6) 29%	6.0	NS
	Male (n = 41) 40%			Female (n = 70) 40%			0.001	NS
	First time patients (n = 39) 37%			Regular patients (n = 76) 41%			0.6	NS

NS: non significant.

3.3. Knowledge of Risk of Other Diseases Associated with Periodontal Disease

An overwhelming number of respondents (89%) answered the question "Do you think that periodontal disease affects your overall health?" with "yes". The highest percentage of affirmative responses was obtained in the 41–50 age group (93%). A detailed distribution of the responses is presented in Table 4.

Table 4. Patients' knowledge about the influence of periodontitis on general health status.

Age Group						Chi-Square	p
21–30 ($n = 28$) 90%	31–40 ($n = 41$) 91%	41–50 ($n = 62$) 93%	51–60 ($n = 66$) 87%	61–70 ($n = 47$) 92%	71–80 ($n = 20$) 91%	1.7	NS
Male ($n = 95$) 90%			Female ($n = 159$) 90%			0.001	NS
First time patients ($n = 97$) 90%			Regular patients ($n = 169$) 91%			0.09	NS

NS: non significant.

3.4. Knowledge Regarding Prevention of Periodontal Disease

To assess the awareness regarding periodontal disease prevention, the participants in our study answered the question "Do you think that inadequate oral hygiene may lead to the occurrence of periodontal disease?" More than 90% of the total number of respondents answered affirmatively, and in the youngest age groups (21–30 years, 31–40 years), a positive answer was given by 100% of the respondents. A detailed analysis of the responses is presented in Table 5. Simultaneously, the health-promoting behavior was assessed by asking participants about their daily hygiene habits as well as the use of dental hygiene devices and additional pharmacological agents. The majority of respondents (90%) admitted that they brushed their teeth at least twice a day. A manual toothbrush was used by 78% of the participants. Flossing was reported by 64% of the patients (significantly more women than men, $p = 0.0008$), and interdental brushes were used by only 26% of the respondents (significantly more women, $p = 0.03$). At the same time, 24% of the participants used toothpicks and only 8% used an irrigator. Table 6 contains a detailed analysis of health-promoting activities, separated by gender, age, and whether the patient was visiting the clinic for the first time or was a regular outpatient.

Table 5. Patient's knowledge about the role of optimal oral hygiene in prevention of periodontitis (Do you think that inadequate oral hygiene affects the presence of periodontal diseases?).

Age Group						Chi-Square	p
21–30 ($n = 31$) 100%	31–40 ($n = 43$) 100%	41–50 ($n = 64$) 97%	51–60 ($n = 73$) 92%	61–70 ($n = 46$) 90%	71–80 ($n = 19$) 86%	10.4	NS
Male ($n = 100$) 97%			Female ($n = 165$) 93%			1.9	NS
First time patients ($n = 100$) 93%			Regular patients ($n = 177$) 96%			1.3	NS

NS: non significant.

Table 6. Self-reported oral hygiene in different age, gender and outpatient clinic status patients (data as a percentage).

Oral Hygiene Practice: Percentage of Participants	Gender			Age Group							Patients Status		
	F	M	p	21–30	31–40	41–50	51–60	61–70	71–80	p	First Time	Regular	p
Brush once a day	7	13	NS	10	4	12	10	12	4	NS	12	8	p = 0.02
Brush twice a day	67	71		68	78	64	66	65	64		73	63	
Brush more than twice a day	26	16		22	18	24	24	24	32		15	29	
Manual toothbrush	75	84	NS	65	65	66	86	94	96	p = 0.0003	80	77	NS
Mechanical toothbrush	25	16		35	35	34	14	6	4		20	23	
Dental floss	70	50	p = 0.0008	65	76	73	63	59	36	p = 0.02	61	66	NS
Interdental toothbrushes	31	19	p = 0.03	19	33	23	28	31	18	NS	21	29	NS
Toothpics	24	24	NS	6	16	28	34	22	23	p = 0.03	24	23	NS
Irrigator	10	5	NS	6	9	12	10	2	0	NS	6	8	NS
Mouthwashes	66	66	NS	84	80	66	62	63	45	p = 0.02	61	70	NS
Oral gels	11	5	NS	3	7	12	10	8	9	NS	9	8	NS
Oral ointments	7	4	NS	3	2	4	8	10	9	NS	5	8	NS
Breath fresheners	9	6	NS	0	9	9	11	2	10	NS	7	6	NS
Herbal remedies	18	12	NS	3	22	13	19	20	14	NS	18	16	NS

NS: non significant, p: Chi square test.

4. Discussion

The survey aimed to evaluate the knowledge of patients seeking periodontal care and their involvement in their daily hygiene regimen. In the studied population, we noted knowledge deficits, particularly related to weaker periodontal disease risk factors (stress, diabetes, osteoporosis, obesity) and the genetic factor, which is the determinant of periodontitis. The patients' awareness of the role of plaque bacteria and the effect of smoking on the periodontium was at a relatively high level. The respondents were also aware of the impact of periodontal disease on general health as well as the role of oral hygiene in preventing the disease. At the same time, few of them (26%) used interdental brushes or an irrigator (8%). Supportive pharmacological agents were more popular. Oral rinses were used by 66% of the participants. Knowledge deficits were most visible in the oldest age group (71–80 years). These findings are consistent with the reports of other researchers, who suggested that knowledge deficits are associated with lower education levels and the age of patients [31,32]. However, according to the analysis of the collected survey data, patients of all age groups need education in the discussed field, not only in terms of the causes of periodontal disease but also its prevention at home.

Home oral hygiene involves using a toothbrush, dental floss, toothpicks, and other devices to remove plaque and food particles from the surface of the teeth. Individual oral hygiene is often considered a key factor in controlling periodontal disease, thus providing an enormous benefit to public health. Despite the lack of direct evidence in the form of randomized clinical trials to confirm the relationship between oral hygiene and periodontal disease, maintaining optimal oral hygiene is a fundamental principle of periodontal disease prophylaxis [33]. Home hygiene, causal treatment, and maintenance therapy are keystones in disease prevention [34], while neglecting oral hygiene leads to the accumulation of plaque, dental calculus, and development of gingivitis [35]. Brushing teeth twice a day with fluoride toothpaste is a basic hygiene procedure performed in developed countries. In the studied population, only 7% of women and 13% of men reported brushing their teeth only once or less frequently per day. This was also the case for 12% of first-time patients and 8% of regular outpatients at the Clinic. The percentage of flossers was also high: 64%. Using dental floss was reported by 50% of men and 70% of women, and interdental brushes by 19% of men and 31% of women. Toothpicks were most popular among those over 40 years of age. As many as 92% of the respondents treated previously at the Outpatient Clinic brushed their teeth twice or more times a day, 66% of whom used floss, while 29% used interdental brushes and 8% reported using an irrigator. The percentage in each case was higher than for patients waiting for their first periodontal visit.

A survey on oral hygiene in the entire Polish population was conducted by Górska and Górski in 2018 (survey in 10 cities). The use of dental floss was reported by 57% of the respondents, interdental brushes by 12%, an irrigator by 8%, and mouthwash by 67% [36]. These results are similar to ours, particularly in terms of the use of an irrigator and mouthwashes. Fewer respondents reported using dental floss and interdental brushes. This is largely related to the fact that the survey was focused on the general population rather than those seeking professional periodontal care. Self-reported oral hygiene was much worse in the Italian population, in which only 23.5% of respondents brushed their teeth twice or more times a day, and daily flossing was reported by 13.3% of people. The recommendation of the Italian authorities to brush one's teeth regularly twice a day and attend check-up visits to the dentist once a year was met by only 12% of the respondents [37].

In the Lithuanian population, over a 20-year time period (1994–2014), the 20–64 age group demonstrated an improvement in the frequency of oral hygiene procedures. There, the percentage of men brushing their teeth at least twice a day increased from 15% to 32% and, in women, from 33% to 59% [38]. Portuguese self-reported oral hygiene surveys reached similar values to the European average. In the examined Portuguese population, 73% of the respondents brushed their teeth at least twice a day (78% of women and 69% of men). Flossing was reported by 29% of women and 18% of men [39].

Effective plaque removal at home plays a key role in the prevention and treatment of periodontal disease. Cleaning the interdental spaces is also very important [40]. In this case, the most effective hygienic aids are interdental space brushes as they remove more plaque than floss or toothpicks [41]. In periodontal patients, these devices should be the first choice for interdental cleaning. The use of interdental cleaning utensils can be considered an indicator of active knowledge of periodontal disease prevention [42].

Individually tailored educational programs related to improvements in oral hygiene may encourage patients to clean the interdental spaces more frequently and maintain a high level of commitment and behavior change. Such programs improve long-term adherence to oral hygiene in periodontal treatment [43]. Optimal oral hygiene leads not only to a change in periodontal indices but also influences the general condition of patients with diabetes and hypertension. Four oral hygiene sessions with a dental hygienist were sufficient to maintain stable blood pressures and significantly lower glycosylated hemoglobin levels at the fourth session [44]. It was proven that a higher level of knowledge about periodontal disease, its pathogenesis, and consequences led to internal motivation and an improvement in oral hygiene, especially in the interdental spaces [45].

When analyzing the results of the presented experiment, the limitations of our survey should also be considered. The study group consisted of patients seeking professional periodontal help at the Outpatient Clinic at the Medical University. The knowledge of this group of patients cannot be compared to the entire Polish population, including those without symptoms of periodontal disease. Another limitation of our work was the size of the assessed group. Despite the fact that our survey lasted over a year, only 302 people decided to complete our questionnaire. The likely reason for this was the need to fill out multiple forms before the periodontal visit, which is particularly cumbersome for the elderly. In our survey, we did not ask about education and socioeconomic status. Although additional questions could provide new information and dependencies, we wanted to avoid the survey being too long. We did not correlate periodontal status with the level of patients' knowledge, which allowed the research to remain anonymous and a larger group of respondents to be gathered.

It is also important to recognize that patients' knowledge is not the only factor affecting oral health; other aspects described by health behavior models are equally important in motivating patients to change their hygiene habits. These evidence-based psychological models are connected, inter alia, with self-efficacy, motivation, counselling, decision balance (relationship of perceived benefits and behavioral barriers), perceived susceptibility, and normative beliefs [46–48]. Knowledge is only a prerequisite, but it is necessary to improve patients' health-seeking behaviors.

5. Conclusions

In our work, we demonstrated that patients have an insufficient level of knowledge related to the risk factors and prevention of periodontal disease, especially through effective interdental cleaning. The collected data indicate the need for further education on periodontal disease among patients attending the Outpatient Clinic for Periodontal Diseases of the Medical University of Bialystok and in the general Polish population. Awareness of the extent of OHL among patients will enable the identification of key issues connected with oral health education interventions. The effective education of patients should result in more successful prevention and treatment of periodontal diseases.

Author Contributions: Conceptualization, E.D. and M.P.; Methodology, E.D.; Software, R.M.; Validation, M.P., E.D. and R.M.; Formal Analysis, R.M. and M.J.; Investigation, M.J.P., K.G., N.P. and T.T.; Data Curation, E.D.; Writing—Original Draft Preparation, E.D.; Writing—Review and Editing, M.P.; Supervision, M.P.; Project Administration, E.D.; Funding Acquisition, E.D. All authors have read and agreed to the published version of the manuscript.

Funding: The authors and their respective institution funded the study (Medical University of Bialystok, ul. Kilińskiego 1, 15-089 Bialystok, Poland).

Institutional Review Board Statement: The study was compliant with the 1975 Helsinki Declaration and its 2000 amendments. The Ethical Committee of Medical University of Bialystok approved this study (R-I-002/80/2016).

Informed Consent Statement: Patient consent was waived due to the fact that the survey was anonymous. Each survey began with a statement: The survey aims to assess the knowledge of the causes of periodontal disease. The survey is anonymous. The questionnaire will be only used for collective analysis. There is no need to complete the survey. By completing the questionnaire, you agree to participate in the study.

Data Availability Statement: The datasets used and/or analyzed during the current study are available from the corresponding author on reasonable request.

Conflicts of Interest: The authors declare that they have no conflict of interest.

References

1. Albandar, J.M. Epidemiology and Risk Factors of Periodontal Diseases. *Dent. Clin. N. Am.* **2005**, *49*, 517–532. [CrossRef] [PubMed]
2. Marcenes, W.; Kassebaum, N.J.; Bernabé, E.; Flaxman, A.; Naghavi, M.; Lopez, A.; Murray, C.J. Global burden of oral conditions in 1990–2010: A systematic analysis. *J. Dent. Res.* **2013**, *92*, 592–597. [CrossRef] [PubMed]
3. Dye, B. The Global Burden of Oral Disease: Research and Public Health Significance. *J. Dent. Res.* **2017**, *96*, 361–363. [CrossRef] [PubMed]
4. Billings, M.; Holtfreter, B.; Papapanou, P.N.; Mitnik, G.L.; Kocher, T.; Dye, B.A. Age-dependent distribution of periodontitis in two countries: Findings from NHANES 2009 to 2014 and SHIP-TREND 2008 to 2012. *J. Clin. Periodontol.* **2018**, *45* (Suppl. 20), S130–S148. [CrossRef]
5. Frencken, J.E.; Sharma, P.; Stenhouse, L.; Green, D.; Laverty, D.; Dietrich, T. Global epidemiology of dental caries and severe periodontitis—A comprehensive review. *J. Clin. Periodontol.* **2017**, *44*, S94–S105. [CrossRef] [PubMed]
6. Fisher, J.; Selikowitz, H.-S.; Mathur, M.; Varenne, B. Strengthening oral health for universal health coverage. *Lancet* **2018**, *392*, 899–901. [CrossRef]
7. Dickson-Swift, V.; Kenny, A.; Farmer, J.; Gussy, M.; Larkins, S. Measuring oral health literacy: A scoping review of existing tools. *BMC Oral Health* **2014**, *14*, 148. [CrossRef]
8. Cabellos-García, A.C.; Martínez-Sabater, A.; Castro-Sánchez, E.; Kangasniemi, M.; Juárez-Vela, R.; Gea-Caballero, V. Relation between health literacy, self-care and adherence to treatment with oral anticoagulants in adults: A narrative systematic review. *BMC Public Health* **2018**, *18*, 1157. [CrossRef]
9. Baskaradoss, J.K. Relationship between oral health literacy and oral health status. *BMC Oral Health* **2018**, *18*, 172. [CrossRef]
10. Wehmeyer, M.M.H.; Corwin, C.L.; Guthmiller, J.M.; Lee, J.Y. The impact of oral health literacy on periodontal health status. *J. Public Health Dent.* **2014**, *74*, 80–87. [CrossRef]
11. Borrell, L.; Papapanou, P.N. Analytical epidemiology of periodontitis. *J. Clin. Periodontol.* **2005**, *32* (Suppl. 6), 132–158. [CrossRef] [PubMed]
12. Kornman, K.S. Mapping the Pathogenesis of Periodontitis: A New Look. *J. Periodontol.* **2008**, *79*, 1560–1568. [CrossRef] [PubMed]
13. Genco, R.J.; Borgnakke, W.S. Risk factors for periodontal disease. *Periodontol. 2000* **2013**, *62*, 59–94. [CrossRef] [PubMed]
14. Williams, R.C.; Offenbacher, S. Periodontal medicine: The emergence of a new branch of periodontology. *Periodontol. 2000* **2000**, *23*, 9–12. [CrossRef] [PubMed]
15. Kumar, P.S. From focal sepsis to periodontal medicine: A century of exploring the role of the oral microbiome in systemic disease. *J. Physiol.* **2017**, *595*, 465–476. [CrossRef] [PubMed]
16. Genco, R.J.; Sanz, M. Clinical and public health implications of periodontal and systemic diseases: An overview. *Periodontol. 2000* **2020**, *83*, 7–13. [CrossRef] [PubMed]
17. Tonetti, M.S.; Van Dyke, T.E. Working group 1 of the joint EFP/AAP workshop. Periodontitis and atherosclerotic cardiovascular disease: Consensus report of the Joint EFP/AAP Workshop on Periodontitis and Systemic Diseases. *J. Clin. Periodontol.* **2013**, *40* (Suppl. 14), S24–S29. [CrossRef]
18. Chapple, I.L.C.; Genco, R. Working group 2 of the joint EFP/AAP workshop. Diabetes and periodontal diseases: Consensus report of the Joint EFP/AAP Workshop on Periodontitis and Systemic Diseases. *J. Clin. Periodontol.* **2013**, *40* (Suppl. 14), S106–S112. [CrossRef]
19. Sanz, M.; Kornman, K. Working group 3 of the joint EFP/AAP workshop. Periodontitis and adverse pregnancy outcomes: Consensus report of the Joint EFP/AAP Workshop on Periodontitis and Systemic Diseases. *J. Clin. Periodontol.* **2013**, *40* (Suppl. 14), S164–S169. [CrossRef]
20. Genco, R.J.; Graziani, F.; Hasturk, H. Effects of periodontal disease on glycemic control, complications, and incidence of diabetes mellitus. *Periodontol. 2000* **2020**, *83*, 59–65. [CrossRef]
21. D'Aiuto, F.; Gkranias, N.; Bhowruth, D.; Khan, T.; Orlandi, M.; Suvan, J.; Masi, S.; Tsakos, G.; Hurel, S.; Hingorani, A.; et al. Systemic effects of periodontitis treatment in patients with type 2 diabetes: A 12 month, single-centre, investigator-masked, randomised trial. *Lancet Diabetes Endocrinol.* **2018**, *6*, 954–965, Erratum in *Lancet Diabetes Endocrinol.* **2019**, *3*, e3. [CrossRef]

22. Butera, A.; Lovati, E.; Rizzotto, S.; Segù, M.; Scribante, A.; Lanteri, V.; Chiesa, A.; Granata, M.; Ruggero, R.Y.B. Professional and Home-Management in non -surgical periodontal therapy to evaluate the percentage of glycated hemoglobin in type 1 diabetes patients. *Int. J. Clin. Dent.* **2021**, *14*, 41–53.
23. Marconcini, S.; Giammarinaro, E.; Cosola, S.; Oldoini, G.; Genovesi, A.; Covani, U. Effects of Non-Surgical Periodontal Treatment on Reactive Oxygen Metabolites and Glycemic Control in Diabetic Patients with Chronic Periodontitis. *Antioxidants* **2021**, *10*, 1056. [CrossRef] [PubMed]
24. Herrera, D.; Molina, A.; Buhlin, K.; Klinge, B. Periodontal diseases and association with atherosclerotic disease. *Periodontol. 2000* **2020**, *83*, 66–89. [CrossRef] [PubMed]
25. Bobetsis, Y.A.; Graziani, F.; Gürsoy, M.; Madianos, P.N. Periodontal disease and adverse pregnancy outcomes. *Periodontol. 2000* **2020**, *83*, 154–174. [CrossRef]
26. Jepsen, S.; Suvan, J.; Deschner, J. The association of periodontal diseases and metabolic syndrome and obesity. *Periodontol. 2000* **2020**, *83*, 125–153. [CrossRef]
27. Zhang, J.; Xu, C.; Gao, L.; Zhang, D.; Li, C.; Liu, J. Influence of anti-rheumatic agents on the periodontal condition of patients with rheumatoid arthritis and periodontitis: A systematic review and meta-analysis. *J. Periodont. Res.* **2021**, *56*, 1099–1115. [CrossRef]
28. Sobocki, B.K.; Basset, C.A.; Bruhn-Olszewska, B.; Olszewski, P.; Szot, O.; Kaźmierczak-Siedlecka, K.; Guziak, M.; Nibali, L.; Leone, A. Molecular mechanisms leading from periodontal disease to cancer. *Int. J. Mol. Sci.* **2022**, *23*, 970. [CrossRef]
29. Lee, J.-H.; Jeong, S.-N. Chronic periodontitis and acute respiratory infections: A nationwide cohort study. *Appl. Sci.* **2021**, *11*, 9493. [CrossRef]
30. Dioguardi, M.; Crincoli, V.; Laino, L.; Alovisi, M.; Sovereto, D.; Mastrangelo, F.; Russo, L.L.; Muzio, L.L. The role of periodontitis and periodontal bacteria in the onset and progression of Alzheimer's disease: A systematic review. *J. Clin. Med.* **2020**, *9*, 495. [CrossRef]
31. El-Qaderi, S.; Quteish Ta'ani, D. Assessment of periodontal knowledge and periodontal status of an adult population in Jordan. *Int. J. Dent. Hyg.* **2004**, *2*, 132–136. [CrossRef] [PubMed]
32. Mårtensson, C.; Söderfeldt, B.; Andersson, P.; Halling, A.; Renvert, S. Factors behind change in knowledge after a mass media campaign targeting periodontitis. *Int. J. Dent. Hyg.* **2006**, *4*, 8–14. [CrossRef] [PubMed]
33. Hujoel, P.P.; Cunha-Cruz, J.; Loesche, W.J.; Robertson, P.B. Personal oral hygiene and chronic periodontitis: A systematic review. *Periodontol. 2000* **2005**, *37*, 29–34. [CrossRef] [PubMed]
34. Page, R.C.; Offenbacher, S.; Schroeder, H.E.; Seymour, G.J.; Kornman, K.S. Advances in the pathogenesis of periodontitis: Summary of developments, clinical implications and future directions. *Periodontol. 2000* **1997**, *14*, 216–248. [CrossRef]
35. Löe, H.; Theilade, E.; Jensen, S.B. Experimental gingivitis in man. *J. Periodontol.* **1965**, *36*, 177–187. [CrossRef]
36. Górska, R.; Górski, B. Self-reported oral status and habits related to oral care in adult Poles: A questionnaire study. *Dent. Med. Probl.* **2018**, *55*, 313–320. [CrossRef]
37. Villa, A.; Kreimer, A.R.; Polimeni, A.; Cicciù, D.; Strohmenger, L.; Gherlone, E.; Abati, S. Self-reported oral hygiene habits among dental patients in Italy. *Med. Princ. Pract.* **2012**, *21*, 452–456. [CrossRef]
38. Raskiliene, A.; Kriaucioniene, V.; Siudikiene, J.; Petkeviciene, J. Self-reported oral health, oral hygiene and associated factors in Lithuanian adult population, 1994–2014. *Int. J. Environ. Res. Public Health* **2020**, *17*, 5331. [CrossRef]
39. Melo, P.; Marques, S.; Silva, O.M. Portuguese self-reported oral-hygiene habits and oral status. *Int. Dent. J.* **2017**, *67*, 139–147. [CrossRef]
40. Claydon, N.C. Current concepts in toothbrushing and interdental cleaning. *Periodontol. 2000* **2008**, *48*, 10–22. [CrossRef]
41. Drisko, C.L. Periodontal self-care: Evidence-based support. *Periodontol. 2000* **2013**, *62*, 243–255. [CrossRef] [PubMed]
42. Deinzer, R.; Micheelis, W.; Granrath, N.; Hoffmann, T. More to learn about: Periodontitis-related knowledge and its relationship with periodontal health behaviour. *J. Clin. Periodontol.* **2009**, *36*, 756–764. [CrossRef] [PubMed]
43. Jönsson, B.; Öhrn, K.; Oscarson, N.; Lindberg, P. The effectiveness of an individually tailored oral health educational programme on oral hygiene behaviour in patients with periodontal disease: A blinded randomized-controlled clinical trial (one-year follow-up). *J. Clin. Periodontol.* **2009**, *36*, 1025–1034. [CrossRef] [PubMed]
44. Kim, N.-H.; Lee, G.-Y.; Park, S.-K.; Kim, Y.-J.; Lee, M.-Y.; Kim, C.-B. Provision of oral hygiene services as a potential method for preventing periodontal disease and control hypertension and diabetes in a community health centre in Korea. *Health Soc. Care Community* **2018**, *26*, e378–e385. [CrossRef]
45. Gunpinar, S.; Meraci, B. Periodontal health education session can improve oral hygiene in patients with gingivitis: A masked randomized controlled clinical study. *J. Periodontol.* **2022**, *93*, 218–228. [CrossRef]
46. Clarkson, J.E.; Young, L.; Ramsay, C.R.; Bonner, B.C.; Bonetti, D. How to influence patient oral hygiene behavior effectively. *J. Dent. Res.* **2009**, *88*, 933–937. [CrossRef]
47. Yevlahova, D.; Satur, J. Models for individual oral health promotion and their effectiveness: A systematic review. *Aust. Dent. J.* **2009**, *54*, 190–197. [CrossRef]
48. Newton, J.T.; Asimakopoulou, K. Managing oral hygiene as a risk factor for periodontal disease: A systematic review of psychological approaches to behaviour change for improved plaque control in periodontal management. *J. Clin. Periodontol.* **2015**, *42* (Suppl. 16), S36–S46. [CrossRef]

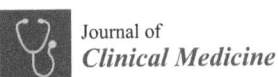

Article

Comparison of the Treatment Efficacy of Endo—Perio Lesions Using a Standard Treatment Protocol and Extended by Using a Diode Laser (940 nm)

Elżbieta Dembowska [1], Aleksandra Jaroń [2], Aleksandra Homik-Rodzińska [1], Ewa Gabrysz-Trybek [3], Joanna Bladowska [4] and Grzegorz Trybek [2,*]

[1] Department of Periodontology, Pomeranian Medical University, 70-111 Szczecin, Poland; elzbieta.dembowska@pum.edu.pl (E.D.); zperio@pum.edu.pl (A.H.-R.)
[2] Department of Oral Surgery, Pomeranian Medical University in Szczecin, 70-111 Szczecin, Poland; jaronola@gmail.com
[3] Department of Diagnostic Imaging and Interventional Radiology, Pomeranian Medical University, 71-242 Szczecin, Poland; ewa_gabrysz@wp.pl
[4] Department of General and Interventional Radiology and Neuroradiology, Wroclaw Medical University, 50-369 Wrocław, Poland; Joanna.bladowska@umed.wroc.pl
* Correspondence: g.trybek@gmail.com

Abstract: Marginal and periapical periodontal diseases cause massive destruction of tooth tissues and surrounding tissues, such as alveolar bone and maxillary sinus floor, visible on radiographs. Lesions involving the apical and marginal periodontium are endo—perio (EPL) lesions. This study aimed to compare the treatment efficacy of endo—perio lesions using a standard treatment protocol and a standard diode laser-assisted treatment protocol. The 12 patients were divided into the study (a) and control (b) group. Periodontal indices, tooth vitality and mobility, occlusal status, and radiographic diagnosis were evaluated. Standard EPL treatment was then performed—without (a) and with (b) the use of diode laser (940 nm). Again, after six months, the above-mentioned parameters were evaluated and compared. The treatment of endo—perio lesions is a significant challenge for modern dentistry. Diode lasers are increasingly used in addition to traditional treatment methods. The conventional use of a 940 nm diode laser with an average power of 0.8 W in pulsed mode allows for the depth of periodontal pockets to be reduced. In addition, the use of a diode laser has a significant effect on tooth mobility and reduces bone loss.

Keywords: endo—perio lesions; diode laser; CBCT; periodontitis

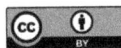

1. Introduction

Marginal and periapical periodontal diseases cause massive destruction of the tooth's tissues, and surrounding tissues, such as alveolar bone and the floor of the maxillary sinus, visible on radiographs [1]. Lesions that involve apical and marginal periodontium are endo—perio lesions (EPL). According to the 2017 classification, this type of lesion affects people with and without periodontal disease [2]. Advanced periodontitis results in the loss of connective tissues and increased depth of periodontal pockets. Secondary changes begin in the pulp of the tooth. Initially, the pulp is in a reversible inflammation state, but irreversible inflammation develops over time. The two are closely related structurally and functionally. Three main connection pathways are responsible for the occurrence of EPL: the main canals of the dental roots, the lateral and accessory canals, and the dentinal canals [2–7].

In 2017, a new classification of endo—periodontal lesions was formulated by Herrera et al. (Table 1). The authors divided the lesions into two groups: endo—periodontal lesions with root damage and without root damage. This new concept has changed the clinical approach, because the primary source, endodontic or periodontal, is not relevant to treatment. The diagnosis of an endo−periodontal lesion must answer whether to preserve the tooth or remove it. In the evaluation, there are three types of diagnosed EPL tooth: hopeless, which is classified for removal; bad; or favorable, which should be cured [2].

Table 1. Endo−perio lesion (EPL) according to Herrera et al. [2].

Endo−periodontal lesion with root damage	Root fracture or cracking	
	Root canal or pulp chamber perforation	
	External root resorption	
Endo−periodontal lesion without root damage	Endo−periodontal lesion in periodontitis patients	Grade 1—narrow deep periodontal pocket in 1 tooth surface
		Grade 2—wide deep periodontal pocket in 1 tooth surface
		Grade 3—deep periodontal pockets in more than 1 tooth surface
	Endo−periodontal lesion in non-periodontitis patients	Grade 1—narrow deep periodontal pocket in 1 tooth surface
		Grade 2—wide deep periodontal pocket in 1 tooth surface
		Grade 3—deep periodontal pockets in more than 1 tooth surface

Treatment of endo−periodontal lesions involves the elimination of pathogens found in periodontal pockets and infected root canals [2,3,8]. The bacteria that are found in both of these environments are very similar. This similarity between bacteria is related to specific conditions, and the occurrence in anaerobic environments [9]. Some studies have shown that most bacteria are located in the outer 300 μm of dentinal tubules. These sites may be reservoirs from which the bacterial recolonization of treated root surfaces can arise [10]. Pathogens found in these types of lesions include *Streptococcus*, *Peptostreptococcus*, *Eubacterium*, *Bacteroides*, and *Fusobacterium*. A study published in 2020 showed that endo−perio lesions can be observed in the endodontium and periodontium, mainly *Tannerella forsythia*, *Porphyromonas gingivalis*, and *Aggregatibacter actinomycetemcomintans* [5].

Treatment in EPL should be two-pronged—periodontal and endodontic. These approaches are mechanical non-surgical periodontal treatment, consisting of surface root planning (SRP) or SRD (surface root debridement). The area, after being cleaned, is prepared to receive the new adhesion. Periodontal surface and root debridement can be performed using hand instruments and ultrasonic scalars. A comparison of manual and ultrasonic instrumentation use indicates that it is not statistically significant [11,12].

The goal of the endodontic algorithm is to eliminate bacteria that are present in the root canals [13,14]. Many proposals and protocols for decontamination and root canal preparation with laser devices have been presented in the literature. The first conventional protocols are CLE (conventional laser endodontics), aPAD (antimicrobial photo-activated disinfection), and LAI (laser-activated irrigation). In recent years, erbium lasers operating with short SSP pulses, low power, PIPS (photon-induced photoacoustic streaming), and SWEEPS (shock wave enhanced emission photoacoustic streaming) have been introduced to endodontic treatment. Treatment is performed using special tips with tailpieces in the presence of irrigation solutions: 17% sodium edetate (EDTA) and 5.25% sodium hypochlorite (NaOCl). They were proven to be very effective, without causing thermal effects on dental hard tissues [15]. The mechanism of their antibacterial action is primarily due to the thermal effects of radiation. Due to the different wavelengths emitted, diode lasers differ in their absorption range in water, which affects the penetration depth of the radiation into the tubules, from 400 to 1000 μm [16,17].

The laser therapy in periodontal pockets is able to eradicate pathogens and avoid surgical treatment.

The above considerations inspired the authors to address this topic.

This study aimed to compare the effectiveness of treating endo−perio lesions using a standard treatment protocol and a standard treatment protocol augmented with a diode laser. Null hypothesis—there is no difference in the efficacy of treating endo−perio lesions using a standard treatment protocol and a standard treatment protocol augmented with a diode laser.

2. Materials and Methods

This study was designed as a randomized and controlled 6-month clinical trial. The study protocol was approved by the Ethics Commission of the Medical University (no. KB-0012/29/17) and was conducted in full accordance with ethical principles, including the WHO Helsinki Declaration (2008 version).

2.1. Subject Selection

Sixteen patients of the Department of Periodontology, Medical University, with endo−perio lesions were enrolled in the pilot study. All patients were diagnosed with stage III periodontitis [18]. Each subject gave informed consent after explaining the study protocol, risks, and benefits. Two patients in both groups were excluded from the study due to missed appointments. Both groups had the same number of teeth—six molars in the study group (G1) and the control group (G2). Seven men and five women aged between 35 and 58 years (mean ± SD 46.5 ± 11.5) participated in the study. The inclusion and exclusion criteria for the study are shown in Table 2.

Table 2. Inclusion and exclusion criteria for enrolled patients.

Inclusion Criteria	Exclusion Criteria
• Patients diagnosed with periodontitis, Grade III periodontitis • Presence of endo−periodontal lesions without root damage • Presence of at least 20 teeth • Patients without increased tooth mobility • Patients without occlusal problems or after occlusion correction • Motivated patients with good oral hygiene (API < 15%)	• Presence of systemic disease • Patients taking antibiotics or immunosuppressive drugs six months before the study • Pregnancy or lactation • Smoking or alcoholism

The study was conducted according to the computerized random assignment of teeth to either the control ($n = 6$) or study ($n = 6$) group. Periodontal and endodontic treatment was performed in the first group, G1, with the additional use of a diode laser with a wavelength of 940 nm. The same procedures were performed in the control group G2, but without using the diode laser (Figure 1).

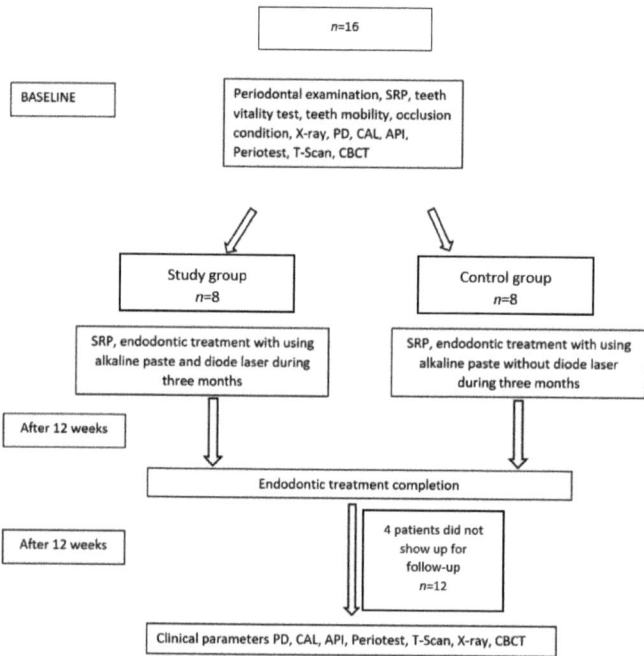

Figure 1. Study scheme.

2.1.1. First Visit

At the first visit, all patients ($n = 12$) were clinically examined for parameters such as periodontal pocket depth (PPD), tooth mobility, vitality test, occlusal status, and X-ray analysis. Periodontal pocket depth (PPD) was examined using a handheld periodontal probe (UNC 15, Hu-Friedy®, Chicago, IL, USA) at six sites. Classified teeth diagnosed with EPP showed no viability when tested with faradic current (PEm-1-type pulpoendometer) and ethyl chloride [19]. In addition, the study teeth were checked with Periotest M (Medizintechnik Gulden®, Modautal, Germany) in both groups before and after treatment. Periotest M is an instrument used to measure tooth mobility [20]. Every patient was checked using the T-scan Novus (Tekscan®, Boston, MA, USA).

In addition, before endodontic and periodontal treatment, cone bean computed tomography (CBCT) was performed to visualize bone defects in the vicinity of the tooth and to gain better insight into the anatomy of the root canal system of the treated tooth.

2.1.2. Treatment

Based on the examination, endodontic and periodontal treatment of the teeth was decided. Scaling and root planning of the teeth were performed using an ultrasonic scaler, and hand curettes were used. Intraoral radiographs (Pax Flex3D, Hwaseong-si, Gyeonggi-do, 18449, Korea) were then taken to classify the teeth, and endodontic treatment was started under anesthesia. The anatomy of the root system was evaluated on CBCT images before endodontic treatment (Figure 2), and endodontic treatment was performed using a microscope (Leica®, Wetzlar, Germany). A two-dimensional image was taken with the instruments in the canals (Figure 3). It was helpful to determine the working lengths of the canals, which were confirmed using a Raypex 5 endometer (VDW®, München, Germany). The rotary preparation was preceded by manually preparing the glide path using stainless steel hand instruments for a #20 file. The canals were prepared with 2% sodium hypochlorite, EDTA, and distilled water, using the crown-down method with the Endostar E3 Basic rotary system (Endostar®, Warszawa, Poland).

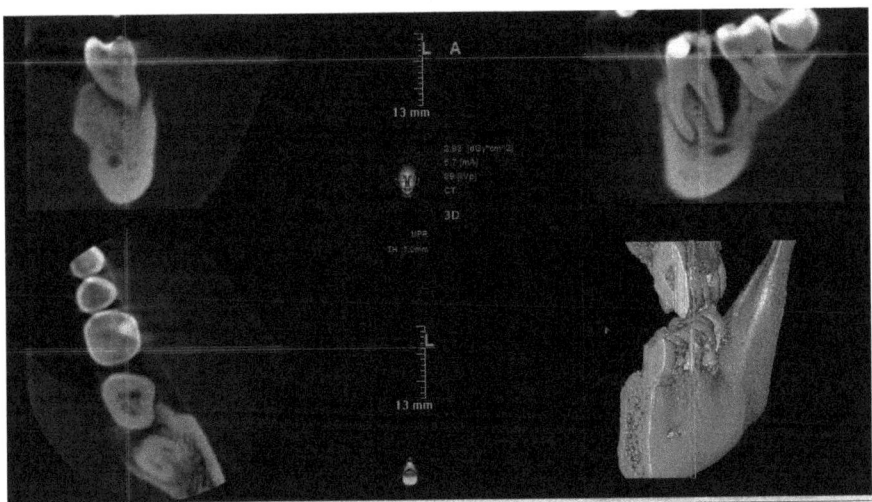

Figure 2. Baseline CBCT.

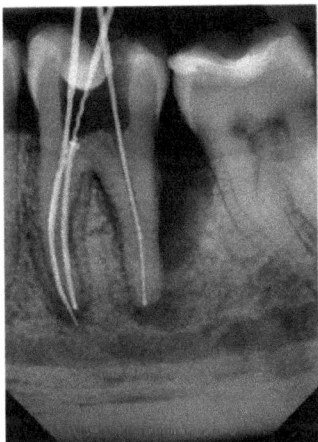

Figure 3. 2D image during endodontic treatment.

After complete canal preparation, the Epic X diode laser (Biolase®, Foothill Ranch, CA, USA) at 940 nm was used in group one. Disinfection was performed with sodium hypochlorite and the diode laser in a pulsed wave, with an operation input of 20 ms and output of 20 ms, average power of 0.8 W, pulse width of 20 ms, and timer of 10 s. The fiber of the diode laser tip with a diameter of 0.2 mm was introduced, which was shorter by 2 mm than the working length of the canals. There were three repetitions of disinfection per channel, with 10-s pauses between the repetitions. Calcium hydroxide paste Calcipast (Cerkamed®, Stalowa Wola, Poland) was applied to the canals between visits, and the teeth were temporarily sealed with Ketac Fil glass-ionomer cement (3M ESPE®, Maplewood, MN, USA).Root debritment was performed in each periodontal pocket. An EPIC X 940 nm laser (Biolase®, Foothill Ranch, CA, USA) with inactive tips was used to disinfect the interdental pockets without prior rinsing of the pockets. Pulse operation was completed with an input of 20 ms and output of 20 ms, average power per pulse of 0.8 W, and pulse energy of 32 mJ. The power density was 1132 W/cm^2. The disinfection procedure used

300 µm diameter inactive quartz tips (E3-7). Each interproximal site was disinfected every 10 s. The fiber was inserted to the full depth of the pockets, for three repetitions in each pocket, with 10-s intervals between [8,21–23]. Disinfection of the pockets and canals was performed twice a month for three months. During all laser operations in the canals and periodontal pockets, the fiber was in continuous motion at a speed of 2 mm/s. After three months, it was decided to fill the canals with gutta-percha cones (Gutta Percha Points, Endostar®, Warszawa, Polska) with an AH Plus sealer (Denstply®, Charlotte, NC, USA) by lateral condensation. All of the laser parameters are shown in Table 3.

Table 3. Laser parameters used during disinfection in periodontal pockets and root canals.

Localization	Fiber	Tip-Spot cm^2	Pulse Width	% on Time	Average/Pulse Power W	Peak Power Dentisity W/cm^2	Average Power Dentisity W/cm^2	Total Energy mJ
Periodontal pocket (10 s)	300 µm	0.0007	input 20 ms/output 20 ms	50%	0.8/1.6	2264	1132	8
Root canal	200 µm	0.0003	input 20 ms/output 20 ms	50%	0.8/1.6	5093	2546	8

The same steps were performed in the control group, but without the diode laser.

After three months, the root canals were filled with gutta-percha cones (Gutta Percha Points, Endostar®, Warszawa, Polad) with AH Plus sealer (Denstply®, Charlotte, NC, USA).

After another three months, periodontal parameters, mobility, and CBCT were performed in both groups. Three-dimensional images were processed into special models to check the change of EPL volume.

Using CBCT, which was taken before and after treatment, STL (stereolithographic) models were made [14,15]. These models depicted the shape of the bone defects (Figures 4 and 5). The effects of the completed treatment were also evaluated.

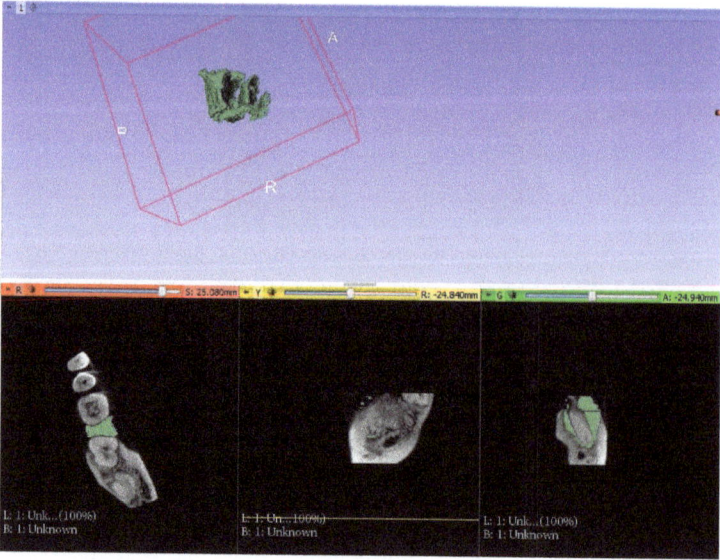

Figure 4. STL model before treatment.

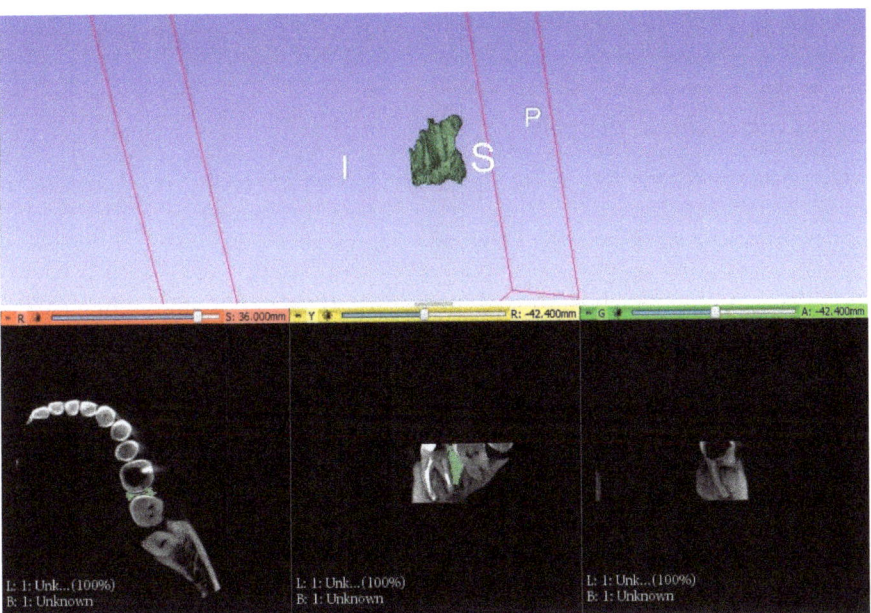

Figure 5. STL model after treatment.

The CT scan was manually segmented in 3D Slicer software to visualize the lesion volume and bone defect regeneration. The files that resulted from the segmentation process were imported into Mini Magics 2.0 software to measure the bone defect volume [24–26].

2.2. Statistical Analysis

The STATA program (Version 15) was used for the statistical analysis. Pocket depth, mobility, and bone volume change were compared between the study and control groups. The significance of differences in the study and control groups at baseline and after treatment (after six months) was determined. Differences were considered statistically significant when the *p*-value was less than 0.05, and a trend at the limit of statistical significance was found when the *p*-value was 0.051–0.099.

3. Results

Baseline Characteristics

Statistical analysis showed a similarity in treatment initiation between the control and study groups. No statistical differences were found in terms of gender, age, and number of teeth (Table 4).

There were no significant statistical differences between the study and control groups in the pre-treatment examination, evaluating the six sites measuring the pocket depth. The groups were similar to each other. Before treatment, the pocket depth in the study group averaged 6.1 mm, and the deepest pocket was 13 mm (Table 5).

Table 4. Study group characteristics.

Sex	Group 1 (G1)	(%)	Group 2 (G2)	(%)	Summary
1 (MALE)	4	66.67%	3	50.00%	7
2 (FEMALE)	2	33.33%	3	50.00%	5
SUMMARY	6		6		12
Chi^2 Pearsons	0.34		df = 1		$p = 0.55819$
Fisher's exact					$p = 1.0000$
R rang Spearman	0.17		t = 0.54233		$p = 0.59947$
NUMBER OF MOLAR	G1		G2		SUMMARY
16	0	0.00%	1	16.67%	1
27	1	16.67%	1	16.67%	2
36	4	66.67%	1	16.67%	5
37	1	16.67%	1	16.67%	2
46	0	0.00%	1	16.67%	1
47	0	0.00%	1	16.67%	1
SUMMARY	6		6		12
Chi^2 Pearson	4.80		df = 5		$p = 0.44078$
R rang Spearman	0.15		t = 0.48224		$p = 0.64001$

Table 5. Periodontal pocket depths (mm) before (B) and after (A) treatment in the study group (G1) around classified teeth.

Localization Patient	Bucc. Mes. B/A (mm)		Bucc. Mid. B/A (mm)		Bucc. Dis. B/A (mm)		Ling. Mes. B/A (mm)		Ling. Mid. B/A (mm)		Ling. Dis. B/A (mm)		AVG. B/A (mm)	AVG. Diff. (mm)
1	5	4	5	3	10	7	4	3	4	3.5	13	10		
2	4	3	6	2	7	3.5	4	3	5	4	5	4		
3	5	4	5	3	4	3	5	3	5	2	5	4	6.1/4.25	1.88
4	8	4.5	6	4.5	6	4	7	6	5	4.5	5	4		
5	11	5	8	8	6	4	8	6	5	4.5	9.5	5		
6	6	5	6	3.5	5	3.5	6	4.5	6	4	5	4		

Bucc.—buccal; Ling.—lingual; Mes.—mesial; Dis.—distal; Mid.—middle; AVG.—average; Diff.—difference.

After treatment, the mean value of pocket depth was 4.22 mm, and the deepest pocket was 10 mm (Table 6). In the control group, the mean PD value was initially 6.03 mm, and the deepest pocket was 12 mm (Table 5). After treatment, the mean PD was 5.80 mm, and the deepest pocket was 10.5 mm (Table 6). The mean difference in PD was 1.88 mm in the treatment group and 0.23 mm in the control group. Significant statistical differences were found by comparing the measurements for all pocket depth sites in the study group before and after treatment. The Student's test and Wilcoxon test were performed. However, significant statistical differences were found in the control group in only one pocket depth site. Due to the significant reduction in pocket depth in the study group, a significant difference was also found in the mean pocket depth values between the study and control groups (Table 7).

Table 6. Periodontal pocket depths before (B) and after (A) treatment in the control group (G2) around classified teeth.

Localization Patient	Bucc. Mes. B/A (mm)		Bucc. Mid. B/A (mm)		Bucc. Dis. B/A (mm)		Ling. Mes. B/A (mm)		Ling. Mid. B/A (mm)		Ling. Dis. B/A (mm)		AVG. B/A (mm)	AVG. Diff. (mm)
1	5	5	6	5.5	7	7	5.5	5	6	6	8	7.5		
2	4	4	4	4	6	5.5	4.5	4.5	5	5	6.5	6.5		
3	5.5	5	8	8	7	6.5	6	5.5	6	5.5	7.5	7	6.03/5.77	0.26
4	5	5	6	6	5.5	5.5	4.5	4.5	5	5	6	5.5		
5	12	10.5	3.5	3.5	6	5.5	7.5	7	4	4	5	5		
6	8	8	6.5	6.5	7	7	7	6.5	5	5	6	5.5		

Bucc.—buccal; Ling.—lingual; Mes.—mesial; Dis.—distal; Mid.—middle; AVG.—average; Diff.—difference.

Table 7. Statistical differences between periodontal pocket depths before (B) and after (A) treatment in the study (G1) and control (G2) groups.

G1	Variable	Average B	SD B±	Variable	Average A	SD A ±	St-p	Wilc. p
1	BUCC. DIS. 1	6.5	2.59	BUCC. DIS. 2	4.25	0.76	0.046	0.028
2	BUCC. MID. 1	6	1.1	BUCC. MID. 2	4	2.12	0.013	0.043
3	BUCC. MES. 1	6.33	2.07	BUCC. MES. 2	4.17	1.44	0.002	0.028
4	LING. DIS. 1	5.67	1.63	LING. DIS. 2	4.08	1.28	0.005	0.028
5	LING. MID. 1	5	0.63	LING. MID. 2	3.67	0.88	0.021	0.028
6	LING. MES. 1	7.25	3.31	LING. MES. 2	5.17	2.40	0.016	0.028
G2	Variable	Average B	SD B±	Variable	Average A	SD A±	St-p	Wilc.p
1	BUCC. DIS. 1	6.58	2.97	BUCC. DIS. 2	6.25	2.49	0.235	
2	BUCC. MID. 1	5.67	1.66	BUCC. MID. 2	5.58	1.66	0.363	
3	BUCC. MES. 1	6.42	0.66	BUCC. MES. 2	6.17	0.75	0.076	0.109
4	LING. DIS. 1	5.83	1.25	LING. DIS. 2	5.92	1.07	0.872	0.500
5	LING. MID. 1	5.17	0.75	LING. MID. 2	4.92	0.8	0.203	
6	LING. MES. 1	6.50	1.1	LING. MES. 2	6.08	1.07	0.042	0.068

Bucc.—buccal; Ling.—lingual; Mes.—mesial; Dis.—distal; Mid.—middle; SD—standard deviation; St-p—Student; Wilc.p—Wilcoxon.

The mean value of Periotest in the study group before treatment was +14.08, and after treatment was +7.87 (Table 8). In the control group, the mean value before treatment was +14.77, and after treatment was +11.42 (Table 9). These results indicate that in the study group, the teeth decreased the mean mobility from 1° to 0°, which means physiological mobility. There was no statistically significant difference between the measurements before treatment in both groups during the statistical analysis. In the second measurement, there was a trend at the limit of statistical significance between the two groups in the Mann−Whitney test (Table 10).

Table 8. Periotest measurements before (B) and after (A) treatment in the study group (G1).

Patient/Periotest Measurements	Before Treatment	After Treatment	Average Mobility B	Max Mobility B	Average Mobility A	Max Mobility A
1	+5	+3				
2	+3.9	+3.6				
3	+20	+10	14.08	22	7.87	12.4
4	+22	+12.4				
5	+15.6	+8.6				
6	+18	+9.6				

Table 9. Periotest measurements before (B) and after (A) treatment in the control group (G2).

Patient/Periotest Measurements	Before Treatment	After Treatment	Average Mobility B	Max Mobility B	Average Mobility A	Max Mobility A
1	+15	+10				
2	+6	+5				
3	+15	+14	14.77	23	11.42	18
4	+23	+18				
5	+13.6	+11				
6	+16	+10.5				

Table 10. Comparison of Periotest measurements in the study (G1) and control (G2) groups after treatment using the Mann−Whitney test.

Group	Amount of Teeth	Average	SD	M-W p
1	6	7.87	3.76	0.092
2	6	11.42	4.34	

M-W—Mann−Whitney test; SD—standard deviation.

As imaged by the STL models, the measurement of bone loss was performed in both groups before treatment, and no statistical difference was found in both groups. After treatment, checking the STL models in the study group, the lesions decreased by an average of 52.5% (Table 11), and in the control group, the lesions decreased by 27% (Table 12).

Table 11. Changes of bone volume (mm^3) in study group (G1) before (B) and after (A) treatment.

Number of Tooth	36	36	37	36	36	27	Average Volume B/A (mm^3)
Volume before treatment (mm^3)	654.4	650	498	300	220	205	
Volume after treatment (mm^3)	309	260	220	140	110	115	421.23/192.3
Change in percent (%)	52.8	60	65	53	50	44	

Table 12. Changes of bone volume (mm^3) in control group (G2) before (B) and after (A) treatment.

Number of Tooth	46	47	36	37	16	27	Average Volume B/A (mm^3)
Volume before treatment (mm^3)	287.3	450	650	700	300	520	
Volume after treatment (mm^3)	207.1	310	400	580	245	360	484.55/350.4
Change in percent (%)	28	31	38	17	18	30.7	

There was a statistically significant difference between the two groups after treatment between the study and control groups' results. This was shown by the Mann–Whitney test and Student's t-test (Table 13).

Table 13. Comparison of bone loss (mm^3) after treatment in the study (G1) and control (G2) groups using Student's t-test and Mann–Whitney test.

Group	Amount of Teeth	Average	SD	ST p	M-W p
1	6	192.3	83.0		
2	6	350.4	133.1	0.033	0.037

M-W—Mann–Whitney test; SD—standard deviation; ST—Student's t-test.

4. Discussion

The use of a diode laser is becoming increasingly popular in periodontal treatment. SRP is often assisted by laser therapy and is very effective for treating periodontal pockets, removing bacteria, and eliminating inflammation [27]. Lasers reduce the depth of periodontal pockets colonized by anaerobic bacteria, responsible for bone loss. This reduces bone lysis and improves tooth retention. The laser-activated irrigation (LAI) method is a straightforward protocol for rinsing and disinfecting the root canal. A fiber optic applicator with a diameter of 200–400 µ is placed approximately 4 mm from the apex. The procedure is performed in successive canals, rinsing is performed only at the end of the applicator, a minimal amount of rinsing solution is used, and the laser energy is directed directly into the dentinal tubules [21,28,29]. Moving the fiber minimizes the risk of thermal complications and allows the radiation to reach the lateral canal surfaces. The combination of diode laser, 5.25% NaOCl solution, and 17% EDTA solution allows for 100% elimination of *Enterococcus faecalis* [15,22]. Diode lasers provide effective removal of bacteria and toxins. In addition to bactericidal and detoxifying effects, diode lasers can accelerate wound healing, facilitate collagen synthesis, accelerate angiogenesis, and enable hemostasis [30,31]. Diode lasers are highly effective at removing the epithelium using a thermal mechanism [23,32]. Most studies on the efficacy of a diode laser as SRP and endodontic treatment support traditional methods with bactericidal effects, soft tissue debridement, and photobiomodulation [27,33–36]. Increasingly, the 940 nm diode laser is being used in dental practice to optimize periodontal and endodontic treatment efficacy. The 940 nm laser has an affinity for hemoglobin and melanin molecules. Its effectiveness is higher due to the fiber's access to furcation areas, deep pockets, and root cavities [30,31]. It should be noted that the combination treatment is actually more effective in decontaminating the periodontal pocket, and it can also be assumed that recolonization is slower. The diode laser removes the mucosal epithelium more precisely than traditional hand tools, while the underlying connective tissue remains intact. According to some authors, lasers do not have apparent therapeutic effects [27]. Another work, a meta-analysis by Quadri [33], indicates that lasers give better therapeutic outcomes. The results of clinical studies on the use of diode lasers as an adjunct to the SRP procedure vary in the choice of parameters, e.g., wavelength, and the power ranges from 0.84, 1, 2, to 2.5 W in CW or pulsed mode. In some studies, the treatments were performed once or several times in a sequence of treatments. For this reason, the results reported in the available clinical studies on periodontal pocket treatment are difficult to compare and analyze [7,8,22,35–37]. In our study, we found a statistically significant reduction in pocket depth in the study group. In addition, diode lasers are beginning to be used as an aid in endodontic treatment for root canal disinfection. This is very helpful for reaching small dentinal canals and removing the smear layer. Diode lasers are available in a broad spectrum of wavelengths from 800 to 1064 nm, differing in their absorption properties. The 940 nm laser has an affinity for hemoglobin and melanin molecules. In addition, the benefits of diode laser and traditional SRP procedures in the treatment algorithm are associated with more significant bactericidal activity, a curettage effect, and a bio stimulatory effect. It should be noted that the combined treatment is actually more effective in decontaminating the pocket, and it can also be assumed that recolonization is slower [38]. Cone-beam computed tomography is also increasingly used in daily practice. The three-dimensional image is more precise than the two-dimensional image, and allows for more than one imaging layer to be visualized. A problem with the use of CBCT can be inexperience, thus incorrectly reading the image related to the artifact and gray tones [39,40]. This observation supports the use of traditional treatment methods with diode laser support in EPP to increase the efficiency of tissue regeneration and thus tooth maintenance, stopping the development of periodontitis. These processes should continue to be observed in 3D images.

This study has some limitations. Unfortunately, because this is a pilot study, the study group was not large. Due to the promising results obtained in our research, we plan to continue this study. Unfortunately, another limitation was the failure to conduct sample size calculations before beginning the study. The authors intend to conduct such a study in the future on a larger group, counting the power of the study and sample size calculations. Three-dimensional assessment of bone atrophy in treated teeth was evaluated in terms of its volume. For a more precise evaluation in further studies, we plan to compare the three-dimensional meshes obtained from STL files, their detailed evaluation in each dimension, and to determine the treatment effect on horizontal and vertical atrophy of alveolar bone [41].

5. Conclusions

The treatment of endo–perio lesions is a significant challenge for modern dentistry. In addition to traditional treatment methods, diode lasers are increasingly being used. The additional use of a 940 nm diode laser with an average power of 0.8 W in pulsed mode reduces periodontal pocket depth. In addition, the use of a diode laser has a significant impact on tooth mobility and reduces bone loss.

Author Contributions: Conceptualization, E.D. and A.H.-R.; methodology, E.D. and A.H.-R.; software, A.J. and G.T.; validation, E.D., G.T., A.H.-R. and A.J.; formal analysis, E.D., G.T., A.H.-R. and A.J.; investigation, E.D., A.H.-R.; resources, E.D., G.T., A.H.-R., A.J., E.G.-T. and J.B.; data curation, E.D., G.T., A.H.-R. and A.J; writing—original draft preparation, E.D., G.T., A.H.-R. and A.J; writing—review and editing, G.T., A.J., E.G.-T. and J.B.; visualization, E.D., G.T. and A.J; supervision, E.D. and

G.T.; project administration, E.D. and G.T. All authors have read and agreed to the published version of the manuscript.

Funding: This research received no external funding.

Institutional Review Board Statement: The study was conducted in accordance with the Declaration of Helsinki, and was approved by the Institutional Review Board Ethics Commission of the Pomeranian Medical University in Szczecin, Poland (No: KB-0012/29/17).

Informed Consent Statement: Informed consent was obtained from all subjects involved in the study.

Data Availability Statement: Data are available upon request.

Conflicts of Interest: The authors declare no conflict of interest.

References

1. Kuligowski, P.; Jaroń, A.; Preuss, O.; Gabrysz-Trybek, E.; Bladowska, J.; Trybek, G. Association between Odontogenic and Maxillary Sinus Conditions: A Retrospective Cone-Beam Computed Tomographic Study. *J. Clin. Med.* **2021**, *10*, 2849. [CrossRef] [PubMed]
2. Herrera, D.; Retamal-Valdes, B.; Alonso, B.; Feres, M. Acute periodontal lesions (periodontal abscesses and necrotizing periodontal diseases) and endo-periodontal lesions. *J. Periodontol.* **2018**, *89* (Suppl S1), S85–S102. [CrossRef]
3. Rotstein, I.; Simon, J.H.S. Diagnosis, prognosis and decision-making in the treatment of combined periodontal-endodontic lesions. *Periodontol. 2000* **2004**, *34*, 165–203. [CrossRef]
4. Gautam, S.; Galgali, S.R.; Sheethal, H.S.; Priya, N.S. Pulpal changes associated with advanced periodontal disease: A histopathological study. *J. Oral Maxillofac. Pathol.* **2017**, *21*, 58–63. [CrossRef]
5. Das, A.C.; Sahoo, S.K.; Parihar, A.S.; Bhardwaj, S.S.; Babaji, P.; Varghese, J.G. Evaluation of role of periodontal pathogens in endodontic periodontal diseases. *J. Fam. Med. Prim. Care* **2020**, *9*, 239–242.
6. Zehnder, M.; Gold, S.I. HasselgrenG.Pathologicinteractions in pulpal and periodontaltissues. *J. Clin. Periodontol.* **2002**, *29*, 663–671. [CrossRef] [PubMed]
7. Fenol, A.; Boban, N.C.; Jayachandran, P.; Shereef, M.; Balakrishnan, B.; Lakshmi, P. A Qualitative Analysis of Periodontal Pathogens in Chronic Periodontitis Patientsafter Nonsurgical Periodontal Therapy with and without Diode Laser Disinfection Using Benzoyl-DL Arginine-2-Naphthylamide Test: A Randomized Clinical Trial. *Contemp. Clin. Dent.* **2018**, *9*, 382–387.
8. Yadwad, K.J.; Veena, H.R.; Patil, S.R.; Shivaprasad, B.M. Diode laser therapy in the management of chronicperiodontitis—A clinico-microbiologicalstudy. *Interv. Med. Appl. Sci.* **2017**, *9*, 191–198.
9. Lopes, E.M.; Passini, M.R.Z.; Kishi, L.T.; Chen, T.; Paster, B.J.; Gomes, B.P.F.A. Interrelationship between the Microbial Communities of the Root Canals and Periodontal Pockets in Combined Endodontic-Periodontal Diseases. *Microorganisms* **2021**, *9*, 1925. [CrossRef]
10. Ossmann, A.; Kranz, S.; Andre, G.; Völpel, A.; Albrecht, V.; Fahr, A.; Sigusch, B.W. Photodynamic killing of Enterococcus faecalis in dentinal tubules using mTHPC incorporated in liposomes and invasomes. *Clin. OralInvestig.* **2015**, *19*, 373–384. [CrossRef]
11. Amid, R.; Kadkhodazadeh, M.; Fekrazad, R.; Hajizadeh, F.; Ghafoori, A. Comparison of the effect of hand instruments, anultrasonicscaler, and anerbium-dopedyttrium aluminium garnet laser on rootsurfaceroughness of teeth with periodontitis: A profilometerstudy. *J. Periodontal Implant Sci.* **2013**, *43*, 101–105. [CrossRef]
12. Moritz, A.; Gutknecht, N.; Doertbudak, O.; Goharkhay, K.; Schoop, U.; Schauer, P.; Sperr, W. Bacterialreduction in periodontalpocketsthroughirradiation with a diode laser: A pilot study. *J. Clin. Laser Med. Surg.* **1997**, *15*, 33–37. [CrossRef] [PubMed]
13. Bartols, A.; Bormann, C.; Werner, L.; Schienle, M.; Walther, W.; Dörfer, C.E. A retrospectiveassessment of differentendodontictreatmentprotocols. *PeerJ* **2020**, *8*, e8495. [CrossRef] [PubMed]
14. Friedman, S.; Mor, C. The success of endodontic therapy—Healing and functionality. *J. Calif. Dent. Assoc.* **2004**, *32*, 493–503.
15. Olivi, G. Laser use in endodontics: Evolution from direct laser irradiation to laser-activatedirrigation. *J. Laser Dent.* **2013**, *21*, 58–71.
16. Pradhan, S.; Karnik, R. Laser endodontictherapyusing 940 nmdiode laser. Temperaturerise on externalrootsurface—Part, I. *Laser* **2010**, *2*, 1–3.
17. Naghavi, N.; Rouhani, A.; Irani, S.; Naghavi, N.; Banihashemi, E. Diode Laser and Calcium Hydroxide for Elimination of Enterococcus Faecalis in Root Canal. *J. Dent. Mater. Tech.* **2014**, *3*, 55–60.
18. Caton, J.G.; Armitage, G.; Berglundh, T.; Chapple, I.; Jepsen, S.; Kornman, K.S.; Mealey, B.L.; Papapanou, P.N.; Sanz, M.; Tonetti, M.S. A new classification scheme for periodontal and peri-implant diseases and conditions—Introduction and key changes from the 1999 classification. *J. Periodontol.* **2018**, *89* (Suppl. S1), S1–S8. [CrossRef]
19. Trybek, G.; Aniko-Włodarczyk, M.; Preuss, O.; Jaroń, A. Assessment of Electrosensitivity of the Pulp of the Mandibular Second Molar after Surgical Removal of an Impacted Mandibular Third Molar. *J. Clin. Med.* **2021**, *10*, 3614. [CrossRef]

20. Shaktawat, A.S.; Verma, K.G.; Goyal, V.; Jasuja, P.; Sukhija, S.J.; Mathur, A. Antimicrobial efficacy of 980 nm diode laser on Enterococcus feacalis in conjunction with various irrigation regimes in infected root canals: An in vitro study. *J. Indian Soc. Pedod. Prev. Dent.* **2018**, *36*, 347–351. [CrossRef]
21. Moura-Netto, C.; Palo, R.M.; Camargo, S.E. Influence of prior 810-nm-diode intracanal laser irradiation on hydrophilic resin-based sealer obturation. *Braz. Oral Res.* **2012**, *26*, 323–329. [CrossRef] [PubMed]
22. Gutknecht, N. Lasers in endodontics. *J. Laser Health Acad.* **2008**, *4*, 1–5.
23. Theodoro, L.H.; Caiado, R.C.; Longo, M.; Novaes, V.C.; Zanini, N.A.; Ervolino, E.; de Almeida, J.M. Effectiveness of the diode laser in the treatment of ligature-induced periodontitis in rats: A histopathological, histometric, and immunohistochemical study. *Lasers Med. Sci.* **2015**, *30*, 1209–1218. [CrossRef]
24. Gutknecht, N.; Franzen, R.; Schippers, M.; Lampert, F. Bactericidal effect of a 980-nm diode laser in the root canal wall dentin of bovine teeth. *J. Clin. Laser Med. Surg.* **2004**, *22*, 9–13. [CrossRef] [PubMed]
25. DiVito, E.; Crippa, R.; Iaria, G. iwsp.: Lasers in endodontics. *Laser* **2012**, *4*, 10–18.
26. Available online: www.slicer.org (accessed on 15 May 2021).
27. Aoki, A.; Mizutani, K.; Takasaki, A.A.; Sasaki, K.M.; Nagai, S.; Schwarz, F.; Yoshida, I.; Eguro, T.; Zeredo, J.L.; Izumi, Y. Current status of clinical laser applications in periodontal therapy. *Gen. Dent.* **2008**, *6*, 674–687.
28. George, R.; Meyers, I.A.; Walsh, L.J. Laser activation of endodonticirrigants with improvedconical laser fibertips for removingsmearlayer in the apical third of the root canal. *J. Endod.* **2008**, *34*, 1524–1527. [CrossRef]
29. Sippus, J.; Gutknecht, N. Deepdisinfection and tubularsmearlayerremoval with Er: YAG usingphoton-inducedphotoacoustic streaming (PIPS) contra laser-activatedirrigation (LAI) technics. *Laser Dent. Sci.* **2019**, *3*, 37–42. [CrossRef]
30. Crispino, A.; Figliuzzi, M.M.; Iovane, C.; Del Giudice, T.; Lomanno, S.; Pacifico, D.; Fortunato, L.; Del Giudice, R. Effectiveness of a diode laser in addition to non-surgicalperiodontaltherapy: Study of intervention. *Ann. Stomatol.* **2015**, *6*, 15–20.
31. Sgolastra, F.; Severino, M.; Gatto, R.; Monaco, A. Effectiveness of diode laser as adjunctive therapy to scaling root planning in the treatment of chronic periodontitis: A meta-analysis. *Lasers Med. Sci.* **2013**, *28*, 1393–1402. [CrossRef]
32. Romanos, G.E.; Henze, M.; Banihashemi, S.; Parsanejad, H.R.; Winckler, J.; Nentwig, G.H. Removal of epithelium in periodontalpocketsfollowing diode (980 nm) laser application in the animal model: An in vitro study. *Photomed. Laser Surg.* **2004**, *22*, 177–183. [CrossRef]
33. Zare, D.; Haerian, A.; Molla, R.; Vaziri, F. Evaluation of the effects of diode (980 nm) laser on gingival inflammation after nonsurgical periodontal therapy. *J. Lasers Med. Sci.* **2014**, *5*, 27–31.
34. Qadri, T.; Javed, F.; Johannsen, G.; Gustafsson, A. Role of diode lasers (800–980 nm) as adjuncts to scaling and root planing in the treatment of chronic periodontitis: A systematic review. *Photomed. Laser Surg.* **2015**, *33*, 568–575. [CrossRef] [PubMed]
35. Dukić, W.; Bago, I.; Aurer, A.; Roguljić, M. Clinical effectiveness of diode laser therapy as an adjunct to non-surgical periodontal treatment: A randomized clinical study. *J. Periodontol.* **2013**, *84*, 1111–1117. [CrossRef] [PubMed]
36. Kamma, J.J.; Vasdekis, V.G.; Romanos, G.E. The effect of diode laser (980 nm) treatment on aggressive periodontitis: Evaluation of microbial and clinical parameters. *Photomed. Laser Surg.* **2009**, *27*, 11–19. [CrossRef]
37. Caruso, U.; Nastri, L.; Piccolomini, R.; d'Ercole, S.; Mazza, C.; Guida, L. Use of diode laser 980 nm as adjunctivetherapy in the treatment of chronicperiodontitis. A randomizedcontrolledclinicaltrial. *New Microbiol.* **2008**, *31*, 513–518. [PubMed]
38. Saydjari, Y.; Kuypers, T.; Gutknecht, N. Laser Application in Dentistry: Irradiation Effects of Nd:YAG 1064 nm and Diode 810 nm and 980 nm in Infected Root Canals-A Literature Overview. *Photomed. Laser Surg.* **2016**, *34*, 336–344. [CrossRef] [PubMed]
39. Alshehri, M.A.; Alamri, H.M.; Alshalhoob, M.A. Zastosowanie CBCT w praktyce stomatologicznej–Systematyczny przegląd piśmiennictwa. *Dent. Trib. Pol. Ed.* **2012**, *10*, 1–5.
40. Jaroń, A.; Gabrycz-Trybek, E.; Bladowska, J.; Trybek, G. Correlation of Panoramic Radiography, Cone-Beam Computed Tomography, and Three-Dimensional Printing in the Assessment of the Spatial Location of Impacted Mandibular Third Molars. *J. Clin. Med.* **2021**, *10*, 4189. [CrossRef]
41. Metlerski, M.; Grocholewicz, K.; Jaroń, A.; Lipski, M.; Trybek, G. Comparison of Presurgical Dental Models Manufactured with Two Different Three-Dimensional Printing Techniques. *J. Healthc. Eng.* **2020**, 8893338. [CrossRef]

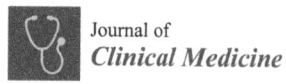

Article

Association between Oral Health Status and Relative Handgrip Strength in 11,337 Korean

Ji-Eun Kim [1], Na-Yeong Kim [1], Choong-Ho Choi [1,2] and Ki-Ho Chung [1,2,*]

[1] Department of Preventive and Public Health Dentistry, Chonnam National University School of Dentistry, Gwangju 61186, Korea; angel761@chonnam.ac.kr (J.-E.K.); 216622@chonnam.ac.kr (N.-Y.K.); hochoi@chonnam.ac.kr (C.-H.C.)
[2] Dental Science Research Institute, Chonnam National University, Gwangju 61186, Korea
* Correspondence: prevention@chonnam.ac.kr; Tel.: +82-62-530-5858

Abstract: Grip strength is a simple indicator of physical strength and is closely associated with systemic health. Conversely, oral health has also been reported to have an important association with systemic health. The present study aimed to assess the effect of oral health status on relative handgrip strength. The data pertaining to 11,337 participants were obtained by means of the seventh Korea National Health and Nutrition Survey (2016 to 2018). Oral health status was evaluated on the basis of the presence of periodontitis and number of remaining teeth (PT, present teeth). Relative handgrip strength was evaluated by means of a digital dynamometer and the value pertaining to the lower 25% of measurements was used as the quartile by gender. The association between oral health status and relative handgrip strength was evaluated by means of multiple regression analysis and multiple logistic regression analysis with covariate correction. Analysis of the crude model revealed a significant association in the group of patients with periodontal disease (odds ratio = 1.69, 95% confidence interval: 1.51–1.89). However, analysis with adjusted covariates revealed that the association was not statistically significant. Moreover, statistical analysis after adjustment for covariates revealed a consistent correlation between PT and relative handgrip strength as categorical and continuous variables. Hence, the present study observed a significant association between oral health status and relative handgrip strength among the Korean adult population.

Keywords: KNHANES; periodontitis; present teeth; relative handgrip strength

Citation: Kim, J.-E.; Kim, N.-Y.; Choi, C.-H.; Chung, K.-H. Association between Oral Health Status and Relative Handgrip Strength in 11,337 Korean. *J. Clin. Med.* **2021**, *10*, 5425. https://doi.org/10.3390/jcm10225425

Academic Editors: Susanne Schulz and Gianrico Spagnuolo

Received: 6 October 2021
Accepted: 18 November 2021
Published: 20 November 2021

Publisher's Note: MDPI stays neutral with regard to jurisdictional claims in published maps and institutional affiliations.

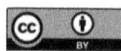

Copyright: © 2021 by the authors. Licensee MDPI, Basel, Switzerland. This article is an open access article distributed under the terms and conditions of the Creative Commons Attribution (CC BY) license (https://creativecommons.org/licenses/by/4.0/).

1. Introduction

Advancements in the field of science have led to an increase in human lifespan, and emphasis on the quality of life is important for the pursuit of a healthy life. Correspondingly, physical function plays an important role in the quality of life [1] and handgrip strength is widely used to conveniently evaluate physical functions [2,3]. Handgrip strength is divided into two categories: absolute handgrip strength and relative handgrip strength. The latter is computed by dividing absolute handgrip strength by the individual's body mass index (BMI). Relative handgrip strength has been recommended to address the disturbance in muscle strength attributable to body mass as well as the health risks associated with weight gain and muscle weakness [4,5]. Moreover, recent studies have demonstrated the association between relative handgrip strength and systemic diseases. A study by Lawman et al. [6] reported the association between handgrip strength and biomarkers of cardiovascular disease using the data obtained from the National Health and Nutrition Examination Survey (2011–2012). Another study by Yi et al. [7] reported the association between handgrip strength and metabolic syndrome using the data obtained from the Korea National Health and Nutrition Survey (KNHANES) (2014–2015). Furthermore, a prospective cohort study of Japanese subjects by Manda et al. [8] reported that handgrip strength could be used to predict the incidence of prediabetes.

Similarly, oral health is closely related not only to an individual's physical fitness [9], but also to systemic diseases. Periodontal disease, one of the most common oral diseases, is a chronic inflammatory disease that can affect humans throughout life [10]. A previous study by Falcao and Bullón [11] observed that the effects of periodontal disease were not limited to the oral cavity alone. The aforementioned study observed associations between periodontal disease and several systemic health conditions and diseases, including cardiovascular disease, diabetes, rheumatoid arthritis, and respiratory disease. Previous studies have reported that the overall nutritional status and quality of life improved with the improvement in chewing ability, which represents the oral health status [12]. In addition, other studies have reported that comfortable chewing warrants the functionality of more than 20 remaining teeth (PT, present teeth) [13]. Moreover, the association between dental occlusion and physical fitness has been reported by Yamaga et al. [14], and another study by Kamdem et al. [15] reported that PT and masticatory function were associated with diabetes. In accordance with the results reported by the aforementioned studies, oral health is very important and periodontal disease and PT are representative indicators of the oral health status [16,17].

In literature, only a limited number of studies have reported the association between handgrip strength and oral health status. The relationship between absolute handgrip strength and PT in the Korean population was reported by Shin [18]. Furthermore, the same association was reported by a similar study with a smaller sample size [16] and another study that performed the statistical analysis after adjustment for a few covariates [19]. However, few studies have confirmed the association between periodontal disease and PT (indicators of oral health status) and the relative handgrip strength (indicator of healthy functioning of the body).

Hence, the purpose of the current study was to assess the association between oral health and relative handgrip strength in adults $\geq$19 years of age. To the best of our knowledge, this is the first domestic study that analyzed the relationship between periodontal disease and PT and relative handgrip strength after adjusting for various covariates in a representative sample of the general population.

2. Materials and Methods

2.1. Study Population

The current study obtained data pertaining to the time period from 2016 to 2018 by means of the seventh KNHANES. Among a total of 24,269 prospective subjects (8150, 8127, and 7992 participants pertaining to the years 2016, 2018, and 2018, respectively), the present study excluded 12,932 subjects who did not undergo oral and handgrip strength evaluations or had missing covariates. The final sample included 11,337 adult participants $\geq$19 years of age (Figure 1).

The current study was approved by the Research Ethics Review Committee of the Korea Centers for Disease Control and Prevention (2018-01-03-P-A). Written informed consent was obtained from all the subjects prior to the survey.

2.2. Handgrip Strength

Handgrip strength was evaluated by means of a digital dynamometer (Digital grip strength dynamometer, T.K.K 5401, Takei Kikai Kogyo Co., Ltd., Tokyo, Japan). In accordance with the guidelines for evaluation [20], the measurement was performed in a standing position and both hands were crossed three times.

For evaluation, the current study employed relative handgrip strength that was computed by dividing the respective maximum handgrip strength of the dominant hand by the corresponding BMI and expressed as kg_{BMI}.

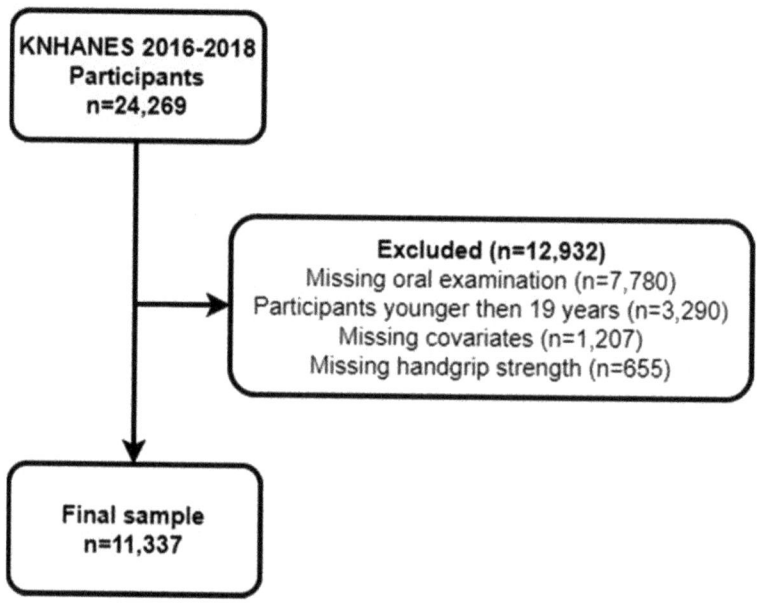

Figure 1. Flow chart of the selection process.

The reference value used for the categorization of low relative handgrip strength was based on the results reported by previous research [21]. The value pertaining to the lower 25% of measurements was used as the quartile by gender.

2.3. Oral Examination

The oral examinations were performed, and results were documented by a trained dentist, according to the guidelines of KNHANES [22]. Periodontitis was diagnosed using the Community Periodontal Index (CPI) [23], which was determined using the WHO CPI probe. The scores were marked as follows: 0: healthy periodontal tissue; 1: periodontal tissue with bleeding on probing; 2: periodontal tissue with calculus formation; 3: periodontal tissue with pocket depth (PD) of 4.0–5.0 mm; and 4: periodontal tissue with PD > 5 mm. It was divided into two categories: Yes, for codes ≥ 3 (codes 3 and 4) and no, for codes below 3 (codes 0, 1, and 2). The PT was calculated by adding up all the remaining teeth (maximum of 28 teeth), excluding the third molars. Subsequently, the subjects were classified into three groups on the basis of the same: 0–9 teeth, 10–19 teeth, and 20–28 teeth.

2.4. Covariates

The general characteristics pertaining to the subjects included gender, age, educational level, and household income. The variables concerning general health behaviors included smoking (nonsmoker, former smoker, current smoker), alcohol consumption (nondrinker, alcohol consumption once per month, alcohol consumption $\geq$ twice per month), exercise (moderate-intensity physical activity for a minimum duration of 2 h 30 min, or high-intensity physical activity for a minimum duration of 1 h 15 min, or a combination of moderate- and high-intensity physical activity per week), BMI (weight/height^2), and presence of comorbidities (number of diagnosed cases of chronic diseases such as hypertension, diabetes, stroke, myocardial infarction or angina pectoris, arthritis, and cancer). Variables pertaining to oral health behaviors included the frequency of brushing teeth per day, use of oral hygiene products (use of dental floss, interdental toothbrush, mouth rinse, electric toothbrush, and other products), chewing problems, speaking problems, dental visits during the past year, and self-perceived oral health status.

2.5. Statistical Analyses

KNHANES is a complex sample survey and data analysis was performed in consideration of the stratification variable, cluster variable, and weight, owing to the complex sample design. The subjects were categorized on the basis of their respective relative handgrip strength. The sociodemographic characteristics of the participants were analyzed using the t-test or chi-square test. The present study employed multiple regression analysis to confirm the association between relative handgrip strength as a continuous variable and PT as a continuous and categorical variable. Moreover, the association between lower relative handgrip strength and PT or categorical periodontal disease as continuous and categorical variables among the subjects with handgrip strength below the lower quartile was assessed using multiple logistic regression analysis. Adjustment for the variables pertaining to general characteristics, general health behaviors, and oral health behaviors was performed to determine the odds ratio (OR) of oral health status and relative handgrip strength. The statistical significance was set at $p < 0.05$. In the present study, SAS 9.4 program (SAS Institute, Cary, NC, USA) was used to perform the statistical analysis.

3. Results

3.1. General Characteristics of the Participants

The general characteristics of the subjects are presented in Table 1. The present study involved a total of 11,337 participants with an average age of 49.81 ± 0.31 years. The group with low relative handgrip strength, which included the subjects with handgrip strength below the lower quartile, had greater age, lower educational levels, lower household income, no exercise routine, obesity, greater number of comorbidities, fewer PT, and a higher proportion of patients with periodontal disease, compared to the group with high relative handgrip strength, which included the subjects with handgrip strength above the lower quartile (top 75%).

Table 1. General characteristics of the subjects.

Variables	Total (n = 11,337)	High Relative Handgrip Strength (n = 8846)	Low Relative Handgrip Strength (n = 2491)	p-Value
General characteristics				
Age	49.81 ± 0.31	47.05 ± 0.28	59.67 ± 0.52	<0.0001 [a]
19–39	3399 (29.98)	3008 (34.00)	391 (15.70)	<0.0001
40–64	5426 (47.86)	4570 (51.66)	856 (34.36)	
≥65	2512 (22.16)	1268 (14.33)	1244 (49.94)	
Educational level				
Primary	2036 (17.96)	1046 (11.82)	990 (39.74)	<0.0001
Middle	1083 (9.55)	778 (8.79)	305 (12.24)	
High	3742 (33.01)	3121 (35.28)	621 (24.93)	
College +	4476 (39.48)	3901 (44.10)	575 (23.08)	
Household income				
Lowest quartile	1964 (17.32)	1125 (12.72)	839 (33.68)	<0.0001
Lower middle quartile	2740 (24.17)	2084 (23.56)	656 (26.33)	
Upper middle quartile	3241 (28.59)	2690 (30.41)	551 (22.12)	
Highest quartile	3392 (29.92)	2947 (33.31)	445 (17.86)	

Table 1. Cont.

Variables	Total (n = 11,337)	High Relative Handgrip Strength (n = 8846)	Low Relative Handgrip Strength (n = 2491)	p-Value
		General health behaviors		
Smoking				
Nonsmoker	6912 (60.97)	5266 (59.53)	1646 (66.08)	<0.0001
Former smoker	2395 (21.13)	1853 (20.95)	542 (21.76)	
Current smoker	2030 (17.91)	1727 (19.52)	303 (12.16)	
Alcohol consumption				
Nondrinker	2979 (26.28)	1946 (22.00)	1033 (41.47)	<0.0001
Once per month	3233 (28.52)	2572 (29.08)	661 (26.54)	
≥Twice per month	5125 (45.21)	4328 (48.93)	797 (32.00)	
Exercise				
No	6377 (56.25)	4720 (53.36)	1657 (66.52)	<0.0001
Yes	4960 (43.75)	4126 (46.64)	834 (33.48)	
BMI (kg/m²)				
<18.5	426 (3.76)	399 (4.51)	27 (1.08)	<0.0001
18.5 to <25	6989 (61.65)	5974 (67.53)	1015 (40.75)	
≥25	3922 (34.59)	2473 (27.96)	1449 (58.17)	
Comorbidity				
0	7431 (65.55)	6421 (72.59)	1010 (40.55)	<0.0001
1	2402 (21.19)	1686 (19.06)	716 (28.74)	
≥2	1504 (13.27)	739 (8.35)	765 (30.71)	
		Oral health behaviors		
Frequency of brushing teeth per day				
≤1	1086 (9.58)	672 (7.60)	414 (16.62)	<0.0001
2	4365 (38.50)	3321 (37.54)	1044 (41.91)	
≥3	5886 (51.92)	4853 (54.86)	1033 (41.47)	
Use of oral hygiene products				
0	5156 (45.48)	3697 (41.79)	1459 (58.57)	<0.0001
1	3975 (35.06)	3250 (36.74)	725 (29.10)	
≥2	2206 (19.46)	1899 (21.47)	307 (12.32)	
Chewing problem				
Comfortable	8940 (78.86)	7267 (82.15)	1673 (67.16)	<0.0001
Uncomfortable	2397 (21.14)	1579 (17.85)	818 (32.84)	
Speaking problem				
Comfortable	10,533 (92.91)	8405 (95.01)	2128 (85.43)	<0.0001
Uncomfortable	804 (7.09)	441 (4.99)	363 (14.57)	
Dental visits during the past year				
No	7165 (63.20)	5395 (60.99)	1770 (71.06)	<0.0001
Yes	4172 (36.80)	3451 (39.01)	721 (28.94)	
Self-perceived oral health status				
Good	7033 (62.04)	5704 (64.48)	1329 (53.35)	<0.0001
Poor	4304 (37.96)	3142 (35.52)	1162 (46.65)	

Table 1. Cont.

Variables	Total (n = 11,337)	High Relative Handgrip Strength (n = 8846)	Low Relative Handgrip Strength (n = 2491)	p-Value
		Oral health status		
PT	24.84 ± 0.08	25.51 ± 0.07	22.41 ± 0.19	<0.0001 [a]
0–9	437 (3.85)	212 (2.40)	225 (9.03)	<0.0001
10–19	940 (8.29)	525 (5.93)	415 (16.66)	
20–28	9960 (87.85)	8109 (91.67)	1851 (74.31)	
Periodontitis				
No	7849 (69.23)	6338 (71.65)	1511 (60.66)	<0.0001
Yes	3488 (30.77)	2508 (28.35)	980 (39.34)	
Relative handgrip strength (kg_{BMI})	1.29 ± 0.01	1.40 ± 0.00	0.88 ± 0.01	<0.0001 [a]

All values are presented as the mean ± standard error or frequency (n, weighted %). p-values were obtained by means of the chi-square test. [a] p-value was obtained by means of the t-test.

3.2. Association between PT and Relative Handgrip Strength as a Continuous Variable

The effects of PT as a continuous and categorical variable on relative handgrip strength as a continuous variable are shown in Table 2. Analysis of the crude model with PT as a continuous variable revealed that increase in PT by one tooth effected significant corresponding increase in the relative handgrip strength by 0.014 kg_{BMI} ($p < 0.0001$). Furthermore, analysis of the model adjusted for covariates revealed that despite the decrease in regression coefficient, increase in PT by one tooth effected significant corresponding increase in the relative handgrip strength by 0.003 kg_{BMI} ($p < 0.0001$).

Table 2. Multivariate regression analysis for PT and relative handgrip strength.

Independent Variables	Crude		Adjusted	
	β	p-Value	β	p-Value
PT (continuous)	0.014	<0.0001	0.003	<0.0001
PT (categorical)				
0~9	−0.183	<0.0001	−0.040	0.0056
10~19	−0.179	<0.0001	−0.038	0.0006
20~28		Ref.		

β: regression coefficient. p-values were obtained by means of logistic regression analysis. Adjusted for general characteristics (gender, age, educational level, and household income), general health behaviors (smoking, alcohol consumption, exercise, and comorbidity), oral health behaviors (frequency of brushing teeth per day, use of oral hygiene products, chewing problem, speaking problem, dental visits during the past year, and self-perceived oral health status), and oral health status (periodontitis).

Regarding the effects of PT as a categorical variable, analysis of the crude model revealed significantly lower relative handgrip strength in the group with fewer teeth than in the group with 20–28 teeth (10–19: −0.179, $p < 0.0001$; 0–9: −0.183, $p < 0.0001$). Moreover, analysis of the model adjusted for covariates revealed a negative correlation (10–19: −0.038, $p = 0.0006$; 0–9: −0.040, $p = 0.0056$).

3.3. Association between Oral Health Status and Low Relative Handgrip Strength among the Subjects with Handgrip Strength Below the Lower Quartile (Lower 25%)

The results of multivariate logistic regression analysis of the effects of oral health status on the risk of low relative handgrip strength among the subjects with handgrip strength below the lower quartile (lower 25%) are shown in Table 3. Analysis of the crude model revealed a significant association between periodontal disease and the risk of lower relative handgrip strength (OR = 1.69, 95% confidence interval [CI]: 1.51–1.89). However, analysis of the model adjusted for covariates did not reveal the same association.

Table 3. Multivariate logistic regression analysis of oral health status and relative handgrip strength.

Independent Variables	Crude OR (95% CI)	Adjusted OR (95% CI)
Periodontitis		
Yes	1.69 (1.51–1.89)	1.02 (0.89–1.16)
No	1	1
PT (continuous)	0.91 (0.90–0.92)	0.97 (0.96–0.99)
PT (categorical)		
0~9	4.33 (3.45–5.44)	1.29 (1.00–1.67)
10~19	3.41 (2.83–4.10)	1.34 (1.10–1.62)
20 ~ 28	1	1

OR: odds ratio, 95% CI: 95% confidence interval. Adjusted for general characteristics (gender, age, educational level, and household income), general health behaviors (smoking, alcohol consumption, exercise, and comorbidity), oral health behaviors (frequency of brushing teeth per day, use of oral hygiene products, chewing problem, speaking problem, dental visits during the past year, and self-perceived oral health status), and oral health status (periodontitis or PT).

Analysis of the crude model with PT as a continuous variable revealed that increase in PT by one tooth effected a corresponding decrease in the OR regarding the risk of low handgrip strength by 0.91 times. Moreover, analysis of the model adjusted for covariates revealed an association between the variables with an OR of 0.97 (CI: 0.96–0.99). Analysis of the model adjusted for covariates with PT as a categorical variable revealed a significant association between PT and the risk of lower relative grip strength among the subjects with PT of 10–19 (OR = 1.34, CI: 1.10–1.62) and 0–9 (OR = 1.29 CI: 1.00–1.67), compared to those with PT of 20–28 (ref).

4. Discussion

The current study confirmed the association between oral health status and relative handgrip strength through analysis of national representative data after adjusting for several covariates. Moreover, no previous Korean study has analyzed the association between oral health status, evaluated by means of PT and the presence/absence of periodontal disease, and relative handgrip strength after adjusting for several covariates. The current results indicate a significant association between oral health status and relative handgrip strength in the Korean adult population.

Handgrip strength is a representative measurement item that can be used to evaluate internal strength. In addition, recent studies have reported a correlation between grip strength and mobility, chronic disease morbidity, disability in old age, and total mortality [24,25]. In the current study, handgrip strength was measured in a standing position. This method of evaluation can assess muscle strength of the core and lower body [6]. Hence, the results can reflect the overall body strength. Moreover, disturbance in muscle strength according to the respective body mass could be excluded through the utilization of relative handgrip strength. Several previous studies have employed relative handgrip strength for evaluations. A study by Alley et al. [3] reported that relative handgrip strength was better suited for the evaluation of weakness than absolute handgrip strength. Moreover, a study by Lawman et al. [6] reported that relative handgrip strength is a useful tool that can be employed in the public health evaluation of muscle mass. Accordingly, the present study endeavored to reflect the exact status of physical fitness of the subjects using relative handgrip strength.

The present regression model, adjusted for covariates, revealed a correlation between PT and relative handgrip strength and showed that the effect of PT was continuous and categorical on relative handgrip strength. With regard to the association between PT as a continuous variable and relative handgrip strength, the current results established that relative handgrip strength significantly increased with the corresponding increase in PT in all models. Among the three categories of subjects with PT of 0–9, 10–19, and 20–28, the groups with fewer teeth displayed a tendency to have lower relative handgrip strength than the group with a higher number of teeth. A study by Shin [18] stated that assessment of the relationship between number of teeth and absolute handgrip strength in Korean adults revealed a significant association between greater number of remaining teeth and greater absolute handgrip strength. The aforementioned results imply that the current results are concurrent with the results of previous studies.

Conversely, with reference to the logistic regression model that assessed the relative handgrip strength as a categorical variable and evaluated the effect of periodontal disease on relative handgrip strength, the association between periodontal disease and relative handgrip strength was confirmed through analysis of the crude model. A previous study by Eremenko et al. [19] reported a relationship between clinical adhesion loss and relative handgrip strength and the results were concurrent with the current results. Nonetheless, analysis of the model adjusted for covariates did not reveal any significant results. Furthermore, a previous systematic review [11] has reported that periodontal disease is associated with several other factors. Consequently, other covariates pertaining to the subjects might have a greater influence on the results of the present study.

The current study observed an association between PT and relative handgrip strength, regardless of the status of continuous or categorical variable, as PT was a categorical variable in the crude model and the model adjusted for covariates. A study of Chinese individuals below the age of 60 years by Zhou et al. [26] employed the average number of missing teeth as the cut-off value for tooth loss and reported an association between tooth loss and relative handgrip strength. The abovementioned results were similar to the current results. The present study was based on two previous studies: a study by Elias et al. [13], which considered the presence of a minimum of 20 teeth as the criterion for masticatory function, and a study by Peres et al. [27], which considered the presence of 10 or fewer natural teeth as the criterion for masticatory function. Thus, the authors are of the opinion that better reflection of oral health status of the subjects was achieved through the categorization of subjects on the basis of PT into three classes, i.e., 0–9, 10–19, and 20–28. In addition, the current results confirm the association between PT and relative handgrip strength as categorical and continuous variables, respectively [16,18,19,26,28,29]. Analysis of the model adjusted for covariates with PT as a categorical variable revealed that the OR pertaining to the group with PT of 0–9 was slightly lower than that of the group with PT of 10–19. The authors are of the opinion that the current analysis involved subjects with a wide range of age and gender differences, such as menopause-related differences (occurrence or absence) in women, which might have influenced the outcomes, despite the adjustments for age and gender. The current study tried to understand the general trends in relation to oral health and relative handgrip strength in the Korean adult population. The scenario warrants further research to confirm the association between variables by categorizing the subjects on the basis of age and gender.

The putative mechanisms concerning the association between oral health and handgrip strength are diverse and remain ambiguous. Recently, a systematic review reported that oral health status and physical fitness and had a bidirectional relationship [9]. A study by Yamaguchi et al. [30] reported a strong association between tooth loss and thickness of the muscle mass with reference to the main masticatory muscle. Furthermore, a study of Japanese population by Yoshino et al. [31] reported that masticatory force was associated with handgrip strength. Additionally, it has been reported that the masticatory discomfort attributable to tooth loss affects the nutritional status, owing to improper dietary habits [12]. In addition, previous studies have reported that the consumption of branched-chain amino acids is associated with handgrip strength [32]. Hence, the direct or indirect effect of tooth loss on physical strength can explain this association with handgrip strength to a certain extent.

According to an alternative putative mechanism, periodontal disease and handgrip strength share common risk factors, such as systemic inflammatory conditions. A previous study by Visser et al. [33] reported that muscle mass and muscle strength in the elderly were related to the concentrations of interleukin-6 and tumor necrosis factor-α. High levels of the aforementioned inflammatory factors were observed in patients with periodontal disease [11].

The present study has certain limitations. The current study was cross-sectional in nature and a causal relationship between the factors could not be determined. Confirmation of the causal relationship between the two factors warrants a longitudinal study.

Nevertheless, the results of the present study correspond to the entire national population, as the oral health status and relative handgrip strength of 11,337 adults was assessed using large-scale data. Moreover, to the best of our knowledge, this is the first study to confirm the association between relative handgrip strength, which denotes physical strength, and oral health status, which was assessed by way of PT and periodontal disease, through analyses after adjustment for the same covariate.

5. Conclusions

The current study verified a significant association between oral health status, evaluated using periodontal disease and PT, and handgrip strength, which represents physical strength, among Korean adults. Promotion and maintenance of oral health is necessary to preserve physical strength, which is essential for a healthy life.

Author Contributions: Conceptualization, N.-Y.K., K.-H.C. and C.-H.C.; writing—original draft preparation, J.-E.K. and K.-H.C. All authors contributed extensively to the work presented in this paper. All authors have read and agreed to the published version of the manuscript.

Funding: This study was financially supported by the Chonnam National University (Grant number: 2021–2155).

Institutional Review Board Statement: The institutional review board (IRB) at the Korea Center for Disease Control and Prevention approved the seventh KNHANES, 2016–2018 (2018-01-03-P-A). All procedures were conducted according to the ethical principles of the Declaration of Helsinki.

Informed Consent Statement: Informed consent was obtained from all subjects involved in the study.

Data Availability Statement: The dataset analyzed for this study can be found at https://knhanes.kdca.go.kr/knhanes/eng/index.do (accessed on 18 November 2021).

Conflicts of Interest: The authors declare no conflict of interest.

References

1. Rizzoli, R.; Reginster, J.-Y.; Arnal, J.-F.; Bautmans, I.; Beaudart, C.; Bischoff-Ferrari, H.; Biver, E.; Boonen, S.; Brandi, M.-L.; Chines, A. Quality of life in sarcopenia and frailty. *Calcif. Tissue Int.* **2013**, *93*, 101–120. [CrossRef]
2. Roberts, H.C.; Denison, H.J.; Martin, H.J.; Patel, H.P.; Syddall, H.; Cooper, C.; Sayer, A.A. A review of the measurement of grip strength in clinical and epidemiological studies: Towards a standardised approach. *Age Ageing* **2011**, *40*, 423–429. [CrossRef] [PubMed]
3. Alley, D.E.; Shardell, M.D.; Peters, K.W.; McLean, R.R.; Dam, T.-T.L.; Kenny, A.M.; Fragala, M.S.; Harris, T.B.; Kiel, D.P.; Guralnik, J.M. Grip strength cutpoints for the identification of clinically relevant weakness. *J. Gerontol. Ser. A Biomed. Sci. Med. Sci.* **2014**, *69*, 559–566. [CrossRef] [PubMed]
4. Choquette, S.; Bouchard, D.; Doyon, C.; Sénéchal, M.; Brochu, M.; Dionne, I.J. Relative strength as a determinant of mobility in elders 67–84 years of age. a nuage study: Nutrition as a determinant of successful aging. *J. Nutr. Health Aging* **2010**, *14*, 190–195. [CrossRef]
5. Studenski, S.A.; Peters, K.W.; Alley, D.E.; Cawthon, P.M.; McLean, R.R.; Harris, T.B.; Ferrucci, L.; Guralnik, J.M.; Fragala, M.S.; Kenny, A.M. The FNIH sarcopenia project: Rationale, study description, conference recommendations, and final estimates. *J. Gerontol. Ser. A Biomed. Sci. Med. Sci.* **2014**, *69*, 547–558. [CrossRef] [PubMed]
6. Lawman, H.G.; Troiano, R.P.; Perna, F.M.; Wang, C.-Y.; Fryar, C.D.; Ogden, C.L. Associations of relative handgrip strength and cardiovascular disease biomarkers in US adults, 2011–2012. *Am. J. Prev. Med.* **2016**, *50*, 677–683. [CrossRef] [PubMed]
7. Yi, D.; Khang, A.R.; Lee, H.W.; Son, S.M.; Kang, Y.H. Relative handgrip strength as a marker of metabolic syndrome: The Korea National Health and Nutrition Examination Survey (KNHANES) VI (2014–2015). *Diabetes Metab. Syndr. Obes. Targets Ther.* **2018**, *11*, 227. [CrossRef]
8. Manda, C.M.; Hokimoto, T.; Okura, T.; Isoda, H.; Shimano, H.; Wagatsuma, Y. Handgrip strength predicts new prediabetes cases among adults: A prospective cohort study. *Prev. Med. Rep.* **2020**, *17*, 101056. [CrossRef]

9. Bramantoro, T.; Hariyani, N.; Setyowati, D.; Purwanto, B.; Zulfiana, A.A.; Irmalia, W.R. The impact of oral health on physical fitness: A systematic review. *Heliyon* **2020**, *6*, e03774. [CrossRef]
10. Li, P.; He, L.; Sha, Y.q.; Luan, Q.x. Relationship of metabolic syndrome to chronic periodontitis. *J. Periodontol.* **2009**, *80*, 541–549. [CrossRef]
11. Falcao, A.; Bullón, P. A review of the influence of periodontal treatment in systemic diseases. *Periodontology 2000* **2019**, *79*, 117–128. [CrossRef] [PubMed]
12. Lee, I.C.; Yang, Y.H.; Ho, P.S.; Lee, I.C. Chewing ability, nutritional status and quality of life. *J. Oral Rehabil.* **2014**, *41*, 79–86. [CrossRef] [PubMed]
13. Elias, A.; Sheiham, A. The relationship between satisfaction with mouth and number and position of teeth. *J. Oral Rehabil.* **1998**, *25*, 649–661. [CrossRef] [PubMed]
14. Yamaga, T.; Yoshihara, A.; Ando, Y.; Yoshitake, Y.; Kimura, Y.; Shimada, M.; Nishimuta, M.; Miyazaki, H. Relationship between dental occlusion and physical fitness in an elderly population. *J. Gerontol. Ser. A Biol. Sci. Med. Sci.* **2002**, *57*, M616–M620. [CrossRef] [PubMed]
15. Kamdem, B.; Seematter-Bagnoud, L.; Botrugno, F.; Santos-Eggimann, B. Relationship between oral health and Fried's frailty criteria in community-dwelling older persons. *BMC Geriatr.* **2017**, *17*, 174. [CrossRef]
16. Hämäläinen, P.; Rantanen, T.; Keskinen, M.; Meurman, J.H. Oral health status and change in handgrip strength over a 5-year period in 80-year-old people. *Gerodontology* **2004**, *21*, 155–160. [CrossRef] [PubMed]
17. Lamster, I.B.; Asadourian, L.; Del Carmen, T.; Friedman, P.K. The aging mouth: Differentiating normal aging from disease. *Periodontology 2000* **2016**, *72*, 96–107. [CrossRef]
18. Shin, H.S. Handgrip strength and the number of teeth among Korean population. *J. Periodontol.* **2019**, *90*, 90–97. [CrossRef]
19. Eremenko, M.; Pink, C.; Biffar, R.; Schmidt, C.O.; Ittermann, T.; Kocher, T.; Meisel, P. Cross-sectional association between physical strength, obesity, periodontitis and number of teeth in a general population. *J. Clin. Periodontol.* **2016**, *43*, 401–407. [CrossRef]
20. Korea Disease Control and Prevention Agency. Guidelines for the 7th National Health and Nutrition Examination Survey (2016–2018). Available online: https://knhanes.kdca.go.kr/knhanes/sub04/sub04_02_02.do?classType=4 (accessed on 23 September 2021).
21. Li, D.; Guo, G.; Xia, L.; Yang, X.; Zhang, B.; Liu, F.; Ma, J.; Hu, Z.; Li, Y.; Li, W. Relative handgrip strength is inversely associated with metabolic profile and metabolic disease in the general population in China. *Front. Physiol.* **2018**, *9*, 59. [CrossRef]
22. Woo, G.-J.; Lee, H.-R.; Kim, Y.; Kim, H.-J.; Park, D.-Y.; Kim, J.-B.; Oh, K.-W.; Choi, Y.-H. Data resource profile: Oral examination of the Korea National Health and Nutrition Examination Survey. *J. Korean Acad. Oral Health* **2018**, *42*, 101–108. [CrossRef]
23. World Health Organization. *Oral Health Surveys: Basic Methods*; World Health Organization: Geneva, Switzerland, 2013.
24. McLean, R.R.; Shardell, M.D.; Alley, D.E.; Cawthon, P.M.; Fragala, M.S.; Harris, T.B.; Kenny, A.M.; Peters, K.W.; Ferrucci, L.; Guralnik, J.M. Criteria for clinically relevant weakness and low lean mass and their longitudinal association with incident mobility impairment and mortality: The foundation for the National Institutes of Health (FNIH) sarcopenia project. *J. Gerontol. Ser. A Biomed. Sci. Med. Sci.* **2014**, *69*, 576–583. [CrossRef]
25. Rantanen, T.; Guralnik, J.M.; Foley, D.; Masaki, K.; Leveille, S.; Curb, J.D.; White, L. Midlife hand grip strength as a predictor of old age disability. *JAMA* **1999**, *281*, 558–560. [CrossRef]
26. Zhou, Y.; Gu, Y.; Zhang, Q.; Liu, L.; Wu, H.; Meng, G.; Bao, X.; Zhang, S.; Sun, S.; Wang, X. Association between tooth loss and handgrip strength in a general adult population. *PLoS ONE* **2020**, *15*, e0236010. [CrossRef] [PubMed]
27. Peres, M.A.; Tsakos, G.; Barbato, P.R.; Silva, D.A.; Peres, K.G. Tooth loss is associated with increased blood pressure in adults—a multidisciplinary population-based study. *J. Clin. Periodontol.* **2012**, *39*, 824–833. [CrossRef] [PubMed]
28. Wu, Y.; Pang, Z.; Zhang, D.; Jiang, W.; Wang, S.; Li, S.; Kruse, T.A.; Christensen, K.; Tan, Q. A cross-sectional analysis of age and sex patterns in grip strength, tooth loss, near vision and hearing levels in Chinese aged 50–74 years. *Arch. Gerontol. Geriatr.* **2012**, *54*, e213–e220. [CrossRef] [PubMed]
29. Yun, J.; Lee, Y. Association between oral health status and handgrip strength in older Korean adults. *Eur. Geriatr. Med.* **2020**, *11*, 459–464. [CrossRef]
30. Yamaguchi, K.; Tohara, H.; Hara, K.; Nakane, A.; Kajisa, E.; Yoshimi, K.; Minakuchi, S. Relationship of aging, skeletal muscle mass, and tooth loss with masseter muscle thickness. *BMC Geriatr.* **2018**, *18*, 67. [CrossRef] [PubMed]
31. Yoshino, Y.; Kamiyama, A.; Harikae, N.; Suzuki, M. Relationships among masticatory ability, handgrip strength, and dietary habits in subjects ranging in age from children to elderlies. *J. Jpn. Soc. Mastication Sci. Health Promot.* **2005**, *15*, 2–10.
32. Park, S.; Chae, M.; Park, H.; Park, K. Higher Branched-Chain Amino Acid Intake Is Associated with Handgrip Strength among Korean Older Adults. *Nutrients* **2021**, *13*, 1522. [CrossRef]
33. Visser, M.; Pahor, M.; Taaffe, D.R.; Goodpaster, B.H.; Simonsick, E.M.; Newman, A.B.; Nevitt, M.; Harris, T.B. Relationship of interleukin-6 and tumor necrosis factor-α with muscle mass and muscle strength in elderly men and women: The Health ABC Study. *J. Gerontol. Ser. A Biol. Sci. Med. Sci.* **2002**, *57*, M326–M332. [CrossRef] [PubMed]

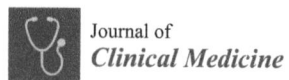

Article

Is Periodontitis a Predictor for an Adverse Outcome in Patients Undergoing Coronary Artery Bypass Grafting? A Pilot Study

Stefan Reichert [1,*], Susanne Schulz [1], Lisa Friebe [1], Michael Kohnert [2], Julia Grollmitz [1], Hans-Günter Schaller [1] and Britt Hofmann [2]

1. Department of Operative Dentistry and Periodontology, Martin-Luther-University Halle-Wittenberg, 06112 Halle (Saale), Germany; susanne.schulz@medizin.uni-halle.de (S.S.); lisa.friebe@hotmail.de (L.F.); julia.grollmitz@uk-halle.de (J.G.); hans.guenter.schaller@uk-halle.de (H.-G.S.)
2. Department of Cardiac Surgery, Mid-German Heart Centre of the University Hospital, 06120 Halle (Saale), Germany; Michael_Kohnert@gmx.de (M.K.); britt.hofmann@uk-halle.de (B.H.)
* Correspondence: stefan.reichert@uk-halle.de; Tel.: +49-345-5573772

Abstract: Periodontitis is a risk factor for atherosclerosis and coronary vascular disease (CVD). This research evaluated the relationship between periodontal conditions and postoperative outcome in patients who underwent coronary artery bypass grafting (CABG). A total of 101 patients with CVD (age 69 years, 88.1% males) and the necessity of CABG surgery were included. Periodontal diagnosis was made according to the guidelines of the Centers for Disease Control and Prevention (CDC, 2007). Additionally, periodontal epithelial surface area (PESA) and periodontal inflamed surface area (PISA) were determined. Multivariate survival analyses were carried out after a one-year follow-up period with Cox regression. All study subjects suffered from periodontitis (28.7% moderate, 71.3% severe). During the follow-up period, 14 patients (13.9%) experienced a new cardiovascular event (11 with angina pectoris, 2 with cardiac decompensation, and 1 with cardiac death). Severe periodontitis was not significant associated with the incidence of new events (adjusted hazard ratio, HR = 2.6; p = 0.199). Other risk factors for new events were pre-existing peripheral arterial disease (adjusted HR = 4.8, p = 0.030) and a history of myocardial infarction (HR = 6.1, p = 0.002). Periodontitis was not found to be an independent risk factor for the incidence of new cardiovascular events after CABG surgery.

Keywords: periodontitis; adjustment risk; adverse effects; cardiovascular disease; coronary artery bypass surgery; morbidity

---

Citation: Reichert, S.; Schulz, S.; Friebe, L.; Kohnert, M.; Grollmitz, J.; Schaller, H.-G.; Hofmann, B. Is Periodontitis a Predictor for an Adverse Outcome in Patients Undergoing Coronary Artery Bypass Grafting? A Pilot Study. *J. Clin. Med.* **2021**, *10*, 818. https://doi.org/10.3390/jcm10040818

Academic Editor: Francisco Mesa
Received: 18 January 2021
Accepted: 10 February 2021
Published: 17 February 2021

Publisher's Note: MDPI stays neutral with regard to jurisdictional claims in published maps and institutional affiliations.

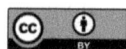

Copyright: © 2021 by the authors. Licensee MDPI, Basel, Switzerland. This article is an open access article distributed under the terms and conditions of the Creative Commons Attribution (CC BY) license (https://creativecommons.org/licenses/by/4.0/).

1. Introduction

Cardiovascular diseases (CVDs) are the number one cause of death globally. In 2016, CVDs represented 31% of all global deaths [1]. According to the 30th German national heart report published in 2018 [2], coronary heart disease (CHD) with 7.9% and acute myocardial infarction with 5.3% were the leading causes of death in Germany. The treatment of patients with CVD is one of the most common medical tasks in developed industrial countries.

Coronary artery bypass grafting (CABG) surgery is a proven cardiac surgery standard procedure for patients with coronary multivessel disease and/or left main coronary stenosis. CABG survival rates depend amongst other things on age. For instance, in patients <70 years, 4-year adjusted survival rate for CABG was 95.0%, in patients 70 to 79 years of age, survival rate was 87.3%, and in patients ≥80 years, survival was 77.4% [3]. Other independent predictors for mortality after CABG are emergency operation, shock, preoperative renal failure, longer total bypass time, intraoperative stroke, postoperative myocardial infarction, gastrointestinal complications, respiratory failure [4], diabetes [5], and peripheral arterial disease (PAD) [6].

Periodontitis is a chronic multifactorial host mediated inflammatory disease associated with dysbiotic plaque biofilms and characterized by progressive destruction of the tooth-supporting apparatus [7,8]. In a lot of cross-sectional and longitudinal studies, a significant association was demonstrated between periodontitis and CVD [9–14] independently of already known risk factors.

Many studies indicate a direct, biologically plausible relationship between periodontitis and CVD. The local host inflammatory response induced by periodontal pathogens promotes the passage of these microorganisms into the blood circulation [15]. Such bacteremia and/or endotoxemia can be caused by invasive dental treatment such as scaling and root planing [16] or even normal daily activities, like tooth brushing, flossing, or food intake [17], and is furthermore associated with the severity of periodontal disease [18]. DNA of key bacteria for periodontitis has been found in both in atheromas [19,20] and heart tissue [21]. In another study, *Aggregatibacter actinomycetemcomitans* was cultured from both specimens taken from periodontal pockets and atheromatous plaque of the same patient [22]. This finding suggests that living bacteria can get from the oral cavity into the coronary arteries and may directly contribute to the pathogenesis of atherosclerosis. In animal experiments, another study showed that *Porphyromonas gingivalis* can invade into heart tissue that has already been damaged by ischemia [23]. This result could indicate that periodontal bacteria not only play a role in the development of atherosclerosis but can also influence the cardiovascular outcome after a primary event.

In a previous study of our group, we investigated the subgingival microbiome in cardiovascular (CV) patients undergoing coronary artery bypass grafting (CABG) in order to identify putative microbial biomarkers for further adverse events after heart surgery. We determined that Saccharibacteria phylum (class: TM7-3, order: CW040, family: F16) was found to be associated with the incidence of secondary CV events ($p = 0.016$) [24]. The present study aims to investigate whether clinical conditions of periodontitis were also associated with the incidence of new cardiovascular events after CABG surgery.

2. Materials and Methods
2.1. Patients with CVD

Out of a population of 308 patients, 102 patients with CHD for whom an CABG surgery was indicated at the department of cardiac surgery of the Mid-German Heart Centre at the University Hospital Halle (Saale) between January and October 2017 were included in the study. A total of 206 patients could not be included in the study because they did not meet the inclusion criteria, a dental examination before the CABG operation was not possible, a cardiac emergency existed, or the patients did not consent to participation in the study. The most common reason for exclusion was that the subjects had fewer than four own teeth. Follow-up data were generated from 101 patients between January 2018 to June 2019 (dropout rate 0.98%). The study design is summarized in Figure 1. An experienced cardiac surgeon diagnosed patients with CHD and checked the inclusion and exclusion criteria. The following inclusion criteria had to be met: age >18 years, at least 60% stenosis of one of the main coronary arteries demonstrated by angiography, presence of at least four teeth. Exclusion criteria were inability to give written informed consent, subgingival scaling and root planing and/or antibiotic therapy during the last 6 months prior to the examination, pregnancy, and the need for antibiotic prophylaxis against endocarditis according to the criteria of the European Society for Cardiology [25]. Moreover, patients with diseases or disorders such as current drug or alcohol abuse that preclude participation in this clinical study according to investigator judgment were excluded.

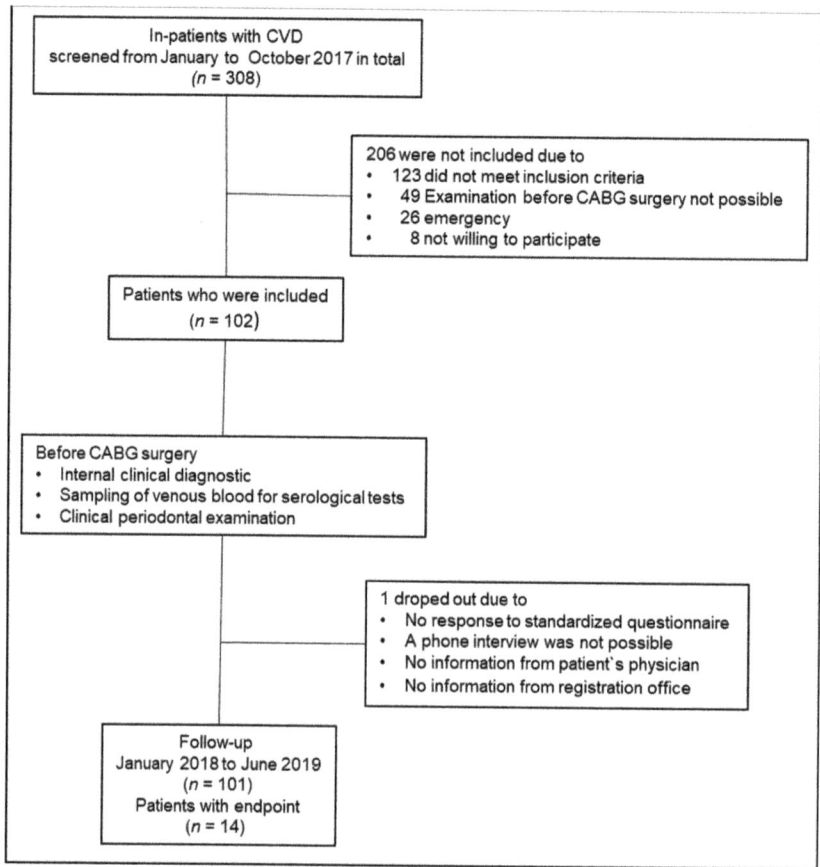

Figure 1. Study design flow chart.

2.2. Demographic Parameters and Clinical and Cardiological Diagnostics

In order to be able to assess the severity of the CVD, the number of coronaries affected was determined (one-, two- or three-vessel disease). In addition, Canadian Cardiovascular Society (CCS) stages for angina pectoris were determined. Baseline variables such as age, smoking status (never, past, current smokers, and pack years) and current or past diseases (e.g., diabetes mellitus, hypertension, peripheral arterial disease (PAD), and dyslipoproteinemia) were assessed as part of the patient's medical history. A person who smoked a minimum of one cigarette per day at the time of questioning was considered to be a current smoker. A past smoker had not smoked for at least one year at the time of the survey. The number of pack years was calculated by multiplying the number of packs of cigarettes smoked per day by the number of years of smoking. Furthermore, all patients underwent detailed clinical and biochemical investigation. For instance, intake of drugs such as lipid lowering drugs, oral anticoagulants, and antiarrhythmics was registered. Serum parameters including international normalized ratio (INR) score, hemoglobin (Hb; mmol/L), hematocrit (1/L), creatinine (μmol/L), urea (mmol/L), glycated hemoglobin (HbA1c; mmol/mol), C-reactive protein (CRP; mg/dL), leukocytes (Gpt/L), and platelets (Gpt/L) were recorded.

2.3. Dental Anamnesis and Examinations

The dental anamnesis and examination was done one day before the CABG surgery. The patients were asked about the frequency of brushing teeth per day and whether they practiced interdental hygiene using dental floss or interdental brushes. Furthermore, the question was asked whether periodontal therapy in form of scaling and root planing had ever been carried out. In order to be able to estimate an increased occurrence of severe periodontitis within a family, the patients were asked whether there was premature tooth loss due to tooth loosening within relatives of the first degree.

Before the dental examination, the study participants were asked to rinse with an antibacterial mouthwash solution (*Chlorhexamed® FORTE alcohol-free 0.2%, GlaxoSmithKline Consumer Healthcare GmbH & Co. KG, Munich, Germany) in order to reduce the risk of bacteremia due to the probing of dental pockets. The clinical dental assessment involved determining the plaque index (PI) [26] and bleeding on probing (BOP) [27]. In the plaque index, four tooth surfaces were evaluated: mesio-buccal, mid-buccal, disto-bucca, and lingual. In the bleeding index, six sites around each tooth (mesio-buccal, mid-buccal, disto-buccal, disto-oral, mid-oral, and mesio-oral) were examined. BOP was only evaluated after a waiting time of 30 s after probing. Furthermore, the number of decayed, filled, and missing teeth was registered as well as the number of teeth with furcation involvement.

The measurements for both maximal clinical probing depth (PD = distance between gingival margin and the apical stop of the probe) and maximum clinical attachment loss (CAL = distance between the cementoenamel junction and the apical stop of the probe) were taken also at six sites around each tooth. The maximum values for each tooth were taken to calculate the overall mean per participant. In order to obtain reproducible results for BOP, PD, and CAL, the two examiners (L.F. and J.G.) were particularly trained in using a pressure-sensitive calibrated dental probe (UNC 15 0.2 N Aesculap, Tuttlingen, Germany). Particular attention was paid to ensuring that the examiner oriented the probe in the direction of the tooth axis. The reading was made exactly to the millimeter. If one measuring point (gingival margin or cementoenamel junction) was between two markers of the measuring scale, the measurement was estimated to 0.5 mm. For the calibration, both examiners determined PD and CAL twice on five periodontal phantom models (phantom model A-PB, frasaco GmbH, Tettnang, Germany) and on five patients. To assess the reproducibility of the double measurements, the Bland–Altman method was used [28]. The difference (d) of the two measurements was calculated and plotted against the mean of the two measurements. The measurements are sufficiently reproducible if 95% of the differences (d) were in the range $d \pm 2 \times s$, where s denotes the standard deviation of the differences. Regarding our two raters, the differences from two measurements for PD and CAL were to 100% in this range $d \pm 2 \times s$. Thus, the examiners L.F. and J.G. were able to generate reproducible measurement results.

The clinical periodontitis case definition was held according to the guidelines of the working group of the Centers for Disease Control and Prevention (CDC) [29]. According to the CDC, a severe periodontitis case was diagnosed if at least ≥ 2 interproximal sites with CAL ≥ 6 mm (not on same tooth) and ≥ 1 interproximal site with PD ≥ 5 mm were present. A moderate periodontitis case was diagnosed if at least ≥ 2 interproximal sites with CAL ≥ 4 mm (not on same tooth) or ≥ 2 interproximal sites with PD ≥ 5 mm (not on one tooth) were present. If no severe or moderate periodontitis was present, periodontitis was diagnosed as mild or absent.

For a more accurate quantification of the root surface affected by attachment loss and quantification of the inflamed epithelial surface, both the periodontal epithelial surface area (PESA) and the periodontal inflamed surface area (PISA) were calculated [30]. For that purpose, a freely downloadable (www.parsprototo.info) Excel spreadsheet was used. In order to calculate PESA, data of CAL and recession were entered. For the calculation of PISA, sites with BOP were recorded additionally.

2.4. Follow-Up

Follow-up data were collected from 101 patients. The follow-up was primarily carried out by telephone interview one year after CABG surgery. If follow-up information could not be obtained, we contacted civil registration offices and requested information about current address or date of death. The postoperative outcome was assessed using the major adverse cardiac and cerebrovascular events (MACCE) criteria established for patients with CHD: 1. no event, 2. myocardial infarction, 3. low cardiac output syndrome, 4. ventricular tachycardia (VT), 5. angina pectoris, 6. renewed revascularization surgery, 7. cardiac decompensation, 8. peripheral circulatory failure, 9. stroke/transient ischemic attack (TIA)/prolonged reversible ischemic neurological deficit (PRIND), 10. cardiac death, 11. stroke death, 12. non-cardiac death.

2.5. Statistics

Statistical analyses were carried out using commercial software (SPSS v.25.0 package, IBM, Chicago, IL, USA). Values of $p < 0.05$ were considered significant. Categorical variables were documented as number and the corresponding percentage in brackets. For comparisons, the chi-squared test was employed. If the expected values in one group were <5, Fisher's exact test was performed. Metric demographic, clinical, and serological data were checked for normal distribution using the Kolmogorov–Smirnov test and the Shapiro–Wilk test. As none of the metric values were normally distributed, they were plotted as median and 25th/75th percentiles. For statistical evaluation, the Mann–Whitney U-test was used. For survival evaluation and in order to generate adjusted hazard ratios (HRs), Cox regression was applied. Classic demographic risk factors for CVD such as age, male gender, and nicotine consumption measured as pack years were included in the regression model. Furthermore, the variable periodontitis was integrated into the model according to the CDC classification and in two further models as PESA and PISA. Finally, after bivariate comparisons, significant variables such as PAD and previous MI were included. Although not significant, atrial fibrillation was included because it occurred twice as often in patients with an event compared to patients without an event. Although statistically significant according to bivariate comparisons, the confounders ingestion of oral anticoagulants or antiarrhythmics and early tooth loss among first-degree relatives were not included in the regression model, as the consumption of oral anticoagulants was strictly correlated with prevalence of atrial fibrillation (Pearson correlation coefficient = 0.872, $p < 0.0001$). Antiarrhythmics were only taken by two patients with event, so inclusion in the Cox model was not statistically meaningful. Of all patients, 43.6% could not answer the question about early tooth loss among first-degree relatives, so this variable was also not included in the regression model.

3. Results

3.1. Incidence of New Cardiovascular Events

No follow-up data could be collected from one patient. Fourteen (13.9%) patients experienced a cardiovascular event within the one-year follow-up after CABG surgery (Figure 1). Eleven patients suffered from angina pectoris, two patients from cardiac decompensation, and one patient died due to a cardiac cause.

3.2. Cross-Section Comparisons

There were no significant differences regarding age, sex ratio, BMI, and nicotine consumption between CVD patients with event and without event (Table 1).

Table 1. Demographic variables in dependence of the occurrence of adverse cardiovascular events one year after CABG surgery.

Variable	Entire Study Cohort n = 101, Median (25th/75th Percentile) or n (%)	Event n = 14, Median (25th/75th Percentile) or n (%)	No event n = 87, Median (25th/75th Percentile) or n (%)	p-Values
age (years)	69.0 (60.0/75.0)	71.0 (60.8/75.3)	69.0 (60.0/74.0)	0.646 *
females	12 (11.9)	2 (14.3)	10 (11.5)	
males	89 (88.1)	12 (85.7)	77 (88.5)	0.671 ***
BMI (kg/m^2)	28.7 (25.6/31.0)	29.7 (25.4/31.8)	28.7 (25.6/30.5)	0.476 *
smoking				
current	22 (21.8)	3 (21.4)	19 (21.8)	
past	42 (41.6)	6 (42.9)	36 (41.4)	
never	37 (36.6)	5 (35.7)	32 (36.8)	0.995 **
pack years	7.5 (0/22.5)	3.0 (0/21.3)	8.0 (0/22.5)	0.686 *

BMI, body mass index; * p calculated with Mann–Whitney U-test; ** p calculated with chi^2-test; *** p calculated with Fisher's exact test.

Patients with event suffered significantly more frequently from PAD and reported more often a previous myocardial infarction (MI). Moreover, they took anticoagulants and antiarrhythmics significantly more frequently. In addition, there was a trend of an elevated number of CVD patients with atrial fibrillation among the event group. (Table 2).

Table 2. Anamnestic and clinical parameters in dependence of the occurrence of adverse cardiovascular events one year after CABG surgery.

Variable	Entire Study Cohort n = 101, Median (25th/75th Percentile) or n (%)	Event n = 14, Median (25th/75th Percentile) or n (%)	No event n = 87, Median (25th/75th Percentile) or n (%)	p-Values
Affected coronaries				
One-vessel disease	5 (5.0)	2 (14.3)	3 (3.4)	
Two-vessel disease	21 (20.8)	3 (21.4)	18 (20.7)	
Three-vessel disease	75 (74.3)	9 (64.3)	66 (75.9)	0.214 **
Angina pectoris grade				
CCS 0	32 (31.7)	7 (50)	25 (28.7)	
CCS I	13 (12.9)	1 (7.7)	12 (13.8)	
CCS II	25 (24.8)	2 (14.3)	23 (26.4)	
CCS III	18 (17.8)	2 (14.3)	16 (18.4)	
CCS IV	13 (12.9)	2 (14.3)	11 (12.6)	0.599 **
History of				
Diabetes mellitus	40 (39.6)	7 (50)	33 (37.9)	0.397 ***
Hypertension	88 (87.1)	14 (100)	74 (85.1)	0.205 ***
Dyslipoproteinemia	81 (80.2)	13 (92.9)	68 (78.2)	0.291 ***
PAD	16 (15.8)	5 (35.7) ↑	11 (12.6)	0.044 ***
CVD	39 (38.6)	5 (35.7)	34 (39.1)	1.00 ***
MI	28 (27,7)	8 (57.1) ↑	20 (23.0)	0.020 ***
stroke/TIA	9 (8.9)	0 (0)	9 (10.3)	0.354 ***
Angina pectoris	75 (74.3)	10 (71.4)	65 (74.7)	0.752 ***
PTCA/stent	15 (14.9)	3 (21.4)	12 (13.8)	0.433 ***
Atrial fibrillation	14 (13.9)	4 (28.6)	10 (11.5)	0.102 ***

Table 2. Cont.

Variable	Entire Study Cohort n = 101, Median (25th/75th Percentile) or n (%)	Event n = 14, Median (25th/75th Percentile) or n (%)	No event n = 87, Median (25th/75th Percentile) or n (%)	p-Values
Blood values				
INR	1.04 (0.99/1.11)	1.04 (0.95/1,12)	1.04 (0.99/1.10)	0.984 *
Hb (mmol/L)	8.8 (8.3/9.4)	8.4 (8.1/9.4)	8.8 (8.3/9.4)	0.437 *
Hematocrit 1/L	0.41 (0.39/0.43)	0.4 (0.38/0.43)	0.41 (0.39/0.43)	0.778 *
Creatinine (μmol/L)	85 (75.5/100)	86.5 (79.5/100.3)	85.0 (74.0/99.0)	0.440 *
Urea (mmol/L)	5.9 (4.5/7.2)	6.8 (5.4/7.6)	5.6 (4.3/6.8)	0.065 *
HbA1C (mmol/mol)	37.6 (31.2/44.4)	39.0 (35.1/52.6)	40.1 (35.9/48.8)	0.769 *
CRP (mg/L)	2.6 (1.2/6.6)	1.4 (0.7/3.9)	2.8 (1.4/6.9)	0.052 *
Leukocytes (Gpt/L)	6.5 (7.6/9.1)	7.2 (5.5/8.5)	7.6 (6.6/9.5)	0.210 *
Platelet (Gpt/L)	238.0 (193.0/269.5)	225.0 (184.0/259.8)	239.0 (193.0/280.0)	0.401 *
Drugs				
Lipid lowering drugs	90 (89.1)	14 (100.0)	76 (87.4)	0.354 ***
Oral anticoagulants	11 (10.9)	4 (28.6) ↑	7 (8.0)	0.044 ***
Antiarrhythmics	2 (2.0)	2 (14.3) ↑	0 (0.0)	0.018 ***

CCS, Canadian Cardiovascular Society; PAD, peripheral arterial disease; CVD, coronary vascular disease; CRP, C-reactive protein; INR, international normalized ratio; Hb, hemoglobin; MI, myocardial infarction; PTCA, percutaneous transluminal coronary angioplasty; TIA, transient ischemic attack; HbA1C, glycated hemoglobin; * p calculated with Mann–Whitney U-test; ** p calculated with chi^2-test; *** p calculated with Fisher's exact test; ↑ significant differences.

Regarding dental conditions, patients with new cardiovascular event reported early tooth loss caused by tooth loosening among first-degree relatives (Table 3) significantly more often. However, 43.6% of all study participants could not answer this question. No other dental parameters such as severe periodontitis, PESA, or PISA were significantly associated with the cardiovascular outcome.

Table 3. Dental conditions in dependence of the occurrence of adverse cardiovascular events one year after CABG surgery. Significant differences are indicated with arrows.

Variable	Entire Study Cohort n = 101, Median (25th/75th Percentile) or n (%)	Event n = 14, Median (25th/75th Percentile) or n (%)	No event n = 87, Median (25th/75th Percentile) or n (%)	p-Values
Dental anamnesis				
tooth brushing/d				
1	15 (14.9)	1 (7.1)	14 (16.1)	
2	80 (79.2)	12 (85.7)	68 (78.2)	
3	6 (5.9)	1 (7.1)	5 (85.7)	0.678 **
Use of floss/interdental brushes	29 (28.7)	5 (35.7)	24 (27.6)	0.563 ***
Previous SRP	12 (11.9)	3 (21.4)	9 (10.3)	0.366 ***
Early tooth loss among first-degree relatives				

Table 3. Cont.

Variable	Entire Study Cohort n = 101, Median (25th/75th Percentile) or n (%)	Event n = 14, Median (25th/75th Percentile) or n (%)	No event n = 87, Median (25th/75th Percentile) or n (%)	p-Values
Yes				
No				
Unknown	26 (25.7)	8 (51.7) ↑	18 (20.7)	
Periodontitis (CDC)				
No or mild	0 (0.0)	0 (0.0)	0 (0.0)	
Moderate	29 (28.7)	3 (21.4)	26 (29.9)	
Severe	72 (71.3)	11 (78.6)	61 (70.1)	0.516 **
Plaque index (%)	1.3 (0.9/1.7)	1.2 (0.8/1.8)	1.3 (1.0/1.7)	0.293 *
Bleeding index (%)	18.0 (10.1/33.3)	19.0 (13.8/37.0)	17.5 (9.6/33.3)	0.220 *
Pocket depth (mm)	3.0 (2.6/3.6)	2.8 (2.6/3.5)	3.0 (2.6/3.6)	0.738 *
% sites with PD				
<3 mm	34.4 (23.3/52.7)	34.8 (23.2/59.1)	34.4 (23.3/52.6)	0.976 *
3–5 mm	56.7 (45.0/67.9)	64.2 (40.7/70.5)	56.3 (45.2/66.7)	0.353 *
>5 mm	1.7 (0/8.3)	1.2 (0/5.9)	1.7 (0/9.1)	0.373 *
Attachment loss (mm)	3.9 (3.1/4.9)	3.9 (3.1/5.0)	3.9 (3.2/5.0)	0.705 *
% sites with CAL				
<3 mm	16.7 (3.9/32.7)	13.5 (3.5/44.3)	19.3 (4.2/32.1)	0.871 *
3–5 mm	59.4 (47.4/68.5)	60.0 (44.3/76.3)	59.4 (48.3/68.2)	0.596 *
>5 mm	12.7 (3.2/33.3)	11.8 (1.8/35.0)	12.7 (3.2/33.3)	0.735 *
PESA (mm^2)	1187.8 (831.4/1617.3)	1393.7 (966.2/1778.6)	1165.2 (812.3/1577.9)	0.453 *
PISA (mm^2)	194.6 (107.6/405.9)	289.7 (164.8/407.9)	191.4 (103.1/419.9)	0.515 *
DMF/T	18 (14.0/22.0)	16.0 (12.0/21.3)	19.0 (14.0/23.0)	0.266 *
Missing teeth	7 (3.0/15.0)	6.0 (2.0/9.8)	7.0 (3.0/17.0)	0.695 *
Teeth with open furcations	0 (0/2.0)	1.0 (0.0/2.0)	0.0 (0.0/2.0)	0.517 *

DMF/T, decayed missing filled/teeth; PD, pocket depth; CAL, clinical attachment loss; PESA, periodontal epithelial surface area; PISA, periodontal inflamed surface area; SRP, scaling and root planing >6 month prior to dental examination, CDC, Centers for Disease Control and Prevention; * p calculated with Mann–Whitney U-test; ** p calculated with chi^2-test; *** p calculated with Fisher's exact test; ↑ significant differences.

3.3. Multivariate Survival Analyses

The possible prognostic value of the periodontal parameters CDC, PESA, and PISA were calculated using Cox regression, taking into account the confounders age, gender, pack years, PAD, previous MI, and atrial fibrillation. For severe periodontitis we observed an increased hazard ratio (HR = 2.6) for the combined endpoint, but this result was not significant ($p = 0.610$). In contrast, PAD and previous myocardial infarction were significantly associated with the combined endpoint. Atrial fibrillation also increased the risk for the combined endpoint with borderline significance (Table 4). If instead of CDC the periodontal parameters PESA or PISA were inserted into the regression model, no significance could be achieved for both variables (PESA: HR = 1.001, $p = 0338$; PISA: HR = 1.0, $p = 0.960$).

Table 4. Hazard ratios (HRs) for new cardiovascular events adjusted for age, gender, pack years, severe periodontitis according to CDC classification, atrial fibrillation, peripheral artery disease (PAD), and previous myocardial infarction (MI).

Confounding Variables	Hazard Ratio	95% CI Lower	CI Upper	p-Values
Age	0.986	0.912	1.067	0.725
Gender (female)	1.601	0.321	7.976	0.566
Pack years	0.960	0.916	1.005	0.082
Severe periodontitis	2.559	0.610	10.743	0.199
Atrial fibrillation	3.701	0.941	14.562	0.061
PAD	4.836	1.162	20.126	0.030
Previous MI	6.056	1.892	19.379	0.002

PAD, peripheral arterial disease; MI, myocardial infarction; CI, confidence interval.

4. Discussion

Periodontitis has a high worldwide prevalence with nearly 40% in the age group of the 35–44-year-olds and nearly 50% in the age group of the 65–74-year-olds [31]. There is increasing evidence that periodontitis can promote the development of systemic diseases such as atherosclerosis and subsequent CVD. Therefore, the aim of our study was to investigate whether periodontitis could influence the cardiovascular outcome after CABG surgery. For periodontitis disease case definition, two different periodontitis classification systems were used in order to compensate disadvantages of a separate system. CDC diagnostics are based on the determination of CAL and PD in interproximal sites. Bleeding upon probing is not taken into account. Three categories of disease, severe, moderate, and no or mild periodontitis, are derived [29]. On the contrary, PESA and PISA are metric variables that can determine the amount of periodontal altered pocket epithelium (PESA) or inflamed pocket epithelium (PISA). It is assumed that in particular the area of the periodontal inflamed tissue may be associated with the systemic inflammatory burden [30].

Among our patients with CVD, the prevalence of severe periodontitis (71.3%, Table 3) was more than two times higher compared to the normal population according to the Fifth German Oral Health Study, which revealed among younger seniors (65 to 74-year-olds) a prevalence of 28.3% [32]. This result may support the importance of severe periodontitis in the pathogenesis of atherosclerosis and CVD. However, we could not show a significant association of severe periodontitis according to CDC definition, PESA, or PISA with the cardiovascular endpoint. For severe periodontitis, only an insignificant trend for the incidence of new cardiovascular events could be shown (Table 4). Thus, we could not demonstrate that severity of periodontitis is a risk factor for a worse postoperative course. The reasons for this result could be manifold. Firstly, it was striking that among our cohort there were no patients in the category of no or mild periodontitis. All study participants had at least moderate periodontitis (Table 3). Therefore, a sharp distinction between periodontally diseased and not diseased was not possible.

The second reason is that both the number of test persons included in our study and the length of the observation period were different in comparison to other studies, which showed a positive association between periodontitis with recurrent cardiovascular events. Dorn et al. [33] investigated 884 survivors of MI and revealed that after an average follow-up of 2.9 years, the mean CAL was associated with recurrent fatal and non-fatal cardiovascular events. Renvert et al. [34] investigated 165 consecutive subjects with acute coronary syndrome (ACS) and 159 medically healthy, matched control subjects regarding periodontal conditions. After an observation period of 3 years, a positive association between alveolar bone loss caused by periodontitis and future ACS events was shown. Since we found at least a trend between severe periodontitis and new cardiovascular events in the present study (Table 4), further studies with more subjects and a longer observation period may be useful.

A third reason may be that other risk factors are more important for the incidence of new cardiovascular events after CABG surgery than periodontitis. In Cox regression, we found a significant positive association between PAD, previous MI, and the cardiovascular endpoint and a trend for atrial fibrillation (Table 4). This result is supported by prior studies. For instance, patients with PAD had poorer long-term survival rates after CABG surgery than patients without PAD [6]. It is assumed that PAD may be a marker of more severe atherosclerosis and subsequent diseases such as CVD. Another possibility is that in spite of successful CABG surgery, the risk of noncardiac mortality may be increased [35]. Another study [36] revealed among patients with PAD a higher incidence of comorbidities in comparison to patients without PAD. Furthermore, a history of MI was associated with increased mortality during the first 30 days after CABG surgery and the incidence of new MI [37]. Other studies have shown a positive association between atrial fibrillation and the outcome of CABG surgery. Preoperative atrial fibrillation was found associated with increased late cardiac morbidity and mortality, poorer long-term survival, higher risk of all-cause mortality, and congestive heart failure [38–40].

A further observation should not go unmentioned. Patients with event reported early tooth loss by tooth loosening among first-degree relatives significantly more often compared to subjects without event (Table 3). This result was not checked in the multivariate survival analysis, as 43.6% of patients could not give an answer to the corresponding question during anamnesis. Furthermore, incorrect information from the patient cannot be ruled out. Nevertheless, this observation may indicate the influence of genetic factors in pathogenesis of periodontitis. This is interesting because periodontitis and CVD share common genetic risk factors. For instance, single nucleotide polymorphisms (SNPs) in long non-coding RNA ANRIL (antisense noncoding RNA in the *INK4* locus) were shown to be associated with both CVD and periodontitis [41]. These risk factors may also be associated with a worse outcome after CABG surgery. This hypothesis should also be tested in further studies.

Limitations of the Study

When interpreting the results of this study, a number of limitations should be noted. First, in comparison to previous studies, the relatively short observation period of one year after CABG has to be mentioned. Secondly, none of the CVD patients included was periodontally healthy. A comparison between CVD patients with and without periodontitis might show a clearer influence of the risk factor periodontitis on the cardiovascular outcome after CABG surgery. However, our patients were aged from 60 to 75 years. In a previous study of our group [42], we determined that among 1002 CVD patients of the same age group, only 2.3% individuals had no periodontitis. Therefore, recruiting CVD patients without periodontitis in the sense of a control group would be very difficult. Thirdly, changes in general conditions, lifestyle habits (in particular smoking status), and possible treatment of periodontitis after CABG might influence the cardiovascular outcome. These factors were not evaluated during follow-up.

5. Conclusions

We obtained a severe trend (HR = 2.6) for periodontitis as one predictor for new adverse events within one year after CABG surgery. In order to obtain a significant result, an extension of the observation time would be useful. We confirmed that PAD and previous MI are putative predictors for a poorer outcome after CABG surgery.

Author Contributions: Conceptualization, S.R., B.H. and S.S.; methodology S.R., B.H. and S.S.; validation, S.R. and S.S.; formal analysis, S.R. and S.S.; investigation, M.K., J.G., L.F. and B.H.; data curation, L.F., J.G., M.K., S.S. and S.R.; writing—original draft preparation, S.R.; writing—review and editing, S.R. and B.H.; supervision, H.-G.S. and B.H.; funding acquisition, S.S. and S.R. All authors have read and agreed to the published version of the manuscript.

Funding: This research was funded by the German Society of Periodontology (DG PARO) and Colgate Palmolive Goldene Apotheke Basel (CP GABA).

Institutional Review Board Statement: The study was conducted according to the guidelines of the Declaration of Helsinki and approved by the Ethics Committee of the Martin Luther University Halle-Wittenberg (date of approval: 2016-11-16). The study is registered in the German Register for Clinical Studies (DRKS) ID: DRKS00015776.

Informed Consent Statement: Informed consent was obtained from all subjects involved in the study.

Data Availability Statement: The data presented in this study are available on request from the corresponding author.

Acknowledgments: We would like to thank all the patients with CVD for their cooperation in this study.

Conflicts of Interest: The authors declare no conflict of interest.

References

1. WHO. Cardiovascular Diseases (CVDs). Available online: https://www.who.int/news-room/fact-sheets/detail/cardiovascular-diseases-(cvds) (accessed on 9 December 2020).
2. Deutsche Herzstiftung e.V. *Deutscher Herzbericht 2018: Heart diseases in the cause of death statistics*; German Heart Foundation e.V.: Frankfurt am Main, Germany, 2018; p. 27.
3. Graham, M.M.; Ghali, W.A.; Faris, P.D.; Galbraith, P.D.; Norris, C.M.; Knudtson, M.L. Survival After Coronary Revascularization in the Elderly. *Circulation* **2002**, *105*, 2378–2384. [CrossRef] [PubMed]
4. Toumpoulis, I.K.; Anagnostopoulos, C.E.; Balaram, S.K.; Rokkas, C.K.; Swistel, D.G.; Ashton, R.C.; Derose, J.J. Assessment of independent predictors for long-term mortality between women and men after coronary artery bypass grafting: Are women different from men? *J. Thorac. Cardiovasc. Surg.* **2006**, *131*, 343–351. [CrossRef]
5. Axelsson, T.A.; Adalsteinsson, J.A.; Arnadottir, L.O.; Helgason, D.; Johannsdottir, H.; Helgadottir, S.; Orrason, A.W.; Andersen, K.; Gudbjartsson, T. Long-term outcomes after coronary artery bypass surgery in patients with diabetes. *Interact. Cardiovasc. Thorac. Surg.* **2020**, *30*, 685–690. [CrossRef] [PubMed]
6. Bonacchi, M.; Parise, O.; Matteucci, F.; Tetta, C.; Moula, A.I.; Micali, L.R.; Dokollari, A.; De Martino, M.; Sani, G.; Grasso, A.; et al. Is Peripheral Artery Disease an Independent Predictor of Isolated Coronary Artery Bypass Outcome? *Hearth Lung Circ.* **2020**, *29*, 1502–1510. [CrossRef]
7. Papapanou, P.N.; Sanz, M.; Buduneli, N.; Dietrich, T.; Feres, M.; Fine, D.H.; Flemmig, T.F.; Garcia, R.; Giannobile, W.V.; Graziani, F.; et al. Periodontitis: Consensus report of workgroup 2 of the 2017 World Workshop on the Classification of Periodontal and Peri-Implant Diseases and Conditions. *J. Periodontol.* **2018**, *89*, S173–S182. [CrossRef]
8. Tonetti, M.S.; Greenwell, H.; Kornman, K.S. Staging and grading of periodontitis: Framework and proposal of a new classification and case definition. *J. Clin. Periodontol.* **2018**, *45*, S149–S161. [CrossRef] [PubMed]
9. Bahekar, A.A.; Singh, S.; Saha, S.; Molnar, J.; Arora, R. The prevalence and incidence of coronary heart disease is significantly increased in periodontitis: A meta-analysis. *Am. Hearth. J.* **2007**, *154*, 830–837. [CrossRef] [PubMed]
10. Blaizot, A.; Vergnes, J.-N.; Nuwwareh, S.; Amar, J.; Sixou, M. Periodontal diseases and cardiovascular events: Meta-analysis of observational studies. *Int. Dent. J.* **2009**, *59*, 197–209. [PubMed]
11. Lockhart, P.B.; Bolger, A.F.; Papapanou, P.N.; Lockhart, P.B.; Bolger, A.F.; Papapanou, P.N.; Osinbowale, O.; Trevisan, M.; Levison, M.E.; Taubert, K.A.; et al. Periodontal disease and atherosclerotic vascular disease: Does the evidence support an independent association: A scientific statement from the American Heart Association. *Circulation* **2012**, *125*, 2520–2544. [CrossRef]
12. Janket, S.-J.; Baird, A.E.; Chuang, S.-K.; Jones, J.A. Meta-analysis of periodontal disease and risk of coronary heart disease and stroke. *Oral Surg. Oral Med. Oral Pathol. Oral Radiol. Endodontol.* **2003**, *95*, 559–569. [CrossRef]
13. Humphrey, L.L.; Fu, R.; Buckley, D.I.; Freeman, M.; Helfand, M. Periodontal disease and coronary heart disease incidence: A sys-tematic review and meta-analysis. *J. Gen. Intern. Med.* **2008**, *23*, 2079–2086. [CrossRef]
14. Dietrich, T.; Sharma, P.; Walter, C.; Weston, P.; Beck, J. The epidemiological evidence behind the association between periodontitis and incident atherosclerotic cardiovascular disease. *J. Periodontol.* **2013**, *84*, S70–S84. [CrossRef] [PubMed]
15. Yun, P.L.W.; Decarlo, A.A.; Chapple, C.C.; Hunter, N. Functional Implication of the Hydrolysis of Platelet Endothelial Cell Adhesion Molecule 1 (CD31) by Gingipains of Porphyromonas gingivalis for the Pathology of Periodontal Disease. *Infect. Immun.* **2005**, *73*, 1386–1398. [CrossRef]
16. Zhang, W.; Daly, C.G.; Mitchell, D.; Curtis, B.H. Incidence and magnitude of bacteraemia caused by flossing and by scaling and root planing. *J. Clin. Periodontol.* **2013**, *40*, 41–52. [CrossRef]
17. Hirschfeld, J.; Kawai, T. Oral inflammation and bacteremia: Implications for chronic and acute systemic diseases involving major organs. *Cardiovasc. Hematol. Disord. Targets* **2015**, *15*, 70–84. [CrossRef] [PubMed]
18. Geerts, S.O.; Nys, M.; De Mol, P.; Charpentier, J.; Albert, A.; Legrand, V.; Rompen, E.H. Systemic Release of Endotoxins Induced by Gentle Mastication: Association With Periodontitis Severity. *J. Periodontol.* **2002**, *73*, 73–78. [CrossRef]

19. Haraszthy, V.I.; Zambon, J.J.; Trevisan, M.; Zeid, M.; Genco, R.J. Identification of periodontal pathogens in atheromatous plaques. *J. Periodontol.* **2000**, *71*, 1554–1560. [CrossRef] [PubMed]
20. Atarbashi-Moghadam, F.; Havaei, S.R.; Havaei, S.A.; Hosseini, N.S.; Behdadmehr, G.; Atarbashi-Moghadam, S. Periopathogens in atherosclerotic plaques of patients with both cardiovascular disease and chronic periodontitis. *ARYA Atheroscler.* **2018**, *14*, 53–57.
21. Ziebolz, D.; Rost, C.; Schmidt, J.; Waldmann-Beushausen, R.; Schöndube, F.A.; Mausberg, R.F.; Danner, B.C. Periodontal Bacterial DNA and Their Link to Human Cardiac Tissue: Findings of a Pilot Study. *Thorac. Cardiovasc. Surg.* **2015**, *66*, 83–90. [CrossRef]
22. Padilla, C.; Lobos, O.; Hubert, E.; Gonzalez, C.; Matus, S.; Pereira, M.; Hasbun, S.; Descouvieres, C. Periodontal pathogens in atheromatous plaques isolated from patients with chronic periodontitis. *J. Periodontal Res.* **2006**, *41*, 350–353. [CrossRef] [PubMed]
23. Shiheido, Y.; Maejima, Y.; Suzuki, J.I. Porphyromonas gingivalis, a periodontal pathogen, enhances myocardial vulnera-bility, thereby promoting post-infarct cardiac rupture. *J. Mol. Cell. Cardiol.* **2016**, *99*, 123–137. [CrossRef] [PubMed]
24. Schulz, S.; Reichert, S.; Grollmitz, J.; Friebe, L.; Kohnert, M.; Hofmann, B.; Schaller, H.G.; Kllawonn, F.; Shi, R. The role of Sacchari-bacteria (TM7) in the oral microbiome as a predictor for secondary cardiovascular events. *Int. J. Cardiol.* **2020**. accept. [CrossRef]
25. Adler, Y.; Charron, P.; Imazio, M.; Badano, L.; Barón-Esquivias, G.; Bogaert, J. ESC Scientific Document Group. *Eur. Heart J.* **2015**, *36*, 2921–2964. [CrossRef]
26. Löe, H.; Silness, J. Periodontal Disease in Pregnancy I. Prevalence and Severity. *Acta Odontol. Scand.* **1963**, *21*, 533–551. [CrossRef]
27. Ainamo, J.; Bay, I. Problems and proposals for recording gingivitis and plaque. *Int. Dent. J.* **1975**, *25*, 229–235.
28. Grouven, U.; Bender, R.; Ziegler, A.; Lange, S. Vergleich von Messmethoden. *DMW Dtsch. Med. Wochenschr.* **2007**, *132*, e69–e73. [CrossRef]
29. Page, R.C.; Eke, P.I. Case Definitions for Use in Population-Based Surveillance of Periodontitis. *J. Periodontol.* **2007**, *78*, 1387–1399. [CrossRef]
30. Nesse, W.; Abbas, F.; Van Der Ploeg, I.; Spijkervet, F.K.L.; Dijkstra, P.U.; Vissink, A. Periodontal inflamed surface area: Quantifying inflammatory burden. *J. Clin. Periodontol.* **2008**, *35*, 668–673. [CrossRef] [PubMed]
31. Nazir, M.; Al-Ansari, A.; Al-Khalifa, K.; Alhareky, M.; Gaffar, B.; Almas, K. Global Prevalence of Periodontal Disease and Lack of Its Surveillance. *Sci. World J.* **2020**, *2020*, 1–8. [CrossRef] [PubMed]
32. Jordan, R.A.; Micheelis, W. *Fünfte Deutsche Mundgesundheitsstudie (DMS V)*, 1st ed.; Deutscher Zahnärzte Verlag DÄV: Köln, Germany, 2016; pp. 396–413.
33. Dorn, J.M.; Genco, R.J.; Grossi, S.G.; Falkner, K.L.; Hovey, K.M.; Iacoviello, L.; Trevisan, M. Periodontal Disease and Recurrent Cardiovascular Events in Survivors of Myocardial Infarction (MI): The Western New York Acute MI Study. *J. Periodontol.* **2010**, *81*, 502–511. [CrossRef]
34. Renvert, S.; Ohlsson, O.; Pettersson, T.; Persson, G.R. Periodontitis: A Future Risk of Acute Coronary Syndrome? A Follow-Up Study Over 3 Years. *J. Periodontol.* **2010**, *81*, 992–1000. [CrossRef]
35. Chu, D.; Bakaeen, F.G.; Wang, X.L.; Dao, T.K.; Lemaire, S.A.; Coselli, J.S.; Huh, J. The Impact of Peripheral Vascular Disease on Long-Term Survival After Coronary Artery Bypass Graft Surgery. *Ann. Thorac. Surg.* **2008**, *86*, 1175–1180. [CrossRef]
36. Van Straten, A.H.M.; Firanescu, C.; Soliman Hamad, M.A. Peripheral vascular disease as a predictor of survival after coronary artery bypass grafting: Comparison with a matched general population. *Ann. Thorac. Surg.* **2010**, *89*, 414–420. [CrossRef] [PubMed]
37. Herlitz, J.; Brandrup, G.; Haglid, M.; Karlson, B.; Albertsson, P.; Lurje, L.; Westberg, S.; Karlsson, T. Death, Mode of Death, Morbidity, and Rehospitalization after Coronary Artery Bypass Grafting in Relation to Occurrence of and Time Since a Previous Myocardial Infarction. *Thorac. Cardiovasc. Surg.* **1997**, *45*, 109–113. [CrossRef] [PubMed]
38. Batra, G.; Ahlsson, A.; Lindahl, B.; Lindhagen, L.; Wickbom, A.; Oldgren, J. Atrial fibrillation in patients undergoing coronary artery surgery is associated with adverse outcome. *Upsala J. Med Sci.* **2019**, *124*, 70–77. [CrossRef] [PubMed]
39. Fengsrud, E.; Englund, A.; Ahlsson, A. Pre- and postoperative atrial fibrillation in CABG patients have similar prognostic impact. *Scand. Cardiovasc. J.* **2016**, *51*, 21–27. [CrossRef]
40. Ngaage, D.L.; Schaff, H.V.; Mullany, C.J.; Sundt, T.M.; Dearani, J.A.; Barnes, S.; Daly, R.C.; Orszulak, T.A. Does preoperative atrial fibrillation influence early and late outcomes of coronary artery bypass grafting? *J. Thorac. Cardiovasc. Surg.* **2007**, *133*, 182–189. [CrossRef] [PubMed]
41. Schaefer, A.S.; Richter, G.M.; Groessner-Schreiber, B.; Noack, B.; Nothnagel, M.; El Mokhtari, N.-E.; Loos, B.G.; Jepsen, S.; Schreiber, S. Identification of a Shared Genetic Susceptibility Locus for Coronary Heart Disease and Periodontitis. *PLoS Genet.* **2009**, *5*, e1000378. [CrossRef] [PubMed]
42. Reichert, S.; Schulz, S.; Benten, A.C.; Lutze, A.; Seifert, T.; Schlitt, M.; Werdan, K.; Hofmann, B.; Wienke, A.; Schaller, H.G. Per-iodontal conditions and incidence of new cardiovascular events among patients with coronary vascular disease. *J. Clin. Periodontol.* **2016**, *43*, 918–925. [CrossRef]

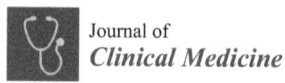

Review

Compromised Teeth Preserve or Extract: A Review of the Literature

Valentina Cárcamo-España [1,*], Nataly Cuesta Reyes [1], Paul Flores Saldivar [1], Eduardo Chimenos-Küstner [2], Alberto Estrugo Devesa [2] and José López-López [2,*]

[1] Department of Oral Medicine, Faculty of Medicine and Health Sciences (Dentistry), University of Barcelona Dental Hospital, University of Barcelona, 08907 Barcelona, Spain
[2] Department of Odontostomatology and Oral Medicine, Faculty of Medicine and Health Sciences (Dentistry), University of Barcelona Dental Hospital, University of Barcelona, 08907 Barcelona, Spain
* Correspondence: vcarcaes13@alumnes.ub.edu (V.C.-E.); 18575jll@gmail.com or jl.lopez@ub.edu (J.L.-L.); Tel.: +34-606-45-73-62 (J.L.-L.)

Abstract: Multiple systems and associated factors have been described in the literature to assess the prognosis of teeth with periodontal disease. Nowadays there is a tendency among clinicians to consider implants as the best solution after tooth extraction, in cases of teeth with a questionable prognosis. However, the value of the natural tooth must be considered, as the proprioception of the periodontal ligament is preserved, and it adapts to stress during functional loads. We first review the literature focusing on analyzing the factors that should guide decision-making to maintain or extract a tooth with a compromised periodontium. Then, we propose a schematic diagram of prognostic indicators to reflect the main factors to consider and the survival rate that each one represents when preserving or extracting a tooth.

Keywords: periodontal tissue; prognosis; permanent teeth; periodontal dentistry

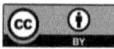

1. Introduction

Oral health care is an essential part of general health and provides people with an increased quality of life [1]. Tooth loss is a serious health problem that affects the functional abilities to chew and speak, psychology, aesthetics, and even social interaction [2]. There is currently no standardized tool to assess the general condition of a tooth and predict whether it is likely to have a long half-life [3].

Prognosis involves "the prediction of the course or outcome of an existing disease, based on empirical information, as well as the ability to recover from the disease" [4]. In dentistry, the predictive probability of dental mortality is based on the stability of the supporting tissues [5]. Various authors postulate that the prognosis is complex, established before treatment, and is supported by clinical and radiographic findings, as well as factors related to the patient, and general factors, such as the systemic condition (diabetes mellitus, smoking habit, motivation, and commitment of the patient) and local factors (factors anatomical, caries, furcation involvement, tooth mobility, periodontal support, pulp involvement, and bone loss) [4]. Prognosis is a dynamic process and should be reassessed, according to the progression of treatment and maintenance of the teeth [3,5].

Understanding the complexity of the prognosis in treatment planning would benefit both the patient and the professional when dealing with other patients facing the same clinical scenario. The development of uniform concepts will facilitate dental education and improve patient care [6].

In recent decades, scientific documentation has positioned implants as the first treatment option in edentulous patients, influencing the decision to extract periodontally compromised teeth [7–10]. In ref. [11], the authors also suggest that proactive or strategic extraction will prevent future bone destruction in a potential area for subsequent implant placement [11]. However, current evidence cannot always support decision-making, especially considering that any extracted tooth will result in alveolar bone resorption, which can occur despite the use of alveolar ridge preservation techniques or immediate implant placement [12–14].

On the other hand, the goal of periodontal therapy is the long-term retention of the natural tooth in a healthy, functional, aesthetically acceptable, and painless state [15]. By way of comparison, when an organ is compromised, measures are taken to prevent further damage or reverse it; however, when it involves a tooth, it is the patients and even some professionals who do not seem to value its preservation [16]. The option of retaining natural teeth, and adopting innovative and cost-effective restorative measures, can provide a practical, pragmatic, and predictable solution over time [17].

The comparison between the preservation of the natural tooth and the placement of an implant is difficult since implants should be considered as a treatment for tooth loss and not as a substitute for the tooth [12]. Clinicians are faced with the dilemma of whether to keep and treat a tooth or extract and replace it with a removable or partially fixed prosthesis. They are the ones who establish the prognosis and carry out the corresponding treatment under their criteria [6].

Based on the foregoing, it may be of interest to have a pattern of action against a tooth of doubtful prognosis; for this, it is important to decide between extracting or not extracting, so the objective of this review was to assess what factors should guide decision-making to maintain or extract a tooth with periodontal involvement with questionable prognosis, and to apply this criterion in a schematic diagram proposed by us.

2. Materials and Methods

An electronic search of the PubMed/MEDLINE database, Cochrane Library, and EBSCOhost (Medline, Cinahl) was performed, using the following search strategy: ((("periodontitis" [MeSH Terms]) AND ("prognosis" [MeSH Terms])) AND ("tooth" [MeSH Terms]), without the restriction of years, to compare the available evidence about the tooth with periodontal involvement and make treatment decisions based on its prognosis. A manual search for missing articles that might not have been found in the electronic and gray literature was performed on the references of the selected articles.

This review is carried out based on the PRISMA criteria, fulfilling 21 criteria [18]. The research question was formulated according to the following PICOS criteria: Patients = people with periodontal compromised teeth and questionable prognosis, Intervention = extract the teeth, Control = maintain the teeth, Outcome = prognosis factors and evaluate the evolution of the periodontally compromised teeth, and Study design = literature review.

Articles related to teeth with periodontal involvement and unfavorable or poor prognosis and clinical studies (observational, descriptive, clinical case reports) in English or Spanish were included in the review. In contrast, animal studies, in-vitro studies, and literature reviews were excluded. The data of the included studies (when available) were collected by three independent authors (V.C.-E., N.C.R. and P.F.S.): authors, year, place where the study was carried out, number of subjects, mean age with standard deviation, sex, design of the study, type of periodontitis [19] (aggressive: $\leq$35 years during the first test of the establishment of the disease with attachment loss $\geq$5 mm and bone loss $\geq$50% in more than 2 sites; chronic: $\geq$10 years during the first test of the establishment of the disease [moderate: 3–4 mm attachment loss and 30–50% bone loss; severe: >5 mm probing depth, >50% bone loss and grade 2 and 3 mobility]), number of teeth with periodontitis, rate of survival or prognosis, factors associated with treatment decision-making, and follow-up (in months). Finally, the information was validated by J.L.-L.

The articles were analyzed for risk of bias using the Newcastle Ottawa Scale (NOS), for the evaluation of cross-sectional studies.

3. Results

The review was carried out from December 2021 to February 2022, both months included. The electronic search in PubMed/MEDLINE, Cochrane Library, EBSCOhost, and a manual search in the bibliography of the selected articles provided 16 articles that met the inclusion criteria [19–34] (Figure 1) (Tables 1 and 2). Most of the articles were observational cross-sectional studies [18–24,28–30] and seven were clinical case reports [25–27,31–34]. The main inclusion criteria of the studies reviewed were that patients diagnosed with periodontitis present records from the initial examination, in addition to an accurate periodontal record of the initial condition, immediately after treatment and annually during the maintenance phase. They evaluated the long-term survival of periodontally compromised teeth and associated factors, in patients treated and in periodontal maintenance, including changes in probing depth (mild: 1–3 mm, moderate: 4–6 mm, and severe $\geq$7 mm), bleeding (mild: <11%, moderate: 11–15% and severe: >15%), and bacterial plaque index (mild: <1, moderate: 1–1.5 and severe: >1.5).

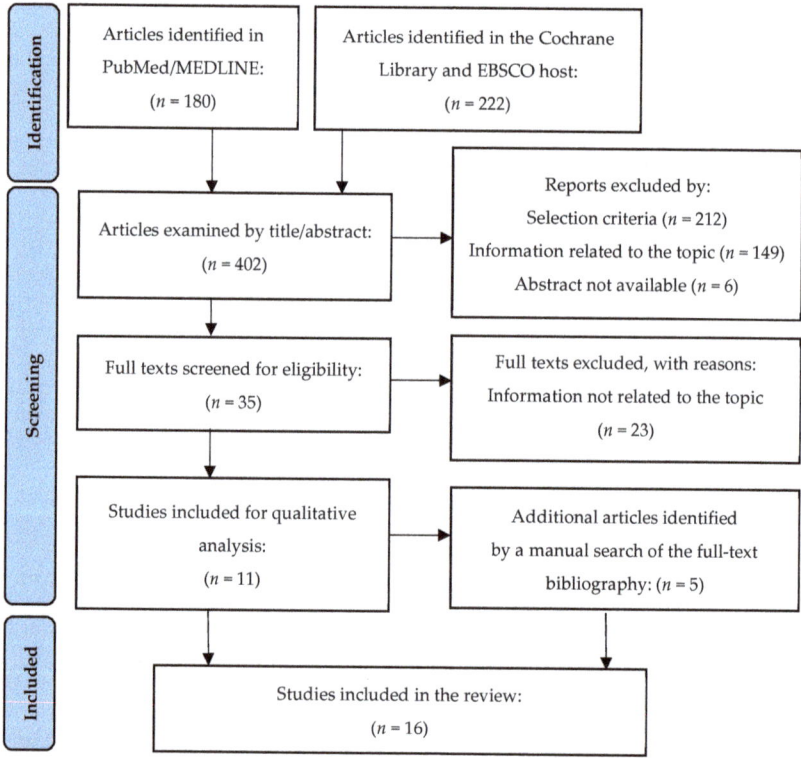

Figure 1. Flowchart showing the synthesis of the bibliographic search, according to the PRISMA guidelines.

Table 1. Summary of observational studies evaluated.

Author/Year/Country	Design/Follow-Up (Months)	No. Patients/Gender/Age (Years)	No. Teeth/Type of Tooth/Type of Periodontitis/Prognosis	Factors Associated with Decision-Making	Reason for Extracting/Preserving
Saminsky, M. et al. (2015) Israel [30]	Cross-sectional 152 ± 25	50 31F/19M 46.6 ± 10.6	1301 M-Pm-C-I ChP NS	Probing depth General health status Smoking habit Periodontal diagnosis Bacterial plaque index Bleeding on probing	151 extracted (96 periodontal causes/55 extensive caries or root fracture)
Goh, V. et al. (2017) China [22]	Cross-sectional 100.4 ± 44.4	65 34F/31M 43.8 ± 11.9	1597 M-Pm-C-I AgP-ChP Good (pdep ≤4 mm)-Fair (pdep ≥5 mm)-Questionable (pdep 6–8 mm), Hopeless (pdep ≥8 mm)-Undetermined	General health status Oral hygiene Use of removable prosthesis Smoking habit Dental visit history Number of teeth Bacterial plaque index Bleeding on probing Probing depth Bone crest level	229 extracted (191 periodontal reasons/23 caries/15 not identifiable by the patient)
De Beule, F. et al. (2017) Belgium [21]	Cross-sectional 197	402 201F/201M 34–88	2559 M* SevP NS	Medical condition Probing Depth Furca engagement Bone loss Gum health Bleeding on probing Tooth type Tooth location	511 extracted (377 periodontal reasons/60 endodontic problems or endo-periodontal lesions/17 fracture/25 caries/1 prosthetic strategy/31 unknown reason)
D'Aiuto, F. et al. (2005) England [20]	Cross-sectional 6	94 50F/44M 46 ± 9	2589 M-Pm-C-I SevP NS	Probing depth Gingival recessions Bacterial plaque index Bleeding on probing Clinical insertion level Furca engagement Tooth mobility Tooth type Smoking habit Periodontal diagnosis	NS

Table 1. Cont.

Author/Year/Country	Design/Follow-Up (Months)	No. Patients/Gender/Age (Years)	No. Teeth/Type of Tooth/Type of Periodontitis/Prognosis	Factors Associated with Decision-Making	Reason for Extracting/Preserving
Graetz, C. et al. (2017) Germany [24]	Cross-sectional 208.8 ± 57.6	57 35F/22M 34.7 ± 8	1505 M-Pm-C-I AgP NS	Probing depth Tooth mobility Radiographic bone loss Furca engagement Smoking habit Tooth type Preoperative antibiotic therapy	232 extracted (prosthetic and periodontal reasons)
Machtei, E. & Hirsch, I. (2007) Israel [28]	Cross-sectional 156	93 59F/34M 45.54 ± 1.13	110 (74 multirooted/36 single root) ChP Hopeless	Probing depth Radiographic bone loss	53 extracted 57 saved (the decision was made by the patient without influence from the dentist)
Bäumer, A. et al. (2011) Germany [19]	Cross-sectional 126	84 68F/16M 30.8 ± 4.1	2154 M*-Pm-C-I AgP NS	Smoking habit History of periodontal disease Dental status Probing depth ≥5 mm Clinical insertion level Bleeding on probing Suppuration on probing Furca engagement Gingival index Bacterial plaque index Educational level Dental care compliance	166 extracted (unknown reason)
Graetz, C. et al. (2011) Germany [23]	Cross-sectional 193 ± 54	68 (34AgP/34ChP) 28F (11AgP/17ChP) 40M (23AgP/17ChP) 33.3 ± 4.1AgP 51.6 ± 7.4ChP	923AgP/874ChP M-Pm-C-I AgP-ChP Good (bone loss <50%)-Questionable (bone loss ≥50%-<70%)-Hopeless (bone loss ≥70%)	Smoking habit Radiographic bone loss ≥50% Probing depth Bacterial plaque index Preoperative antibiotic therapy	142AgP extracted 133ChP extracted (112AgP-48ChP periodontal reasons/the rest due to endodontic involvement, caries, prosthetics, fracture, or unknown reason)

Table 1. Cont.

Author/Year/Country	Design/Follow-Up (Months)	No. Patients/Gender/Age (Years)	No. Teeth/Type of Tooth/Type of Periodontitis/Prognosis	Factors Associated with Decision-Making	Reason for Extracting/Preserving
Martinez-Canut, P. (2015) Spain [29]	Cross-sectional 242.4 ± 28.8	500 344F/156M 22-74	12.830 M*-Pm-C-I AgP-ChP NS	Health condition Smoking habit Bacterial plaque index Probing depth >6 mm Gum recession Furca engagement Tooth mobility 2-3 Radiographic bone loss >50% Root crown ratio 1/1 Root anatomy Periodontal diagnosis	875 extracted (515 periodontal disease/172 non-restorable caries/75 root and/or coronary fracture/26 endodontic complications/85 strategic extraction for prosthetic and orthodontic considerations)

F: female, M: male, AgP: aggressive periodontitis, ChP: chronic periodontitis, SevP: severe periodontitis, EndP: endoperiodontal injury, M: molar tooth, M*: except third molar, Pm: premolar tooth, C: canine tooth, I: incisive tooth, MxLI: maxillary lateral incisor, MdCI: mandibular central incisor, pdep: probing depth, NS: not specified.

Table 2. Summary of clinical case reports evaluated.

Author/Year/Country	Design/Follow-Up (Months)	No. Patients/Gender/Age (Years)	No. Teeth/Type of Tooth/Type of Periodontitis/Prognosis	Factors Associated with Decision-Making	Reason for Extracting/Preserving
Grigorie, M.M. et al. (2021) Romania [25]	Case report 48	1 1F 62	27 M-Pm-C-I ChP Hopeless (pdep >8 mm, with class II or higher furcation involvement and bone loss ≥70%).	Smoking habit Probing depth ≥5 mm Bony vertical defects Furca engagement Tooth mobility Bacterial plaque index Tooth migration Reduced periodontal support Infrabony defect	1 extracted (caries and endodontic complications)

119

Table 2. Cont.

Author/Year/Country	Design/Follow-Up (Months)	No. Patients/Gender/Age (Years)	No. Teeth/Type of Tooth/Type of Periodontitis/Prognosis	Factors Associated with Decision-Making	Reason for Extracting/Preserving
Kavarthapu, A. & Malaiappan, S. (2019) India [27]	Case report 9	1 1F 28	1 M AgP Bad	Probing depth >8 mm Bleeding on probing Bacterial plaque index Grade II furcation involvement Vertical bone loss Purulent discharge Tooth mobility grade 2 Negative pulp vitality Apical radiolucency	The tooth was saved (patient compliance)
Seshima, F. et al. (2016) Japan [31]	Case report 14	1 1M 66	27 M-Pm-C-I ChP NS	Probing depth ≥7 mm Bone loss Bleeding on probing Bacterial plaque index Blood glucose levels Tooth mobility	1 extracted (prophylactic reasons: impacted tooth)
Zafiropoulos, G.G.K. et al. (2011) Germany [33]	Case report 180/84	2 1F/1M 33/39	28/26 M-Pm-C-I ChP NS	Probing depth Bleeding on probing Bacterial plaque index Furca engagement Radiographic bone loss ≥50% Tooth mobility Clinical insertion level Periodontal pathogens	Case 1: all were preserved (the patient rejects any extraction); Case 2: 21 extracted (advanced bone loss and/or dental mobility)
Zucchelli, G. (2007) Italy [34]	Case report 12–36	1 1F 39	1 MxLI EndP NS	Probing Depth Bacterial plaque index Bleeding on probing Clinical insertion level Gingival recession ≥3 mm Bone loss Tooth mobility grade 3 Radiographic radiolucency Negative vitality test Absence of fillings	53 extracted (43 multirooted/10 single root); 57 saved (31 multirooted/26 single root) (unknown reason)

Table 2. Cont.

Author/Year/Country	Design/Follow-Up (Months)	No. Patients/Gender/Age (Years)	No. Teeth/Type of Tooth/Type of Periodontitis/Prognosis	Factors Associated with Decision-Making	Reason for Extracting/Preserving
Tözüm, T.F. et al. (2006) Turkey [32]	Case report 18	1 1M 42	1 MdCI ChP NS	Bacterial plaque index Clinical attachment level ≥6 mm Tooth mobility grade 3 Negative vitality test Probing depth ≥4 mm Radiographic bone loss Extrusion Keratinized gingiva ≥2 mm	1 saved (upon advice from the dentist to consider a new treatment option)
Kamma, J.J. & Baehni, P.C. (2003) Greece [26]	Case report 60	25 14F/11M 34.3 ± 2.5	NS NS AgP NS	Smoking habit Bacterial plaque index Gingival index Bleeding on probing Suppuration on probing Probing depth Clinical insertion level Radiographic bone loss	29 extracted (18 due to furca involvement/the rest unknown reason)

121

A total of 1.445 patients were examined (Table 3), with an age range of 22–88 years. There was a total of 868 women (60.06%) and 577 men (39.93%). Not all studies evaluated the prognosis of teeth with periodontal involvement (31.25%); however, 14 articles (87.5%) mentioned the reasons for deciding whether to extract or preserve it. Of a total of 26.553 teeth with periodontal involvement, 2.597 were extracted, with the periodontal cause being the most common reason (1.610 teeth [61.99%]), followed by prosthetic reasons (455 teeth [17.52%]) such as caries or crown/root fracture, endodontic complications (86 teeth [3.31%]), and due to unknown or unidentifiable causes by the patient (446 teeth [17.17%]). Thus, 23.956 teeth were preserved, including 144 initially scheduled for extraction. Of these 144 teeth that were preserved, 87 (60.41%) of the patients played a main role in changing the prognosis and making decisions in the final treatment, followed by 57 teeth (39.58%) where the reason was unknown.

Table 3. Summary of demographic data and teeth evaluated.

Variable		Total
Gender	Women	868 (60.06%)
	Men	577 (39.93%)
Total patients		1.445
Age range		22–88 years
Total teeth examined		26.553
Teeth extracted		2.597
Periodontal reasons		1.610 (61.99%)
Prosthetic reasons		455 (17.52%
Endodontic complications		86 (3.31%)
Unknown or unidentifiable reason		446 (17.17%)
Teeth preserved (no initial commitment)		23.812
Teeth preserved (with initial commitment)		144
The patient made the final decision		87 (60.41%)
Unknown or unidentifiable reason		57 (39.58%)

In relation to the type of periodontal disease, chronic periodontitis was the most common diseases (nine articles [22,23,25,28–33]), followed by aggressive periodontitis (seven articles [19,22–24,26,27,29]. Only two of the articles [20,21] mentioned that the patients had severe periodontitis. Finally, of the 16 articles selected, only 5 [22,23,25,27,28] mentioned establishing a prognosis before determining treatment, and the longest follow-up time was 242.4 ± 28.8 months [29].

Among the factors considered prior to making the decision to retain or extract a tooth and subsequent treatment planning, the most common was probing depth ≥ 5 mm (16 articles [18–33]), followed by the bacterial plaque index (13 articles [19,20,22,23,25–27,29–34]), bleeding on probing (9 articles [19–22,26,27,30,31,34]), smoking >5 years and consumption of ≥ 10 cigarettes/day (9 articles [19,20,22–26,29,30], grade 2 and 3 tooth mobility (9 articles [20,24,25,27,29,31–34], and class II and III furcation involvement (8 articles [19–21,24,25,27,29,33].

We analyzed the nine cross-sectional observational studies with the Newcastle Ottawa Scale (NOS) (Table 4) and observed that one study had a high risk of bias (50%), three studies had a moderate risk of bias (25%), and five studies had a low risk of bias (0.0–12.5%). In the seven clinical case reports, an assessment of the quality of the evidence was not applied, since blinding of participants and personnel (performance bias) and blinding of outcome assessment (detection bias) were not applicable, associated with incomplete outcome data (attrition bias) and selective reporting (reporting bias).

Table 4. The table shows the risk of bias criteria using the adapted Newcastle Ottawa Scale (NOS) for cross-sectional studies. If the criterion is met, a green dot is placed in the box, otherwise, if it is not met, a red dot is placed. Studies with a total score of 7 or 8 green points were considered a low risk of bias; 6 green dots were considered to be at medium risk of bias; 5 green dots or less were judged to be at high risk of bias.

Item	Saminsky, M. et al., 2015 [30]	Goh, V. et al., 2017 [22]	De Beule, F. et al., 2017 [21]	D'Aiuto, F. et al., 2005 [20]	Graetz, C. et al., 2017 [24]	Machtei, E. & Hirsch, I., 2007 [28]	Bäumer, A. et al., 2011 [19]	Graetz, C. et al., 2011 [23]	Martinez-Canut, P., 2015 [29]
Selection									
1. Is the sample representative of the target average population?	🟢	🟢	🟢	🟠	🟢	🟢	🟢	🟢	🟢
2. Was the sample size justified and satisfactory?	🟢	🟢	🟢	🟠	🟢	🟢	🟢	🟠	🟢
3. It was established which subjects would be included and was the inclusion range satisfactory?	🟢	🟢	🟢	🟢	🟢	🟢	🟢	🟢	🟢
Comparability									
1. Were anthropometric measurements adequately adjusted for age and gender?	🟠	🟢	🟢	🟠	🟢	🟠	🟢	🟢	🟠
2. Were other factors such as race/ethnicity, educational level, habits, probing depth, survival rate, etc. adequately adjusted?	🟠	🟢	🟢	🟢	🟢	🟢	🟢	🟢	🟢
Results									
1. Was the result established independently and with data linkage?	🟢	🟢	🟢	🟢	🟢	🟢	🟢	🟢	🟢
2. Was the result determined by a self-report?	🟢	🟢	🟢	🟢	🟢	🟢	🟢	🟢	🟢
3. The statistical test used to analyze the information is clearly described and appropriate, and the measures of the association presented include confidence intervals and level of probability (*p*-value)?	🟢	🟢	🟢	🟢	🟢	🟢	🟢	🟢	🟢
Total	6	6	7	4	6	7	7	8	7

4. Discussion

The decision to keep or extract a periodontally compromised tooth with a hopeless or questionable prognosis is not always easy to predict. Assigning a long-term prognosis is critical, particularly in the dilemma of performing appropriate rehabilitative treatments after periodontal therapy, especially if it involves major prosthetic rehabilitation or implant placement [35]. Lundgren, D. et al. postulate that postponing the insertion of implants in patients susceptible to periodontitis should be considered strategically, optimizing the longevity of the natural dentitions [36] and facilitating a global solution that can reduce the risks of long-term implant treatment [37]. It has been shown that in teeth with a hopeless prognosis or with an indication for extraction, after periodontal treatment, it is possible to stop the progression of the disease to a certain extent and minimize or even prevent tooth loss [12,20,22,24,30]. We must consider that the population is aging, and patients no longer accept removable dentures; they expect that the dentist's knowledge and skills will allow them to maintain healthy mouths as they age [38]. That is why the demands of the patient must be taken into consideration, but it is the clinician who establishes the treatment plan, in favor or against preserving the tooth. The patient must be fully and adequately informed to have their consent.

After reviewing the selected articles, the decision to keep or extract a tooth depends on several factors, such as the patient's expectations, control of diabetes mellitus, socioeconomic level, age, oral hygiene, depth of periodontal probing, tooth mobility, root anomalies, furcation involvement, commitment to periodontal treatment and maintenance programs, extensive caries, smoking habit, among others [39,40]. Samet, N. et al. [3] established that the risk factors are divided into biological (systemic condition associated with the immune system and healing, alteration of salivary flow, special needs limiting oral hygiene, high count of *Streptococcus mutans* and *Lactobacillus*, family history, missing teeth), behavior (poor oral hygiene or compromised diet, cariogenic diet, low exposure to fluoride, parafunctional habits, commitment and willingness to adhere to a long-term maintenance protocol, smoking habit), and financial/personal (motivation during treatment, economic resources, time availability, attitude to tooth loss, knowledge about its condition and necessary treatments, aesthetic expectations). For example, in the study by Saminsky, M., et al. [30], the main reason when deciding whether or not the tooth should be extracted was periodontal causes; 11.7% of teeth with periodontal pockets of 4–6 mm and 37.7% with $\geq$7 mm were extracted ($p < 0.001$). Most patients (32 of 50) received two or more periodontal support treatments per year and multi-rooted teeth (17.9%) showed a higher risk of being extracted compared to single-rooted teeth (3.6%; $p < 0.001$). Among the patient characteristics, it was observed that age is strongly related to tooth loss, especially in patients $\geq$60 years old (13.9% present risk of extraction; $p < 0.001$). Goh, V., et al. [22] found similar results: sites with probing depth $\geq$6 mm were positively associated with tooth loss ($p < 0.002$), presenting a greater association when treatment was interrupted for several years ($p < 0.001$).

In this review, several articles postulate various treatment options. However, there are no randomized clinical trials available in the dental literature comparing fixed prostheses in teeth with questionable prognoses with fixed prostheses on implants. In addition, an exact comparison is not possible since each tooth is unique and determined by particular factors. For example, in the study by Tözüm, T.F. et al. [32], after performing the endodontic and periodontal treatment of the compromised tooth, the pain subsided, but the mobility persisted (grade 3). Subsequently, the extraction and intentional reimplantation were carried out, applying an autologous platelet gel inside the alveolus. This allowed a significant gain in clinical attachment level and alveolar bone level, and a total reduction in tooth mobility was observed after 18 months, without observing ankylosis or root resorption.

Another factor previously mentioned is that periodontal support therapy is considered to play an important role in tooth preservation, but the cost and efforts involved are rarely considered [41]. Progression of periodontal disease and reinfection of sites, as well as tooth loss, are possible, especially in patients susceptible to periodontitis [12]. Several factors can affect periodontal healing, such as the presence of morphological defects (a three-walled intraosseous defect will heal better than a one- or two-walled defect), tooth mobility, tissue graft treatments, dentist skills, and level of commitment of the patient [38]. In the study by Graetz, C. et al. [24], after periodontal therapy, the initial mean probing depth was 5.8 ± 2.1 mm and decreased to 3.5 ± 1.1 mm; patients who received adjuvant antibiotic therapy due to persistent inflammation showed an initially greater probing depth of 6.35 ± 2.42 mm and bone loss of >70% in 12.5% (70 teeth).

The fate of a tooth is usually influenced by the treatment planning that involves the entire dentition and the patient's preferences, with the decision to extract or maintain it largely depending on the dentist, based on their experience and clinical judgment [39,42,43]. To achieve the ideal treatment, there are several factors to be considered during the treatment planning process. These factors include the main demand of the patient; an adequate analysis of the cost-benefit; and risks associated with oral hygiene, tobacco history, and periodontal disease [44]. Su, H. et al. consider that the factor that seems to have the greatest impact on treatment planning is the level of training of the dentist [6]. Clinicians with more than 15 years of experience prefer to perform extractions more frequently than clinicians with less than 5 years of experience [45]. On the other hand, Baba, N.Z. et al. postulate that the treatment decision should be based on satisfying the patient's wishes and on the importance of evaluating each tooth individually to obtain the treatment with the best result in terms of aesthetics, comfort, function, and cost-effectiveness [46]. In the study by Zafiropoulos, G.G.K., et al. [33], no tooth was extracted in one of the treated patients, since he refused any extraction, opting for 6-monthly maintenance. During the last 4 years of follow-up, the multirooted teeth lost an average of 7.3 mm of clinical attachment, while in the rest of the teeth the loss was only 0.3–0.4 mm. Multirooted teeth with class III furcation involvement had a survival of 8 years.

The placement of implants to replace extracted teeth should be considered acceptable in the case of non-restorable teeth or patients with recurrent periodontal disease, with recurrences after periodontal treatment [46]. Only when the periodontal condition is stabilized and adequate bacterial plaque control is obtained, can the placement of implants be planned as an integral part of the rehabilitation [38]. This should be based on two levels of risk: (1) patient-level: gingival bleeding, the prevalence of residual pockets ≥ 5 mm, number of missing teeth, loss of attachment/support of the bone level concerning the patient's age, systemic and genetic condition [46,47], and environmental factors, such as smoking; (2) site level: the presence of residual periapical lesions, alveolar bone height and quality, gingival biotype, the proximity of the anatomical structure, and condition of neighboring teeth (residual periodontal pockets, gingival bleeding and suppuration, tooth anatomy and position, compromise of furca, presence of iatrogenic factors and tooth mobility) [12,48].

It is necessary to expand research related to periodontal and dental prognosis, establish the dental condition at all times, and develop evidence-based treatment strategies [35]. In some cases, it is necessary to integrate the areas of endodontics, periodontics, and orthodontics, to maintain teeth without changing the long-term prognosis [43,49]. When deciding between keeping or replacing a tooth affected by periodontitis, it is important to consider our ability to understand and treat possible future diseases, such as peri-implantitis [44], in which treatment cannot be guaranteed to be predictable [12]. Therefore, it should be discussed whether or not a tooth with a periodontal disease without major restorative treatments should be extracted, assess the potential for success in periodontal treatment, and seriously question the advisability of replacing the tooth [44].

Another factor to consider is tooth extraction for aesthetic reasons, which will only be considered if the prosthetic restoration can significantly improve the aesthetic result and the satisfaction of the patient's expectations (a key component in the planning of all treatments) [12]. Retaining a tooth may be advantageous in the presence of a thin biotype, unfavorable interproximal bone, or in the presence of a long-standing adjacent implant. It is likely that, after extraction of the tooth with periodontal compromise, the interdental papilla is not present, especially when the distance between the interproximal bone and the proximal contact is greater than 5 mm (>4 mm in thin biotype and >5 mm in thick biotype) [46]. The type of tooth and its position must also be considered; in particular, the molars show less improvement, associated with the complexity of the root anatomy. Martinez-Canut, P. [29] determined that the type of tooth is significantly associated with the risk of tooth loss due to periodontal disease ($p < 0.001$). The risk was multiplied by two in maxillary canines, maxillary incisors, and mandibular lateral incisors; and by seven in maxillary premolars, mandibular central incisors, mandibular canines, and mandibular premolars. In addition, the mandibular first molar was 2.5 times less likely to be lost than the rest of the molars. On the other hand, the absence of adjacent teeth contributed to a better result in teeth with periodontal compromise, since it facilitated the control of bacterial plaque, which must be considered clinically when deciding to extract or maintain a tooth under these conditions [50,51].

The evidence reflects that the decision to keep or extract a tooth must be multifactorial since it is an irreversible process. The periodontal status and the restorability of the affected tooth should be highlighted as the main factors for prognosis. Taking as reference the publications of Avila, G. et al., 2009 [39] and Nunn, M.E. et al., 2012 [35], we propose a schematic diagram of the prognostic indicators, which reflects the factors to be considered and the survival rate that each one represents, when deciding to keep or extract a tooth (Figure 2).

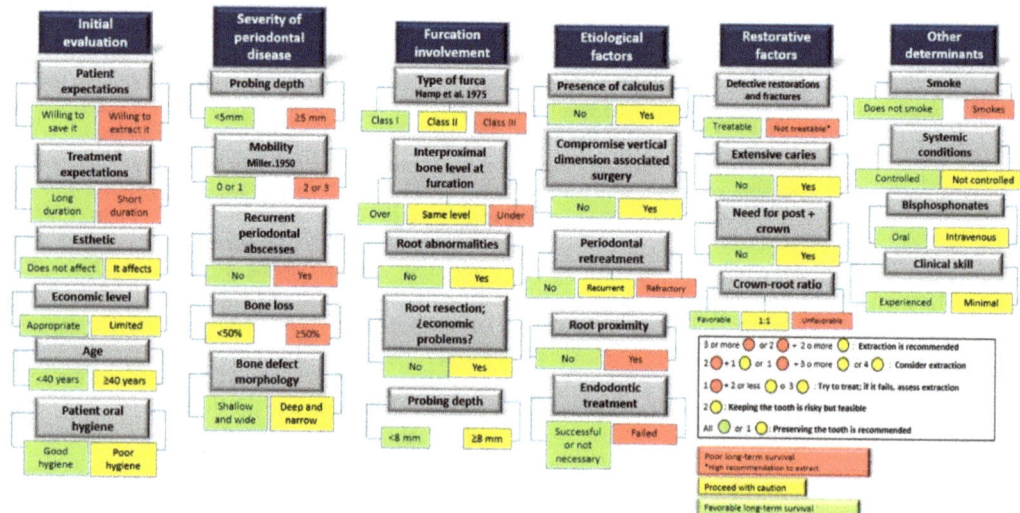

Figure 2. Schematic diagram of the main factors that should guide decision-making to maintain or extract a tooth from a periodontal point of view. Based, with modifications made by the authors, on the schemes initially proposed by Avila, G. et al., 2009 [39]; Nunn, M.E. et al., 2012 [35].

5. Conclusions

In short, and by way of summary, the factors that should guide decision-making to maintain or extract a periodontally compromised tooth include both general patient factors and individual factors of dentition. General factors include biological risk factors, behavioral risk factors, and personal/financial risk factors. Among the individual factors of dentition, we can distinguish periodontal, aesthetic, restorative/endodontic, and prosthetic factors.

Author Contributions: Conceptualization, J.L.-L. and V.C.-E.; investigation, V.C.-E., N.C.R. and P.F.S.; methodology, V.C.-E., N.C.R. and P.F.S.; data curation, V.C.-E.; validation, J.L.-L.; writing—original draft preparation, V.C.-E.; writing—review and editing, V.C.-E., J.L.-L. and E.C.-K.; supervision, J.L.-L., E.C.-K. and A.E.D. All authors have read and agreed to the published version of the manuscript.

Funding: This research received no external funding.

Institutional Review Board Statement: The study was conducted following the Declaration of Helsinki and approved by the Institutional Review Board (or Ethics Committee) of the University of Barcelona.

Informed Consent Statement: Informed consent was obtained from all subjects involved in the study.

Data Availability Statement: Not applicable.

Conflicts of Interest: The authors declare no conflict of interest.

References

1. Polzer, I.; Schimmel, M.; Müller, F.; Biffar, R. Edentulism as part of the general health problems of elderly adults. *Int. Dent. J.* **2010**, *60*, 143–155. [PubMed]
2. De Melo, M.A.; Lino, P.A.; Dos Santos, T.R.; Vasconcelos, M.; Lucas, S.D.; de Abreu, M.H. A 15-year time-series study of tooth extraction in brazil. *Medicine* **2015**, *94*, e1924.

3. Samet, N.; Jotkowitz, A. Classification and prognosis evaluation of individual teeth—A comprehensive approach. *Quintessence Int.* **2009**, *40*, 377–387. [PubMed]
4. Beck, J.D. Risk revisited. *Community Dent. Oral Epidemiol.* **1998**, *26*, 220–225. [CrossRef] [PubMed]
5. Kwok, V.; Caton, J.G. Commentary: Prognosis revisited: A system for assigning periodontal prognosis. *J. Periodontol.* **2007**, *78*, 2063–2071. [CrossRef] [PubMed]
6. Su, H.; Liao, H.; Fiorellini, J.P.; Kim, S. Factors affecting treatment planning decisions for compromised anterior teeth. *Int. J. Periodontics Restor. Dent.* **2014**, *34*, 389–398.
7. Greenstein, G.; Greenstein, B.; Cavallaro, J. Prerequisite for treatment planning implant dentistry: Periodontal prognostication of compromised teeth. *Compend. Contin. Educ. Dent.* **2007**, *28*, 436–446.
8. Pjetursson, B.E.; Tan, W.C.; Tan, K.; Brägger, U.; Zwahlen, M.; Lang, N.P. A systematic review of the survival and complication rates of resin-bonded bridges after an observation period of at least 5 years. *Clin. Oral Implants Res.* **2008**, *19*, 131–141. [CrossRef]
9. Carlsson, G.E. Critical review of some dogmas in prosthodontics. *J. Prosthodont. Res.* **2009**, *53*, 3–10. [CrossRef] [PubMed]
10. Lekholm, U.; Gunne, J.; Henry, P.; Higuchi, K.; Lindén, U.; Bergström, C. Survival of the brånemark implant in partially edentulous jaws: A 10-year prospective multicenter study. *Int. J. Oral Maxillofac. Implants.* **1999**, *14*, 639–645.
11. Kao, R.T. Strategic extraction: A paradigm shift that is changing our profession. *J. Periodontol.* **2008**, *79*, 971–977. [CrossRef] [PubMed]
12. Donos, N.; Laurell, L.; Mardas, N. Hierarchical decisions on teeth vs. implants in the periodontitis-susceptible patient: The modern dilemma. *Periodontol. 2000* **2012**, *59*, 89–110. [CrossRef] [PubMed]
13. Araújo, M.G.; Sukekava, F.; Wennström, J.L.; Lindhe, J. Tissue modeling following implant placement in fresh extraction sockets. *Clin. Oral Implant. Res.* **2006**, *17*, 615–624. [CrossRef]
14. Botticelli, D.; Berglundh, T.; Lindhe, J. Hard-tissue alterations following immediate implant placement in extraction sites. *J. Clin. Periodontol.* **2004**, *31*, 820–828. [CrossRef] [PubMed]
15. Hirschfeld, L.; Wasserman, B. A long-term survey of tooth loss in 600 treated periodontal patients. *J. Periodontol.* **1978**, *49*, 225–237. [CrossRef] [PubMed]
16. Park, H.; Song, H.Y.; Han, K.; Cho, K.; Kim, Y. Number of remaining teeth and health–related quality of life: The korean national health and nutrition examination survey 2010–2012. *Health Qual. Life Outcomes* **2019**, *17*, 1–10. [CrossRef]
17. Meyers, I.A. Herodontics–is there a place for maintaining the apparently hopeless tooth? *Aust. Dent. J.* **2019**, *64*, S71–S79. [CrossRef]
18. Page, M.J.; Moher, D.; Bossuyt, P.M.; Boutron, I.; Hoffmann, T.C.; Mulrow, C.D.; Shamseer, L.; Tetzlaff, J.M.; Akl, E.A.; Brennan, S.E.; et al. PRISMA 2020 explanation and elaboration: Updated guidance and exemplars for reporting systematic reviews. *BMJ* **2021**, *29*, 372. [CrossRef]
19. Bäumer, A.; El Sayed, N.; Kim, T.; Reitmeir, P.; Eickholz, P.; Pretzl, B. Patient-related risk factors for tooth loss in aggressive periodontitis after active periodontal therapy. *J. Clin. Periodontol.* **2011**, *38*, 347–354. [CrossRef]
20. D'Aiuto, F.; Ready, D.; Parkar, M.; Tonetti, M.S. Relative contribution of patient-, tooth-, and site-associated variability on the clinical outcomes of subgingival debridement. I. probing depths. *J. Periodontol.* **2005**, *76*, 398–405. [CrossRef]
21. De Beule, F.; Alsaadi, G.; Perić, M.; Brecx, M. Periodontal treatment and maintenance of molars affected with severe periodontitis (DPSI = 4): An up to 27-year retrospective study in a private practice. *Quintessence Intl.* **2017**, *48*, 391–405.
22. Goh, V.; Hackmack, P.P.; Corbet, E.F.; Leung, W.K. Moderate-to long-term periodontal outcomes of subjects failing to complete a course of periodontal therapy. *Aust. Dent. J.* **2017**, *62*, 152–160. [CrossRef] [PubMed]
23. Graetz, C.; Dörfer, C.E.; Kahl, M.; Kocher, T.; Fawzy El-Sayed, K.; Wiebe, J.F.; Gomer, K.; Rühling, A. Retention of questionable and hopeless teeth in compliant patients treated for aggressive periodontitis. *J. Clin. Periodontol.* **2011**, *38*, 707–714. [CrossRef] [PubMed]
24. Graetz, C.; Sälzer, S.; Plaumann, A.; Schlattmann, P.; Kahl, M.; Springer, C.; Dörfer, C.; Schwendicke, F. Tooth loss in generalized aggressive periodontitis: Prognostic factors after 17 years of supportive periodontal treatment. *J. Clin. Periodontol.* **2017**, *44*, 612–619. [CrossRef]
25. Grigorie, M.M.; Suciu, I.; Zaharia, D.; Ionescu, E.; Chirila, M.; Voiculeanu, M. Hopeless tooth? prognosis and comprehensive treatment. A case report. *J. Med. Life* **2021**, *14*, 287–294. [CrossRef]
26. Kamma, J.J.; Baehni, P.C. Five-year maintenance follow-up of early-onset periodontitis patients. *J. Clin. Periodontol.* **2003**, *30*, 562–572. [CrossRef]
27. Kavarthapu, A.; Malaiappan, S. Management of periodontic–endodontic lesion in aggressive periodontitis-9 months follow-up: Report of a case. *Indian J. Dent. Res.* **2019**, *30*, 149–153.
28. Machtei, E.E.; Hirsch, I. Retention of hopeless teeth: The effect on the adjacent proximal bone following periodontal surgery. *J. Periodontol.* **2007**, *78*, 2246–2252. [CrossRef]
29. Martinez-Canut, P. Predictors of tooth loss due to periodontal disease in patients following long-term periodontal maintenance. *J. Clin. Periodontol.* **2015**, *42*, 1115–1125. [CrossRef]
30. Saminsky, M.; Halperin-Sternfeld, M.; Machtei, E.E.; Horwitz, J. Variables affecting tooth survival and changes in probing depth: A long-term follow-up of periodontitis patients. *J. Clin. Periodontol.* **2015**, *42*, 513–519. [CrossRef]
31. Seshima, F.; Nishina, M.; Namba, T.; Saito, A. Periodontal regenerative therapy in patient with chronic periodontitis and type 2 diabetes mellitus: A case report. *Bull. Tokyo Dent. Coll.* **2016**, *57*, 97–104. [CrossRef] [PubMed]

32. Tözüm, T.F.; Keçeli, H.G.; Serper, A.; Tuncel, B. Intentional replantation for a periodontally involved hopeless incisor by using autologous platelet-rich plasma. *Oral Surg. Oral Med. Oral Pathol. Oral Radiol. Endod.* **2006**, *101*, e119–e124. [CrossRef] [PubMed]
33. Zafiropoulos, G.K.; di Prisco, M.O.; Deli, G.; Hoffmann, O. Maintenance of class III trifurcated molars versus implant placement in regenerated extraction sockets: Long-term results of 2 cases. *J. Oral Implantol.* **2011**, *37*, 141–155. [CrossRef] [PubMed]
34. Zucchelli, G. Long-term maintenance of an apparently hopeless tooth: A case report. *Eur. J. Esthet. Dent.* **2007**, *2*, 390–404.
35. Nunn, M.E.; Fan, J.; Su, X.; Levine, R.A.; Lee, H.; McGuire, M.K. Development of prognostic indicators using classification and regression trees for survival. *Periodontol. 2000* **2012**, *58*, 134–142. [CrossRef]
36. Lundgren, D.; Rylander, H.; Laurell, L. To save or to extract, that is the question. natural teeth or dental implants in periodontitis-susceptible patients: Clinical decision-making and treatment strategies exemplified with patient case presentations. *Periodontol. 2000* **2008**, *47*, 27–50. [CrossRef]
37. Levin, L.; Halperin-Sternfeld, M. Tooth preservation or implant placement: A systematic review of long-term tooth and implant survival rates. *J. Am. Dent. Assoc.* **2013**, *144*, 1119–1133. [CrossRef]
38. Caplan, D.J.; Li, Y.; Wang, W.; Kang, S.; Marchini, L.; Cowen, H.J.; Yan, J. Dental restoration longevity among geriatric and special needs patients. *JDR Clin. Transl. Res.* **2019**, *4*, 41–48. [CrossRef]
39. Avila, G.; Galindo-Moreno, P.; Soehren, S.; Misch, C.E.; Morelli, T.; Wang, H. A novel decision-making process for tooth retention or extraction. *J. Periodontol.* **2009**, *80*, 476–491. [CrossRef]
40. Halperin–Sternfeld, M.; Levin, L. Do we really know how to evaluate tooth prognosis? A systematic review and suggested approach. *Quintessence Int.* **2013**, *44*, 447–456.
41. Pretzl, B.; Wiedemann, D.; Cosgarea, R.; Kaltschmitt, J.; Kim, T.S.; Staehle, H.J.; Eickholz, P. Effort and costs of tooth preservation in supportive periodontal treatment in a german population. *J. Clin. Periodontol.* **2009**, *36*, 669–676. [CrossRef] [PubMed]
42. D'Cruz, L. Dento-legal considerations about an MI approach. *Br. Dent. J.* **2017**, *223*, 199–201. [CrossRef] [PubMed]
43. Diamantatou, T.; Kotina, E.; Roussou, I.; Kourtis, S. Treatment options for anterior teeth with questionable prognosis: Critical factors in determining whether to maintain or extract. *J. Esthet. Restor. Dent.* **2016**, *28*, 157–170. [CrossRef]
44. Moshaverinia, A.; Kar, K.; Chee, W.W. Treatment planning decisions: Implant placement versus preserving natural teeth. *J. Calif. Dent. Assoc.* **2014**, *42*, 859–868. [PubMed]
45. Saghafi, N.; Heaton, L.J.; Bayirli, B.; Turpin, D.L.; Khosravi, R.; Bollen, A. Influence of clinicians' experience and gender on extraction decision in orthodontics. *Angle. Orthod.* **2017**, *87*, 641–650. [CrossRef]
46. Baba, N.Z.; Goodacre, C.J.; Kattadiyil, M.T. Tooth retention through root canal treatment or tooth extraction and implant placement: A prosthodontic perspective. *Quintessence Int.* **2014**, *45*, 405–416.
47. Martu, M.A.; Maftei, G.A.; Luchian, I.; Popa, C.; Filioreanu, A.M.; Tatarciuc, D.; Nichitean, G.; Hurjui, L.-L.; Foia, L.-G. Wound healing of periodontal and oral tissues: Part II-Patho-phisiological conditions and metabolic diseases. *Rom. J. Oral Rehabil.* **2020**, *12*, 30–40.
48. Clark, D.; Levin, L. In the dental implant era, why do we still bother saving teeth? *J. Endod.* **2019**, *45*, S57–S65. [CrossRef]
49. Popa, C.G.; Luchian, I.; Ioanid, N.; Goriuc, A.; Martu, I.; Bosinceanu, D.; Martu, M.A.; Tirca, T.; Martu, S. ELISA Evaluation of RANKL Levels in Gingival Fluid in Patients with Periodontitis and Occlusal Trauma. *Rev. Chim.* **2018**, *69*, 1578–1580. [CrossRef]
50. Lin, J.; Tu, C.; Chen, Y.; Wang, C.Y.; Liu, C.M.; Kuo, M.Y.P.; Chang, P.C. Influence of adjacent teeth absence or extraction on the outcome of non-surgical periodontal therapy. *Int. J. Environ. Res. Public Health.* **2019**, *16*, 4344.
51. Ettinger, R.L. Restoring the ageing dentition: Repair or replacement? *Int. Dent. J.* **1990**, *40*, 275–282. [PubMed]

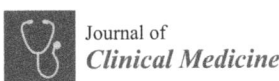

Article

Quantification of Bacteria in Mouth-Rinsing Solution for the Diagnosis of Periodontal Disease

Jeong-Hwa Kim [1,†], Jae-Woon Oh [1,†], Young Lee [2], Jeong-Ho Yun [3], Seong-Ho Choi [4] and Dong-Woon Lee [1,*]

1. Department of Periodontology, Dental Hospital, Veterans Health Service Medical Center, Seoul 05368, Korea; choco1206@naver.com (J.-H.K.); ohsoon1052@naver.com (J.-W.O.)
2. Veterans Medical Research Institute, Veterans Health Service Medical Center, Seoul 05368, Korea; lyou7688@gmail.com
3. Department of Periodontology, College of Dentistry and Institute of Oral Bioscience, Jeonbuk National University, Jeonju 54896, Korea; grayheron@hanmail.net
4. Department of Periodontology, College of Dentistry and Research Institute for Periodontal Regeneration, Yonsei University, Seoul 03722, Korea; SHCHOI726@yuhs.ac
* Correspondence: dongden@daum.net; Tel.: +82-2-2225-1928; Fax: +82-2-2225-1659
† These authors contributed equally to this work.

Abstract: This study aimed to evaluate the feasibility of diagnosing periodontitis via the identification of 18 bacterial species in mouth-rinse samples. Patients (n = 110) who underwent dental examinations in the Department of Periodontology at the Veterans Health Service Medical Center between 2018 and 2019 were included. They were divided into healthy and periodontitis groups. The overall number of bacteria, and those of 18 specific bacteria, were determined via real-time polymerase chain reaction in 92 mouth-rinse samples. Differences between groups were evaluated through logistic regression after adjusting for sex, age, and smoking history. There was a significant difference in the prevalence (healthy vs. periodontitis group) of *Aggregatibacter actinomycetemcomitans* (2.9% vs. 13.5%), *Treponema denticola* (42.9% vs. 69.2%), and *Prevotella nigrescens* (80% vs. 2.7%). Levels of *Treponema denticola*, *Prevotella nigrescens*, and *Streptococcus mitis* were significantly associated with severe periodontitis. We demonstrated the feasibility of detecting periopathogenic bacteria in mouth-rinse samples obtained from patients with periodontitis. As we did not comprehensively assess all periopathogenic bacteria, further studies are required to assess the potential of oral-rinsing solutions to indicate oral infection risk and the need to improve oral hygiene, and to serve as a complementary method for periodontal disease diagnosis.

Keywords: polymerase chain reaction; periodontitis; bacteria

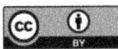

1. Introduction

Subgingival plaque bacteria are the main etiology of periodontitis. Complex interactions between certain pathogens are key in the development of periodontal disease [1]. Microbial complexes in the subgingival biofilm are classified into five groups: red, green, orange, yellow, and purple. In particular, the red group, which is composed of *Tannerella forsythia*, *Treponema denticola*, and *Porphyromonas gingivalis*, has been determined as one of the main causes of periodontal disease [1].

Several studies have shown that the presence and number of these bacteria are related to disease prediction criteria such as probing depth, bone loss, attachment loss, and bleeding on probing [2,3]. Various bacterial species besides those of the red complex have been found to be key in the development and progression of periodontitis; among these species, *P. gingivalis*, *Prevotella intermedia*, and *Aggregatibacter actinomycetemcomitans* have been shown to have the strongest association with periodontal disease [4]. A previous study showed that *P. gingivalis*, *T. denticola*, and *A. actinomycetemcomitans*, when present in saliva, contributed to pocket deepening [5]. In order to detect the bacteria associated with periodontal disease, plaque is usually collected from a specific tooth and analyzed [4,6]. Most studies have analyzed bacterial groups using plaque samples [7].

Multiplex real time-polymerase chain reaction (RT-PCR) allows RT measurement of amplified deoxyribonucleic acid (DNA) using a fluorescent substance. In general PCR, the final product is observed via agarose gel electrophoresis; therefore, accurate bacterial quantification is impossible. However, multiplex RT-PCR can be used to quantitatively analyze the product amplified per PCR cycle.

Mouth-rinsing solutions have been used in various sialochemistry studies [8,9]. Recently, some studies assessing the prevalence and levels of specific bacterial species have been conducted using PCR analysis of mouth-rinsing solutions [10]. However, very few studies have investigated the link between the diagnosis of periodontitis and the oral bacteria present in a mouth-rinsing solution. Additionally, the phosphate-buffered saline solution used in previous studies has been reported to cause discomfort.

The purpose of this study was to examine the correlation between periodontal disease and 18 different bacteria by conducting a RT-PCR analysis of mouth-rinsing solutions and to evaluate the usefulness of this diagnostic method.

2. Materials and Methods

2.1. Patient Selection

Patients who visited the Department of Periodontology at the Veterans Health Service Medical Center between 2018 and 2019 for various reasons underwent routine examination. Due to the lack of prior studies conducted with rinsing solutions, we decided to use this method to compare bacterial species prevalence and levels in healthy patients and patients with severe periodontal disease. After examination, 110 patients were selected to participate in the study.

However, 18 patients refused to participate in the mouth-rinsing test. Hence, 92 patients were finally included in this study. Additionally, five subjects were excluded from the study because their mouth-rinsing solutions were contaminated in the process of transferring the collected samples (Figure 1). The study protocol was approved by the institutional review board of Veterans Health Service Medical Center (BOHUN No. 2018-03-002). All participants provided written informed consent. This study was conducted according to the Helsinki Declaration of 1975 and its later revisions.

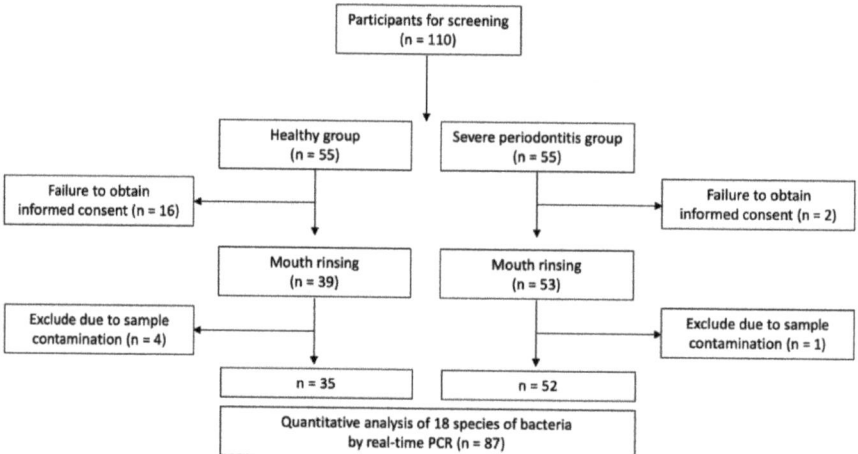

Figure 1. Study flow chart.

2.2. Sample Size Determination

The sample size was calculated using G*Power 3.1 software [11]. Comparisons between the two groups were conducted at a two-sided alpha level of 5% and a power of 90%. It was determined that a sample size of 42 participants per group would provide a power of 90% for the detection of between-group differences. However, considering a drop-out rate of 25%, a sample size of 55 patients per group was finalized.

2.3. Periodontal Examination

Each patient underwent an assessment of the probing depth and gingival recession at six sites per tooth using a periodontal probe (PCP-12, Hu-Friedy, Rotterdam, The Netherlands) by one examiner. Attachment loss was also measured.

After the dental examination, the presence and severity of periodontal disease were determined according to the Centers for Disease Control and Prevention/American Academy of Periodontology definitions [12]. We performed an additional examination using a mouth-rinse solution in both healthy patients and those with severe periodontal disease. Severe periodontitis was defined as two or more interproximal sites with a clinical attachment loss ≥ 6 mm, which are not the same area, and one or more interproximal sites with a probing depth ≥ 5 mm.

2.4. Sample Collection and DNA Extraction

Mouth-rinse samples were collected in the morning after regular brushing. Each subject rinsed their mouth with 10 mL of Easygen gargle (YD Global Life Science, Seongnam, Korea) for 60 s, after which the gargling liquid containing the patient's saliva was collected as previously described [13]. DNA was extracted from the gargle sample using a Qiagen column (DNA Mini Kit, Qiagen, Hilden, Germany), according to the manufacturer's instructions.

2.5. Multiplex Quantitative RT-PCR (qPCR)

The qPCR was performed with the EasyPerio molecular kit (YD Global Lifescience, Seongnam, Korea), according to the manufacturer's instructions. The kit consisted of 8 different oligo mixes and 2 × master mixes. This was designed according to the typical multiplex qPCR method [14]. The CFX96 Touch™ RT-PCR Detection System (Bio-Rad, Hercules, CA, USA) was used for qPCR. The sequential steps in the PCR procedure were as follows: pre-denaturation for 30 s at 95 °C; 40 cycles of 5 s denaturation at 95 °C; and 30 s extension and annealing at 62 °C. Fluorescence scanning was performed after the extension and annealing step. Information on the primers and probes is displayed in Table 1. In this way, DNA of 18 species of bacteria was extracted and analyzed by RT-qPCR. The 18 species of bacteria were the following: *A. actinomycetemcomitans, P. gingivalis, T. forsythia, T. denticola, Fusobacterium nucleatum, P. intermedia, Parvimonas micra, Campylobacter rectus, Eubacterium nodatum, Eikenella corrodens, Streptococcus mitis, Streptococcus mutans, Lactobacillus casei, Staphylococcus aureus, Enterococcus faecalis, Actinomyces viscosus, Prevotella nigrescens*, and *Streptococcus sobrinus*.

2.6. Bacterial Quantification

Standard curves were generated using the 18 plasmids at five different concentrations. The plasmids' DNA contained specific sequences of each microorganism. Each bacterial gene used for plasmid construction is listed in Table 1. The copy numbers of each oral-bacterial DNA were calculated by substituting the cycle threshold values obtained from the qPCR into the quantitative formula obtained through the standard curve.

Table 1. Primers and probes of the 18 species of bacteria analyzed.

Bacteria	Target Gene	Primer/Probe	Sequence (5'-3')	Ref.	Bacteria	Target Gene	Primer/Probe	Sequence (5'-3')	Ref.
Aggregatibacter actinomycetemcomitans	leukotoxin	Forward Reverse Probe	CG********GA AT********CA [FAM]GG********CC[BHQ1]	[15]	Eubacterium nodatum	hypothetical protein	Forward Reverse Probe	TG********GA AA********AT [TR]TT********GG[BHQ2]	[16]
Porphyromonas gingivalis	hemagglutinin	Forward Reverse Probe	AC********GC GC********CT [HEX]CG********GA[BHQ1]	[17]	Eikenella corrodens	prolineiminopeptidase	Forward Reverse Probe	GC********TG GC********TT [Cy5]AC********AT[BHQ2]	[16]
Tannerella forsythia	karilysin protease	Forward Reverse Probe	TG********CC TT********CA [TR]CC********GG[BHQ2]	[18]	Streptococcus mitis	16S ribosomal RNA	Forward Reverse Probe	GT********CG TA********AT [FAM]TA********CC[BHQ1]	[19]
Treponema denticola	OpdB	Forward Reverse Probe	AG********AG GC********AT [Cy5]CG********TC[BHQ2]	[20]	Streptococcus mutans	PTS EII	Forward Reverse Probe	CA********CA TG********CC [HEX]TG********GG[BHQ1]	[21]
Fusobacterium nucleatum	16S ribosomal RNA	Forward Reverse Probe	GG********TC CT********GC [FAM]AA********CG[BHQ1]	[22]	Streptococcus sobrinus	Ftsk	Forward Reverse Probe	GG********CC AC********GG [TR]AG********GC[BHQ2]	[23]
Prevotella intermedia	hemagglutinin	Forward Reverse Probe	CA********AC CA********TC [HEX]CC********AC[BHQ1]	[15]	Lactobacillus casei	att	Forward Reverse Probe	CA********GT AC********CC [Cy5]TG********GT[BHQ2]	[24]
Prevotella nigrescens	gyrase subunit B	Forward Reverse Probe	AG********CT GC********CT [TR]GC********AA[BHQ2]	[16]	Staphylococcus aureus	clumping factor A	Forward Reverse Probe	GC********AA GA********TT [FAM]TG********CA[BHQ1]	[25]
Parvimonas micra	16S ribosomal RNA	Forward Reverse Probe	GA********AG GG********CC [FAM]GG********CA[BHQ1]	[15]	Enterococcus faecalis	gelE-sprE operon	Forward Reverse Probe	GA********TT CG********AC [HEX]GC********GA[BHQ1]	[26]
Campylobacter rectus	GroEL	Forward Reverse Probe	AA********GG TC********GA [HEX]GG********GT[BHQ1]	[16]	Actinomyces viscosus	nanH	Forward Reverse Probe	GC********CG GA********CA [TR]GA********AA[BHQ2]	[21]

2.7. Statistical Analysis

This study evaluated whether there was a significant difference in the prevalence and levels of bacterial species between healthy individuals and those with periodontitis. Sex and smoking history were expressed as frequencies and percentages, and age, as means and standard deviations. The total number of bacteria was reported as median and interquartile range, and the number of each bacterial species was reported after normalization (dividing by the total number of bacteria in each sample). Differences in prevalence between groups were evaluated through logistic regression. Spearman's rank correlation was used to examine the association between the levels of the different target species. Only two species that had at least five complete observations were estimated with the correlation coefficient. Logistic regression models were applied with disease status (healthy or with periodontal disease) as the dependent variable and the bacterial category as the independent variable. The bacterial category comprised three levels. Level 0 represented PCR-negative subjects, while levels 1 and 2 were categorized according to the median of the number of bacterial cells in PCR-positive subjects; levels 1 and 2 were assigned to values less than or greater than the median, respectively.

The Firth's penalized maximum-likelihood bias-reduction method was used to estimate the odds ratio when there was a complete separation [27,28]. All regression analyses were adjusted for known confounders of periodontitis, including age, sex, and smoking history.

Statistical analyses were performed using R 3.5.1 (R Development Core Team; R Foundation for Statistical Computing, Vienna, Austria). *p* values < 0.05 were considered statistically significant.

3. Results

There were 35 individuals in the healthy group and 52 in the severe periodontitis group (Table 2). Figure 2 shows the mean counts of bacteria in the two groups. The number of bacteria of the red, yellow, and orange groups was higher in patients with periodontal disease than in the healthy group. The results of the quantitative analysis of the 18 species of bacteria are shown in Table 3. *S. mitis*, *P. micra*, and *F. nucleatum* were found in all subjects in the healthy group. *P. nigrescens* and *C. rectus* were found in 80% of the subjects in the healthy group. Among bacteria in the red complex group, *P. gingivalis* was found in 45.7%, *T. forsythia* in 74.3%, and *T. denticola* in 42.9% of the subjects in the healthy group. *E. faecalis* and *A. viscosus* were not detected in any of the healthy subjects. Similar to the healthy group, *S. mitis*, *P. micra*, and *F. nucleatum* were found in all subjects in the severe periodontitis group. *P. gingivalis*, *P. nigrescens*, *T. forsythia*, and *T. denticola* were detected in 90.4%, 82.7%, 73.1%, and 69.2% of individuals with severe periodontitis, respectively. After adjusting for age, sex, and smoking history, there were differences in the prevalence of *A. actinomycetemcomitans*, *T. denticola*, and *P. nigrescens* between the healthy group and severe periodontitis group. Among the red complex group bacteria, only *T. denticola* prevalence was significantly different between groups (Table 3).

Table 4 shows the correlations between the different bacterial species in all participants. Correlation coefficients ranged from −1 to 1, with numbers greater than 0 indicating positive correlations and numbers lower than 0 indicating negative correlations. *A. actinomycetemcomitans* and *P. gingivalis* showed a correlation of 0.96 and a *p* value lower than 0.05, indicating a significant positive correlation. *P. gingivalis* had a positive correlation with *E. nodatum* and a negative correlation with *S. mitis*. *T. forsythia* was negatively correlated with *F. nucleatum*, *P. nigrescens*, and *S. mitis*. *F. nucleatum* was positively correlated with *P. nigrescens*, *S. mitis*, and *L. casei*. *P. intermedia* was positively correlated with *P. nigrescens* and *C. rectus*.

Table 5 shows the correlations between bacterial species in the healthy group. *T. forsythia* was positively correlated with *C. rectus* and negatively correlated with *S. mitis*. *T. denticola* was negatively correlated with *S. mitis*.

Table 2. Participant demographics.

Characteristic		Healthy Group (n = 35)	Severe Periodontitis Group (n = 52)
Age (Years, mean ± SD)		39.0 ± 17.9	56.2 ± 15.2
Sex	Male	29 (83%)	44 (85%)
	Female	6 (17%)	8 (15%)
Smoking	Non-smokers	31 (89%)	46 (88%)
	Current smokers	4 (11%)	6 (12%)

Abbreviations: SD, Standard deviation.

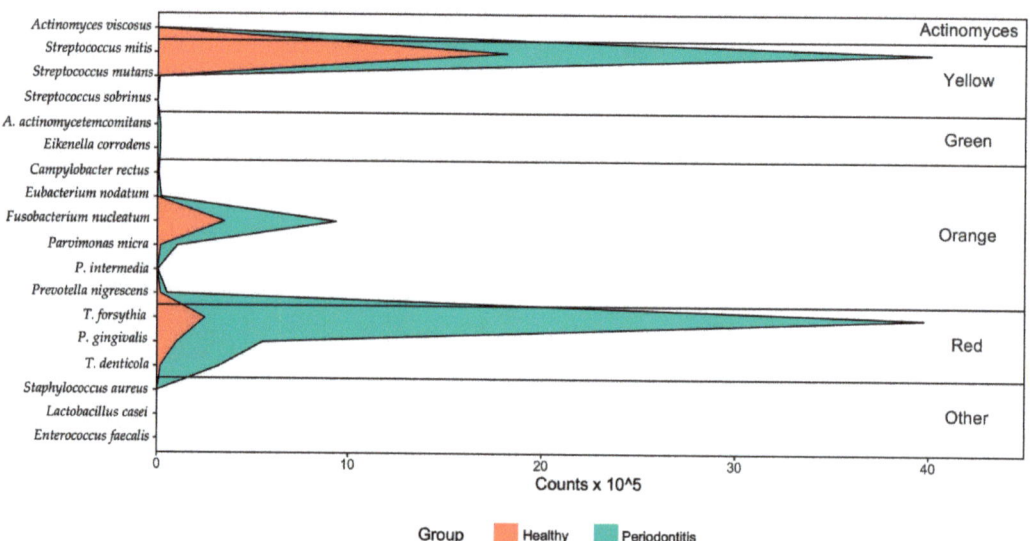

Figure 2. Mean bacterial cells in the healthy group and periodontal disease group.

Table 6 shows the correlations between bacterial species in the periodontal disease group. *P. gingivalis* had a significant positive correlation with *A. actinomycetemcomitans*. *F. nucleatum* was negatively correlated with *T. forsythia*.

Table 7 shows the categorization of the number of bacteria into three levels. *P. gingivalis*, *T. denticola*, *P. micra*, *S. mitis*, *L. casei*, *S. aureus*, *E. nodatum*, and total bacteria were significantly associated with severe periodontitis at certain levels. However, after adjusting for factors such as sex, age, and smoking, only *T. denticola*, *P. nigrescens*, and *S. mitis* were significant. *T. denticola* significance was only noted at level 2, in which the risk of periodontal disease was 7.3 times higher compared to level 0. *P. nigrescens* was significantly associated with severe periodontitis at levels 1 and 2; the risk of periodontal disease at level 2 was 22.5 times higher than that at level 0. *S. mitis* significance was only observed at level 2.

Table 3. Prevalence of target species and their quantities in polymerase chain reaction-positive subjects.

Bacteria	Healthy Group (n = 35)	Severe Periodontitis Group (n = 52)
Aggregatibacter actinomycetemcomitans		
Prevalence, n (%) [a]	1 (2.9)	7 (13.5)
Median bacterial cells proportion (%) (IQR)	0.46 (0.46–0.46)	0.75 (0.46–1.07)
Porphyromonas gingivalis		
Prevalence, n (%)	16 (45.7)	47 (90.4)
Median bacterial cells proportion (%) (IQR)	3.43 (1.74–5.86)	3.83 (2.27–8.28)
Tannerella forsythia		
Prevalence, n (%)	26 (74.3)	38 (73.1)
Median bacterial cells proportion (%) (IQR)	3.07 (0.65–7.74)	26.07 (4.49–50.82)
Treponema denticola		
Prevalence, n (%) [a]	15 (42.9)	36 (69.2)
Median bacterial cells proportion (%) (IQR)	0.59 (0.18–2.34)	2.91 (1.36–5.39)
Fusobacterium nucleatum		
Prevalence, n (%)	35 (100.0)	52 (100.0)
Median bacterial cells proportion (%) (IQR)	18.73 (13.31–23.15)	12.89 (7.23–20.02)
Prevotella intermedia		
Prevalence, n (%)	8 (22.9)	15 (28.8)
Median bacterial cells proportion (%) (IQR)	0.22 (0.05–0.46)	0.11 (0.05–0.19)
Prevotella nigrescens		
Prevalence, n (%) [a]	28 (80.0)	43 (82.7)
Median bacterial cells proportion (%) (IQR)	0.73 (0.4–1.94)	0.47 (0.14–1.23)
Parvimonas micra		
Prevalence, n (%)	35 (100.0)	52 (100.0)
Median bacterial cells proportion (%) (IQR)	0.5 (0.29–0.82)	0.99 (0.45–1.81)
Campylobacter rectus		
Prevalence, n (%)	28 (80.0)	45 (86.5)
Median bacterial cells proportion (%) (IQR)	0.11 (0.06–0.18)	0.08 (0.04–0.13)
Eubacterium nodatum		
Prevalence, n (%)	3 (8.6)	14 (26.9)
Median bacterial cells proportion (%) (IQR)	0.21 (0.12–0.27)	0.71 (0.3–1.34)
Eikenella corrodens		
Prevalence, n (%)	4 (11.4)	15 (28.8)
Median bacterial cells proportion (%) (IQR)	0.07 (0.04–0.45)	0.28 (0.15–0.71)
Streptococcus mitis		
Prevalence, n (%)	35 (100.0)	52 (100.0)
Median bacterial cells proportion (%) (IQR)	73.72 (63.61–79.49)	59.13 (37.87–70.34)
Streptococcus mutans		
Prevalence, n (%)	23 (65.7)	35 (67.3)
Median bacterial cells proportion (%) (IQR)	0.03 (0.02–0.1)	0.03 (0.01–0.15)
Streptococcus sobrinus		
Prevalence, n (%)	1 (2.9)	5 (9.6)
Median bacterial cells proportion (%) (IQR)	0.06 (0.06–0.06)	0 (0–0.01)
Lactobacillus casei		
Prevalence, n (%)	6 (17.1)	18 (34.6)
Median bacterial cells proportion (%) (IQR)	0.01 (0–0.04)	0 (0–0.01)
Staphylococcus aureus		
Prevalence, n (%)	15 (42.9)	4 (7.7)
Median bacterial cells proportion (%) (IQR)	0.02 (0.01–0.14)	0.03 (0–0.07)
Enterococcus faecalis		
Prevalence, n (%)	0 (0.0)	0 (0.0)
Median bacterial cells proportion (%) (IQR)	NA (NA–NA)	NA (NA–NA)
Actinomyces viscosus		
Prevalence, n (%)	0 (0.0)	0 (0.0)
Median bacterial cells proportion (%) (IQR)	NA (NA–NA)	NA (NA–NA)
Total number of cells Prevalence, n (%)	35 (100.0)	52 (100.0)
Median bacterial cells (IQR)	36,126,518 (16,199,034–92,716,204)	108,524,910 (69,243,624.5–177,393,988.25)

Abbreviations: IQR, interquartile range; NA, not available. [a] Significant difference between groups at $p < 0.05$, analyzed using the logistic regression analysis.

Table 4. Interspecies correlations in all subjects.

	Aa	Pg	Tf	Td	Fn	Pi	Pn	Pm	Cr	En	Ec	Sm	Smu	Ss	Lc	Sa	Total
Aa		0.96 *	−0.49	0.3	0.38		0.98 *	0.91 *	0.57			0.07					−0.26
Pg			−0.04	0.25	−0.01	−0.06	0.16	0.23	−0.02	0.57 *	−0.3	−0.34 *	0.16	0.5	−0.05	−0.27	−0.06
Tf				0.19	−0.56 *	−0.21	−0.28 *	0.03	−0.02	0.1	−0.37	−0.87 *	−0.22	−0.54	−0.2	−0.21	0.14
Td					−0.17	0.53 *	0.05	0.61 *	−0.08	0.8 *	−0.24	−0.42 *	−0.02	−0.17	0.34	−0.4	−0.07
Fn						0.21	0.25 *	−0.15	0.18	−0.17	0.07	0.25 *	0.02	0.9 *	0.52 *	0.02	−0.13
Pi							0.53 *	0.14	0.51 *	0.51		0.09	−0.09		0.43		0.32
Pn								0.15	0.23	−0.16	−0.13	0.07	−0.18	0.75	−0.03	−0.32	−0.21
Pm									0.18	0.13	−0.27	−0.23 *	0	0.17	−0.02	−0.23	−0.02
Cr										−0.31	−0.24	0.03	−0.15	0.88 *	0.06	−0.24	−0.16
En												−0.13	0.35	0.3			0.42
Ec												0.24	0.19		−0.17		−0.16
Sm													0.12	0.33	0.04	0.23	−0.03
Smu														−0.12	−0.13	−0.15	−0.09
Ss																	−0.62
Lc																	−0.16
Sa																	−0.21
Total																	

Abbreviations: Aa, *Aggregatibacter actinomycetemcomitans*; Pg, *Porphyromonas gingivalis*; Tf, *Tannerella forsythia*; Td, *Treponema denticola*; Fn, *Fusobacterium nucleatum*; Pi, *Prevotella intermedia*; Pm, *Parvimonas micra*; Cr, *Campylobacter rectus*; En, *Eubacterium nodatum*; Ec, *Eikenella corrodens*; Sm, *Streptococcus mitis*; Smu, *Streptococcus mutans*; Lc, *Lactobacillus casei*; Sa, *Staphylococcus aureus*; Pn, *Prevotella nigrescens*; Ss, *Streptococcus sobrinus*; and * $p < 0.05$.

Table 5. Interspecies correlations in healthy subjects.

	Aa	Pg	Tf	Td	Fn	Pi	Pn	Pm	Cr	En	Ec	Sm	Smu	Ss	Lc	Sa	Total
Aa		0.96 *	−0.81	0.24	0.55		0.98 *	0.92 *	0.56			0.18					−0.34
Pg			−0.03	0.22	0.02	−0.04	0.12	0.22	0	0.57 *	−0.32	−0.3 *	0.14	0.71	−0.05		−0.07
Tf				0.11	−0.67 *	−0.13	−0.34	−0.12	−0.13	0.05	−0.49	−0.88 *	−0.29	0.11	−0.31		0.05
Td					−0.12	0.55	0.07	0.62 *	−0.09	0.78 *	−0.34	−0.33 *	−0.08	−0.17	0.4		−0.16
Fn						0.26	0.33 *	−0.1	0.24	−0.12	0.28	0.43 *	0.38 *	0.33	0.19		0.01
Pi							0.75 *	0.21	0.56 *	0.58		0.15	−0.16				0.36
Pn								0.23	0.4 *	−0.22	−0.14	0.15	−0.15	−0.26	−0.17		−0.23
Pm									0.22	−0.09	−0.32	−0.11	−0.08	−0.37	0.11		−0.12
Cr										−0.32	−0.22	0.12	−0.18	0.95 *	0.22		−0.14
En												−0.13	0.31	0.3			0.45
Ec												0.2	0.18		−0.23		−0.24
Sm													0.12	−0.2	0.24		0.04
Smu														0.01			−0.23
Ss																	−0.49
Lc																	−0.12
Sa																	
Total																	

Abbreviations: Aa, *Aggregatibacter actinomycetemcomitans*; Pg, *Porphyromonas gingivalis*; Tf, *Tannerella forsythia*; Td, *Treponema denticola*; Fn, *Fusobacterium nucleatum*; Pi, *Prevotella intermedia*; Pm, *Parvimonas micra*; Cr, *C. Campylobacter rectus*; En, *Eubacterium nodatum*; Ec, *Eikenella corrodens*; Sm, *S. Streptococcus mitis*; Smu, *Streptococcus mutans*; Lc, *Lactobacillus casei*; Sa, *Staphylococcus aureus*; Pn, *Prevotella nigrescens*; Ss, *Streptococcus sobrinus*; and * $p < 0.05$.

Table 6. Interspecies correlations in subjects with severe periodontitis.

	Aa	Pg	Tf	Td	Fn	Pi	Pn	Pm	Cr	En	Ec	Sm	Smu	Ss	Lc	Sa	Total
Aa		0.96 *	−0.81	0.24	0.55		0.98 *	0.92 *	0.56			0.18					−0.34
Pg			−0.03	0.22	0.02	−0.04	0.12	0.22	0	0.57 *	−0.32	−0.3 *	0.14	0.71	−0.05		−0.07
Tf				0.11	−0.67 *	−0.13	−0.34	−0.12	−0.13	0.05	−0.49	−0.88 *	−0.29	0.11	−0.31		0.05
Td					−0.12	0.55	0.07	0.62 *	−0.09	0.78 *	−0.34	−0.33 *	−0.08	−0.17	0.4		−0.16
Fn						0.26	0.33 *	−0.1	0.24	−0.12	0.28	0.43 *	0.38 *	0.33	0.19		0.01
Pi							0.75 *	0.21	0.56 *	0.58		0.15	−0.16				0.36
Pn								0.23	0.4 *	−0.22	−0.14	0.15	−0.15	−0.26	−0.17		−0.23
Pm									0.22	−0.09	−0.32	−0.11	−0.08	−0.37	0.11		−0.12
Cr										−0.32	−0.22	0.12	−0.18	0.95 *	0.22		−0.14
En												−0.13	0.31	0.3			0.45
Ec												0.2	0.18		−0.23		−0.24
Sm													0.12	−0.2	0.24		0.04
Smu														0.01			−0.23
Ss																	−0.49
Lc																	−0.12
Sa																	
Total																	

Abbreviations: Aa, *Aggregatibacter actinomycetemcomitans*; Pg, *Porphyromonas gingivalis*; Tf, *Tannerella forsythia*; Td, *Treponema denticola*; Fn, *Fusobacterium nucleatum*; Pi, *Prevotella intermedia*; Pm, *Parvimonas micra*; Cr, *Campylobacter rectus*; En, *Eubacterium nodatum*; Ec, *Eikenella corrodens*; Sm, *S. Streptococcus mitis*; Smu, *Streptococcus mutans*; Lc, *Lactobacillus casei*; Sa, *Staphylococcus aureus*; Pn, *Prevotella nigrescens*; Ss, *Streptococcus sobrinus*; and * $p < 0.05$.

Table 7. Association of severe periodontitis according to levels of target species.

	Levels	No of Subjects	No. (%) with Severe Periodontitis	Crude OR (95% CI)	p Value	Adjusted OR (95% CI)	p Value
Aa	0	79	45 (57.0)	1	-	1	-
	1	4	3 (75.0)	1.8 (0.3–18.9)	0.557	13.7 (0.9–389.2)	0.059
	2	4	4 (100.0)	6.8 (0.7–915.8)	0.111	1.6 (0.1–232.1)	0.750
Pg	0	24	5 (20.8)	1	-	1	-
	1	31	23 (74.2)	10.9 (3.1–39.0)	<0.001	3.3 (0.4–26.6)	0.271
	2	32	24 (75.0)	11.4 (3.2–40.6)	<0.001	1.1 (0.1–8.7)	0.942
Tf	0	23	14 (60.9)	1	-	1	-
	1	32	13 (40.6)	0.4 (0.1–1.3)	0.141	0.1 (0.0–1.1)	0.059
	2	32	25 (78.1)	2.3 (0.7–7.5)	0.169	3.7 (0.3–48.1)	0.319
Td	0	36	16 (44.4)	1	-	1	-
	1	25	14 (56.0)	1.6 (0.6–4.4)	0.375	5.3 (0.6–44.8)	0.129
	2	26	22 (84.6)	6.9 (2.0–24.0)	0.002	7.3 (1.1–47.4)	0.035
Fn	1	43	30 (69.8)	1	-	1	-
	2	44	22 (50.0)	0.4 (0.2–1.0)	0.062	1.0 (0.2–4.3)	0.969
Pi	0	64	37 (57.8)	1	-	1	-
	1	11	7 (63.6)	1.3 (0.3–4.8)	0.717	0.7 (0.1–7.6)	0.762
	2	12	8 (66.7)	1.5 (0.4–5.3)	0.568	0.5 (0.1–3.4)	0.504
Pn	0	16	9 (56.2)	1	-	1	-
	1	35	25 (71.4)	1.9 (0.6–6.7)	0.289	120.4 (5.3–2725.4)	0.002
	2	36	18 (50.0)	0.8 (0.2–2.5)	0.677	22.5 (2.0–260.6)	0.012
Pm	1	43	19 (44.2)	1	-	1	-
	2	44	33 (75.0)	3.8 (1.5–9.4)	0.004	4.4 (1.0–20.1)	0.057

Table 7. Cont.

	Levels	No. of Subjects	No. (%) with Severe Periodontitis	Crude OR (95% CI)	p Value	Adjusted OR (95% CI)	p Value
Cr	0	14	7 (50.0)	1	-	1	-
	1	36	25 (69.4)	2.3 (0.6–8.1)	0.203	3.5 (0.5–27.3)	0.226
	2	37	20 (54.1)	1.2 (0.3–4.0)	0.795	1.6 (0.2–11.0)	0.628
En	0	70	38 (54.3)	1	-	1	-
	1	8	5 (62.5)	1.3 (0.3–6.1)	0.694	0.3 (0.1–2.0)	0.227
	2	9	9 (100.0)	16.0 (1.9–2097.0)	0.006	4.3 (0.4–609.5)	0.280
Ec	0	68	37 (54.4)	1	-	1	-
	1	9	6 (66.7)	1.7 (0.4–7.3)	0.490	2.6 (0.2–30.9)	0.441
	2	10	9 (90.0)	7.5 (0.9–62.8)	0.061	13.6 (0.5–380.9)	0.124
Sm	1	43	33 (76.7)	1	-	1	-
	2	44	19 (43.2)	0.2 (0.1–0.6)	0.001	0.1 (0.0–0.8)	0.024
Smu	0	29	17 (58.6)	1	-	1	-
	1	29	18 (62.1)	1.2 (0.4–3.3)	0.788	2.5 (0.4–18.3)	0.354
	2	29	17 (58.6)	1.0 (0.4–2.8)	1	0.4 (0.1–2.5)	0.316
Ss	0	81	47 (58.0)	1	-	1	-
	1	3	3 (100.0)	5.1 (0.5–692.1)	0.205	1.6 (0.1–244.0)	0.755
	2	3	2 (66.7)	1.2 (0.2–13.7)	0.856	1.4 (0.1–193.5)	0.873
Lc	0	63	34 (54.0)	1	-	1	-
	1	12	11 (91.7)	9.4 (1.1–77.0)	0.037	1.4 (0.1–14.1)	0.795
	2	12	7 (58.3)	1.2 (0.3–4.2)	0.780	0.3 (0.0–1.9)	0.192
Sa	0	68	48 (70.6)	1	-	1	-
	1	9	2 (22.2)	0.1 (0.0–0.6)	0.011	0.2 (0.0–2.0)	0.162
	2	10	2 (20.0)	0.1 (0.0–0.5)	0.006	0.4 (0.0–7.4)	0.525

Table 7. Cont.

Levels	No. of Subjects	No. (%) with Severe Periodontitis	Crude OR (95% CI)	p Value	Adjusted OR (95% CI)	p Value
Total						
1	43	18 (41.9)	1	-	1	-
2	44	34 (77.3)	4.7 (1.9–12.0)	0.001	1.4 (0.3–5.8)	0.673

Level 0 indicates polymerase chain reaction (PCR)-negative subjects. Level 1 indicates that the number of bacterial cells is less than the median number in PCR-positive subjects. Level 2 indicates that the number of bacterial cells is equal to or greater than the median number in PCR-positive subjects. Logistic regression analysis was performed after adjusting for known confounders: sex, age, and smoking history. Abbreviations: OR, odds ratio; CI, confidence interval; Aa, *Aggregatibacter actinomycetemcomitans*; Pg, *Porphyromonas gingivalis*; Tf, *Tannerella forsythia*; Td, *Treponema denticola*; Fn, *Fusobacterium nucleatum*; Pi, *Prevotella intermedia*; Pm, *Parvimonas micra*; Cr, *Campylobacter rectus*; En, *Eubacterium nodatum*; Ec, *Eikenella corrodens*; Sm, *Streptococcus mitis*; Smu, *Streptococcus mutans*; Lc, *Lactobacillus casei*; Sa, *Staphylococcus aureus*; Pn, *Prevotella nigrescens*; and Ss, *Streptococcus sobrinus*.

4. Discussion

To the best of our knowledge, this preliminary study is the first to quantify bacteria with PCR in a mouth-rinsing solution, as opposed to a subgingival plaque or saliva sample. Newer diagnostic methods have been developed with more detailed stages and grades corresponding to the related treatment protocol [29]. While periodontal probing is the traditional method used for diagnosing periodontal disease, the detection of periopathogenic bacteria with PCR may potentially serve as an adjunct assessment. Nevertheless, to date, no standardized methods have been proposed for the diagnosis of periodontal disease based on gargled solutions [30].

Several studies on periodontal pathogens have been conducted using RT-PCR analysis. *P. gingivalis*, *T. forsythia*, *T. denticola*, and *P. intermedia* have been reported to be mainly prevalent in Asian populations [31,32]. However, *A. actinomycetemcomitans* prevalence varies widely. In this study, a low *A. actinomycetemcomitans* prevalence was observed. Previous studies have reported even lower levels in this and other previous studies compared to other pathogens [2,33]. In line with the results of previous studies, we found significant differences between the groups of bacteria known to be related to periodontal disease. The prevalence of *A. actinomycetemcomitans*, *T. denticola*, *P. nigrescens*, and *S. mitis* were significantly different between the healthy and periodontal disease groups.

A. actinomycetemcomitans is a common pathogen in aggressive periodontitis, and it is known to have mutually inhibitory effects on *Streptococcus sanguis*, *Streptococcus uberis*, and *A. viscosus* [34]. *A. actinomycetemcomitans* is involved in the pathogenesis of aggressive periodontitis in younger patients [35]. *T. denticola* and *P. nigrescens* are both known to be related to periodontitis. A previous study showed clear evidence of increased immune responses to *T. denticola*, *P. nigrescens*, and *F. nucleatum* in 89 patients with chronic periodontitis [36]. *F. nucleatum* is frequently detected in the subgingival plaque of patients with chronic periodontitis and is often found associated with periodontal pockets. *A. actinomycetemcomitans*, *T. forsythia*, *T. denticola*, and *P. gingivalis* are strongly associated with periodontal disease, disease progression, and treatment failure. *P. intermedia*, *P. micra*, *C. rectus*, *E. nodatum*, *P. nigrescens*, and *F. nucleatum* can also act as pathogens if their concentrations exceed certain thresholds [37].

Periodontal disease is a result of complex interactions between the periodontal pathogens and normal flora [38]. This fact rationalizes the use of mouth-rinsing solution for bacterial analysis, as it provides mixed bacterial samples. Nevertheless, the presence of periodontal pathogens in the gingival crevices by itself does not cause or initiate periodontal inflammation. The bacterial load in an area with periodontal disease is higher than that in a healthy area; these bacteria are called periodontopathic [39]. *P. gingivalis* and *T. forsythia* are some of the main pathogens of periodontitis, but no significant difference was found between the healthy and periodontal disease groups in this study. The distribution, as well as the number of bacterial species varies in diseased and healthy periodontal tissues. In this study, *S. mitis*, a Gram-positive strain present in healthy tissues, had a 100% prevalence in both normal and severe periodontitis groups. *F. nucleatum*, which belongs to the red complex group and is strongly associated with periodontal disease, also had a 100% prevalence in both groups. Therefore, although these bacterial species may be proportionally less dominant, they are present in the oral cavity as a constituent of the normal flora [40]. Our findings revealed a significant positive correlation between *A. actinomycetemcomitans* and *P. gingivalis*. This indicates that both bacterial species affect each other's growth [38]. In addition, *P. gingivalis* and *E. nodatum* also showed a positive correlation, indicating that the higher the number of *P. gingivalis*, the higher the number of *E. nodatum*. Conversely, *T. forsythia* was negatively correlated with *F. nucleatum*, *P. nigrescens*, and *S. mitis*. Hence, these bacteria may inhibit each other's growth.

After dividing bacterial levels according to whether they were above or below the median, and adjusting for confounding factors (e.g., sex, age, and smoking habit), *T. denticola*, *P. nigrescens*, and *S. mitis* were significantly associated with periodontitis. These results indicate that the risk of periodontal disease is increased if the levels of *T. denticola* and *P. nigrescens* are high. It can also be inferred that the higher the level of *S. mitis*, the lower the risk of developing periodontal disease.

This study has some limitations because we could not verify the reproducibility of our results. Moreover, in order for the mouth-rinsing solution analysis to be of diagnostic value, a certain number of bacteria must be detected to indicate disease. Implementation of the new classification system described above was not possible when recruiting participants in this study. We could only divide participants into two groups: healthy and severe periodontitis. Due to the lack of previous studies on diagnostic methods using mouth-rinsing solutions, we tried to evaluate differences between the two groups using the existing classification method. This should be complemented in the next study. There were limitations in adjusting for age, sex, and smoking history, because of the small sample size. Among the correction variables, age is an important variable related to periodontal disease, but in this study, the sample size was not large enough to consider the correction variable, even though it had already been adjusted.

As mentioned earlier, periodontitis is a disease with various factors caused by subgingival bacterial colonies such as *A. actinomycetemcomitans*, *T. forsythia*, and *P. gingivalis*. [41]. However, *P. gingivalis* was not significantly associated with periodontitis after adjustment for confounding factors in this study. *P. gingivalis* has been shown to have a higher prevalence in deep pockets [1,42,43]. Therefore, the results of our study may reflect the low ability of mouth rinsing to sample *P. gingivalis* in these regions. Because the number of bacteria needed to cause periodontal disease may vary depending on the host's immune system, additional research methods are needed, such as comparing with crevicular fluid and gingival biopsy to show reliable results [44].

This study suggests that the analysis of mouth-rinsing solution might be a promising diagnostic method, and further studies with greater sensitivity should be conducted with larger samples to determine its perceived usefulness. Diagnosing the severity of periodontitis by analyzing gargled mouth-rinse solutions is less invasive than collecting plaque samples. We hope that the analysis of mouth-rinsing solutions will become an accepted diagnostic method for periodontal disease. A limitation of this study is that only three peripopathogenic bacteria, among a total of 18 species, exhibited a significant difference between the healthy and periodontal disease groups; nevertheless, the advantages of the detection method are obvious.

In summary, the findings of this study are as follows: (1) similar to previous studies, bacteria known to cause periodontal disease were detected with mouth-rinsing solutions in patients with severe periodontal disease; (2) significant differences were found in the prevalence (healthy vs. periodontal disease group) of *A. actinomycetemcomitans* (2.9% vs. 13.5%), *T. denticola* (42.9% vs. 69.2%), and *P. nigrescens* (80% vs. 82.7%); and (3) *T. denticola*, *P. nigrescens*, and *S. mitis* levels were significantly different between groups in the quantitative analysis.

We did not comprehensively assess all peripopathogenic bacteria in this study; therefore, additional research is required to assess the potential of oral-rinsing solutions to reflect oral-infection risk and the need to improve oral hygiene, as well as to serve as a complementary method for periodontal disease diagnosis. Similar to the results of plaque analysis, which has been conducted in many studies, the results obtained by detecting bacteria in mouth-rinsing solutions show that there is a relationship between specific bacteria and severe periodontal disease. While mouth-rinsing solutions are non-invasive, simple, and capable of detecting a wide range of bacterial species, they are limited by the lack of clear diagnostic criteria. Therefore, in order for this diagnostic method to be effective, research aimed at establishing the criteria for the type and number of bacteria should be conducted. Recently, the concept of the diagnosis of periodontitis has been improved to complement the treatment stage. If this simple diagnostic kit is quantified and developed, it is expected to be helpful in future treatment planning.

Author Contributions: Conceptualization, D.-W.L.; methodology, D.-W.L. and J.-H.Y.; software, Y.L.; validation, J.-W.O. and J.-H.K.; formal analysis, Y.L.; investigation, D.-W.L.; resources, D.-W.L.; data curation, J.-H.K. and J.-W.O.; writing—original draft preparation, J.-H.K. and J.-W.O.; writing—review and editing, D.-W.L.; visualization, J.-H.Y.; supervision, S.-H.C.; project administration, D.-W.L.; funding acquisition, D.-W.L. All authors have read and agreed to the published version of the manuscript.

Funding: This research was funded by VHS Medical Center Research Grant, Republic of Korea, grant number VHSMC18015.

Institutional Review Board Statement: The study was conducted according to the guidelines of the Declaration of Helsinki, and approved by the Institutional Review Board of Veterans Health Service Medical Center (BOHUN No. 2018-03-002).

Informed Consent Statement: Informed consent was obtained from all participants involved in the study.

Data Availability Statement: The datasets generated during the current study are available from the corresponding author on reasonable request.

Conflicts of Interest: The authors declare no conflict of interest.

References

1. Socransky, S.S.; Haffajee, A.D.; Cugini, M.A.; Smith, C.; Kent, R.L., Jr. Microbial complexes in subgingival plaque. *J. Clin. Periodontol.* **1998**, *25*, 134–144. [CrossRef]
2. Papapanou, P.N.; Teanpaisan, R.; Obiechina, N.S.; Pithpornchaiyakul, W.; Pongpaisal, S.; Pisuithanakan, S.; Baelum, V.; Fejerskov, O.; Dahlen, G. Periodontal microbiota and clinical periodontal status in a rural sample in southern Thailand. *Eur. J. Oral Sci.* **2002**, *110*, 345–352. [CrossRef]
3. Pradhan-Palikhe, P.; Mäntylä, P.; Paju, S.; Buhlin, K.; Persson, G.R.; Nieminen, M.S.; Sinisalo, J.; Pussinen, P.J. Subgingival Bacterial Burden in Relation to Clinical and Radiographic Periodontal Parameters. *J. Periodontol.* **2013**, *84*, 1809–1817. [CrossRef]
4. Hyvärinen, K.; Laitinen, S.; Paju, S.; Hakala, A.; Suominen-Taipale, L.; Skurnik, M.; Könönen, E.; Pussinen, P.J. Detection and quantification of five major periodontal pathogens by single copy gene-based real-time PCR. *Innate Immun.* **2009**, *15*, 195–204. [CrossRef]
5. Paju, S.; Pussinen, P.J.; Suominen-Taipale, L.; Hyvönen, M.; Knuuttila, M.; Könönen, E. Detection of Multiple Pathogenic Species in Saliva is Associated with Periodontal Infection in Adults. *J. Clin. Microbiol.* **2008**, *47*, 235–238. [CrossRef] [PubMed]
6. Mineoka, T.; Awano, S.; Rikimaru, T.; Kurata, H.; Yoshida, A.; Ansai, T.; Takehara, T. Site-Specific Development of Periodontal Disease is Associated with Increased Levels of *Porphyromonas gingivalis*, *Treponema denticola*, and *Tannerella forsythia* in Subgingival Plaque. *J. Periodontol.* **2008**, *79*, 670–676. [CrossRef] [PubMed]
7. Torrungruang, K.; Jitpakdeebordin, S.; Charatkulangkun, O.; Gleebbua, Y. *Porphyromonas gingivalis*, *Aggregatibacter actinomycetemcomitans*, and *Treponema denticola*/*Prevotella intermedia* Co-Infection are Associated with Severe Periodontitis in a Thai Population. *PLoS ONE* **2015**, *10*, e0136346. [CrossRef]
8. Yoshizawa, J.M.; Schafer, C.A.; Schafer, J.J.; Farrell, J.J.; Paster, B.J.; Wong, D.T.W. Salivary Biomarkers: Toward Future Clinical and Diagnostic Utilities. *Clin. Microbiol. Rev.* **2013**, *26*, 781–791. [CrossRef] [PubMed]
9. Aguirre, A.; Testa-Weintraub, L.; Banderas, J.; Haraszthy, G.; Reddy, M.; Levine, M. Sialochemistry: A Diagnostic Tool? *Crit. Rev. Oral Biol. Med.* **1993**, *4*, 343–350. [CrossRef]
10. Liguori, G.; Lucariello, A.; Colella, G.; de Luca, A.; Marinelli, P. Rapid identification of Candida species in oral rinse solutions by PCR. *J. Clin. Pathol.* **2006**, *60*, 1035–1039. [CrossRef]
11. Faul, F.; Erdfelder, E.; Buchner, A.; Lang, A.-G. Statistical power analyses using G*Power 3.1: Tests for correlation and regression analyses. *Behav. Res. Methods* **2009**, *41*, 1149–1160. [CrossRef]
12. Eke, P.I.; Page, R.C.; Wei, L.; Thornton-Evans, G.; Genco, R.J. Update of the Case Definitions for Population-Based Surveillance of Periodontitis. *J. Periodontol.* **2012**, *83*, 1449–1454. [CrossRef] [PubMed]
13. Kim, E.-H.; Joo, J.-Y.; Lee, Y.J.; Koh, J.-K.; Choi, J.-H.; Shin, Y.; Cho, J.; Park, E.; Kang, J.; Lee, K.; et al. Grading system for periodontitis by analyzing levels of periodontal pathogens in saliva. *PLoS ONE* **2018**, *13*, e0200900. [CrossRef] [PubMed]
14. Rodríguez, A.; Rodríguez, M.; Córdoba, J.J.; Andrade, M.J. Design of primers and probes for quantitative real-time PCR methods. In *PCR Primer Design*; Humana Press: New York, NY, USA, 2015; Volume 1275, pp. 31–56.
15. Boutaga, K.; van Winkelhoff, A.J.; Vandenbroucke-Grauls, C.M.J.E.; Savelkoul, P.H.M. Periodontal pathogens: A quantitative comparison of anaerobic culture and real-time PCR. *FEMS Immunol. Med. Microbiol.* **2005**, *45*, 191–199. [CrossRef]
16. Elkaïm, R.; Dahan, M.; Kocgozlu, L.; Werner, S.; Kanter, D.; Kretz, J.G.; Tenenbaum, H. Prevalence of periodontal pathogens in subgingival lesions, atherosclerotic plaques and healthy blood vessels: A preliminary study. *J. Periodontal Res.* **2007**, *43*, 224–231. [CrossRef]

17. Boutaga, K.; van Winkelhoff, A.J.; Vandenbroucke-Grauls, C.M.J.E.; Savelkoul, P.H.M. Comparison of real-time PCR and culture for detection of Porphyromonas gingivalis in subgingival plaque samples. *J. Clin. Microbiol.* **2003**, *41*, 4950–4954. [CrossRef] [PubMed]
18. Suzuki, N.; Yoshida, A.; Saito, T.; Kawada, M.; Nakano, Y. Quantitative Microbiological Study of Subgingival Plaque by Real-Time PCR Shows Correlation between Levels of *Tannerella forsythensis* and *Fusobacterium* spp. *J. Clin. Microbiol.* **2004**, *42*, 2255–2257. [CrossRef]
19. Suzuki, N.; Nakano, Y.; Yoshida, A.; Yamashita, Y.; Kiyoura, Y. Real-Time TaqMan PCR for Quantifying Oral Bacteria during Biofilm Formation. *J. Clin. Microbiol.* **2004**, *42*, 3827–3830. [CrossRef] [PubMed]
20. Asai, Y.; Jinno, T.; Igarashi, H.; Ohyama, Y.; Ogawa, T. Detection and Quantification of Oral Treponemes in Subgingival Plaque by Real-Time PCR. *J. Clin. Microbiol.* **2002**, *40*, 3334–3340. [CrossRef]
21. Rawashdeh, R.Y.; Malkawi, H.I.; Al-Hiyasat, A.S.; Hammad, M.M. A fast and sensitive molecular detection of *Streptococcus mutans* and *Actinomyces viscosus* from dental plaques. *Jordan J. Biol. Sci.* **2008**, *1*, 135–139.
22. Yun, J.-H.; Park, J.-E.; Kim, D.-I.; Lee, S.-I.; Choi, S.-H.; Cho, K.-S.; Lee, D.-S. Identification of putative periodontal pathogens in Korean chronic periodontitis patients. *J. Korean Acad. Periodontol.* **2008**, *38*, 143–152. [CrossRef]
23. Yoshida, A.; Suzuki, N.; Nakano, Y.; Kawada, M.; Oho, T.; Koga, T. Development of a 5′ Nuclease-Based Real-Time PCR Assay for Quantitative Detection of Cariogenic Dental Pathogens Streptococcus mutans and Streptococcus sobrinus. *J. Clin. Microbiol.* **2003**, *41*, 4438–4441. [CrossRef]
24. Haarman, M.; Knol, J. Quantitative Real-Time PCR Analysis of Fecal Lactobacillus Species in Infants Receiving a Prebiotic Infant Formula. *Appl. Environ. Microbiol.* **2006**, *72*, 2359–2365. [CrossRef] [PubMed]
25. Sakai, H.; Procop, G.W.; Kobayashi, N.; Togawa, D.; Wilson, D.A.; Borden, L.; Krebs, V.; Bauer, T.W. Simultaneous Detection of Staphylococcus aureus and Coagulase-Negative Staphylococci in Positive Blood Cultures by Real-Time PCR with Two Fluorescence Resonance Energy Transfer Probe Sets. *J. Clin. Microbiol.* **2004**, *42*, 5739–5744. [CrossRef] [PubMed]
26. Granger, K.; Rundell, M.S.; Pingle, M.R.; Shatsky, R.; Larone, D.H.; Golightly, L.M.; Barany, F.; Spitzer, E.D. Multiplex PCR-Ligation Detection Reaction Assay for Simultaneous Detection of Drug Resistance and Toxin Genes from *Staphylococcus aureus*, *Enterococcus faecalis*, and *Enterococcus faecium*. *J. Clin. Microbiol.* **2009**, *48*, 277–280. [CrossRef] [PubMed]
27. Firth, D. Bias Reduction of Maximum Likelihood Estimates. *Biometrika* **1993**, *80*, 27. [CrossRef]
28. Heinze, G.; Schemper, M. A solution to the problem of separation in logistic regression. *Stat. Med.* **2002**, *21*, 2409–2419. [CrossRef]
29. Tonetti, M.S.; Greenwell, H.; Kornman, K.S. Staging and grading of periodontitis: Framework and proposal of a new classification and case definition. *J. Periodontol.* **2018**, *89*, S159–S172. [CrossRef]
30. Park, N.J.; Zhou, X.; Yu, T.; Brinkman, B.M.; Zimmermann, B.G.; Palanisamy, V.; Wong, D.T. Characterization of salivary RNA by cDNA library analysis. *Arch. Oral Biol.* **2007**, *52*, 30–35. [CrossRef]
31. Papapanou, P.N.; Baelum, V.; Luan, W.-M.; Madianos, P.N.; Chen, X.; Fejerskov, O.; Dahlén, G. Subgingival Microbiota in Adult Chinese: Prevalence and Relation to Periodontal Disease Progression. *J. Periodontol.* **1997**, *68*, 651–666. [CrossRef]
32. Kuboniwa, M.; Amano, A.; Kimura, K.R.; Sekine, S.; Kato, S.; Yamamoto, Y.; Okahashi, N.; Iida, T.; Shizukuishi, S. Quantitative detection of periodontal pathogens using real-time polymerase chain reaction with TaqMan probes. *Oral Microbiol. Immunol.* **2004**, *19*, 168–176. [CrossRef] [PubMed]
33. He, J.; Huang, W.; Pan, Z.; Cui, H.; Qi, G.; Zhou, X.; Chen, H. Quantitative analysis of microbiota in saliva, supragingival, and subgingival plaque of Chinese adults with chronic periodontitis. *Clin. Oral Investig.* **2011**, *16*, 1579–1588. [CrossRef]
34. Slots, J. Subgingival microflora and periodontal disease. *J. Clin. Periodontol.* **1979**, *6*, 351–382. [CrossRef]
35. Haubek, D.; Ennibi, O.-K.; Poulsen, K.; Vaeth, M.; Poulsen, S.; Kilian, M. Risk of aggressive periodontitis in adolescent carriers of the JP2 clone of Aggregatibacter (Actinobacillus) actinomycetemcomitans in Morocco: A prospective longitudinal cohort study. *Lancet* **2008**, *371*, 237–242. [CrossRef]
36. Papapanou, P.N.; Neiderud, A.M.; Disick, E.; Lalla, E.; Miller, G.C.; Dahlén, G. Longitudinal stability of serum immunoglobulin G responses to periodontal bacteria. *J. Clin. Periodontol.* **2004**, *31*, 985–990. [CrossRef]
37. Van Winkelhoff, A.J.; Loos, B.G.; van der Reijden, W.A.; van der Velden, U. Porphyromonas gingivalis, Bacteroides forsythus and other putative periodontal pathogens in subjects with and without periodontal destruction. *J. Clin. Periodontol.* **2002**, *29*, 1023–1028. [CrossRef] [PubMed]
38. Kolenbrander, P.E.; Palmer, R.J.; Periasamy, S.; Jakubovics, N.S. Oral multispecies biofilm development and the key role of cell–cell distance. *Nat. Rev. Microbiol.* **2010**, *8*, 471–480. [CrossRef] [PubMed]
39. Socransky, S.S.; Haffajee, A.D. The Bacterial Etiology of Destructive Periodontal Disease: Current Concepts. *J. Periodontol.* **1992**, *63*, 322–331. [CrossRef] [PubMed]
40. Aas, J.A.; Paster, B.J.; Stokes, L.N.; Olsen, I.; Dewhirst, F.E. Defining the Normal Bacterial Flora of the Oral Cavity. *J. Clin. Microbiol.* **2005**, *43*, 5721–5732. [CrossRef]
41. Genco, R.; Kornman, K.; Williams, R.; Offenbacher, S.; Zambon, J.J.; Ishikawa, I.; Listgarten, M.; Michalowicz, B.; Page, R.; Schenkein, H.; et al. Periodontal Diseases: Pathogenesis and Microbial Factors. *J. Am. Dent. Assoc.* **1998**, *129*, 58S–62S. [CrossRef]

42. Kawada, M.; Yoshida, A.; Suzuki, N.; Nakano, Y.; Saito, T.; Oho, T.; Koga, T. Prevalence of Porphyromonas gingivalis in relation to periodontal status assessed by real-time PCR. *Oral Microbiol. Immunol.* **2004**, *19*, 289–292. [CrossRef] [PubMed]
43. Klein, M.I.; Gonçalves, R.B. Detection of Tannerella forsythensis(Bacteroides forsythus) and Porphyromonas gingivalisby Polymerase Chain Reaction in Subjects with Different Periodontal Status. *J. Periodontol.* **2003**, *74*, 798–802. [CrossRef] [PubMed]
44. Lee, N.-H.; Lee, E.; Kim, Y.-S.; Kim, W.-K.; Lee, Y.-K.; Kim, S.-H. Differential expression of microRNAs in the saliva of patients with aggressive periodontitis: A pilot study of potential biomarkers for aggressive periodontitis. *J. Periodontal Implant. Sci.* **2020**, *50*, 281–290. [CrossRef] [PubMed]

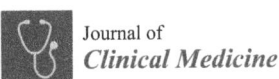

Article

Heterogeneity of Blood Vessels and Assessment of Microvessel Density-MVD in Gingivitis

Ciprian Roi [1], Pușa Nela Gaje [2], Raluca Amalia Ceaușu [2], Alexandra Roi [3,*], Laura Cristina Rusu [3], Eugen Radu Boia [4], Simina Boia [5], Ruxandra Elena Luca [6] and Mircea Riviș [1]

1. Department of Anesthesiology and Oral Surgery, Multidisciplinary Center for Research, Evaluation, Diagnosis and Therapies in Oral Medicine, "Victor Babeș" University of Medicine and Pharmacy, 300041 Timisoara, Romania; ciprian.roi@umft.ro (C.R.); rivis.mircea@umft.ro (M.R.)
2. Department of Microscopic Morphology and Histology, Angiogenesis Research Center, "Victor Babeș" University of Medicine and Pharmacy, 300041 Timisoara, Romania; gaje.nela@umft.ro (P.N.G.); ra.ceausu@umft.ro (R.A.C.)
3. Department of Oral Pathology, Multidisciplinary Center for Research, Evaluation, Diagnosis and Therapies in Oral Medicine, "Victor Babeș" University of Medicine and Pharmacy, 300041 Timisoara, Romania; laura.rusu@umft.ro
4. Department of Ear Nose and Throat, "Victor Babeș" University of Medicine and Pharmacy Timisoara, 300041 Timisoara, Romania; eugen.boia@umft.ro
5. Department of Periodontology, "Victor Babeș" University of Medicine and Pharmacy Timisoara, 300041 Timisoara, Romania; simina.boia@umft.ro
6. Department of Oral Rehabilitation and Dental Emergencies, "Victor Babeș" University of Medicine and Pharmacy, 300041 Timisoara, Romania; luca.ruxandra@umft.ro
* Correspondence: alexandra.moga@umft.ro; Tel.: +40-748-245-993

Abstract: Gingivitis is a very common oral disease highly prevalent in adults that, if left untreated, can progress to periodontitis. It involves a complex and slow interaction between the host response and the oral microbiome represented by the dental plaque. The inflammation of the gingiva is associated with the activation of pathological angiogenesis and the existence of a high number of newly formed blood vessels quantified as microvessel density (MVD). The present study includes a number of 51 gingival biopsies from patients with different gingival indexes (GI): GI = 0, $n = 12$; GI = 1, $n = 15$; GI = 2, $n = 16$; and GI = 3, $n = 8$, processed and stained with the routine hematoxylin–eosin method. The inflammatory infiltrate was scored, the blood vessels were detected with anti-CD34 antibody, and MVD was determined. Inflammatory changes were observed in 39 of the 51 cases included in our study. CD34 + vessels with normal morphological appearance were observed in all 12 cases of health gingiva. In cases of inflammatory lesions, the morphology of the blood vessels showed changes with the evolution of gingival lesions. In severe inflammation, a particular aspect was observed in the vessels, such as the presence of the phenomenon of intussusception. MVD increases with the severity of gingival lesions, with the highest density being observed in severe inflammation.

Keywords: gingivitis; MVD; angiogenesis; CD34

1. Introduction

Periodontal health is defined by Chapple as a "state free from inflammatory periodontal disease that allows an individual to function normally and avoid consequence (mental or physical) due to current or past disease" [1]. The periodontal health of an individual can be assessed by the clinical absence of diseases such as gingivitis, periodontitis, or other periodontal disorders.

On the other hand, periodontal disorders are very common and may impact up to 90% of the world's population. Gingivitis is a pathological condition often associated with bacterial biofilm that is generally reversible upon a rigorous reinstatement of oral hygiene procedures [2]. Despite the fact that it is considered to be the "route" towards the development of periodontitis, affecting a considerably high number of patients, this pathology is often disregarded [3–5].

The study conducted by Lang et al. [3] is based on identifying the presence of gingivitis as a key risk factor in the incidence of periodontal disease, revealing their association in approximately 37% of the gingivitis cases and showing a definite progression to periodontitis and loss of teeth thereafter. A patient diagnosed with gingivitis can revert to a complete state of oral health, while once diagnosed with periodontitis, even following successful therapy, further lifelong supportive care is required to prevent the recurrence of the disease [6]. The heterogeneity of this condition is also highlighted during the treatment protocol, revealing a percentage of the diagnosed gingivitis cases that do not respond properly to standard mechanical treatment [7] and the healing of the tissue exhibiting normal biological conditions is absent [8].

The classification of gingival diseases is made by taking into consideration the presence or absence of dental plaque. Dental plaque-induced gingival diseases may occur on a periodontium with no attachment loss or with attachment loss that is stable and not progressing [9].

Angiogenesis in the oral mucosa diseases, and implicitly gingivitis, is a negative prognostic factor that potentiates the manifestations of the disease and worsens its progression. The process is defined as the formation of new blood vessels from pre-existing ones. It involves endothelial cell migration and proliferation, and the further formation and organization of tubular structures that in time will bond, resulting in a final form of stable blood vessels. Through this process, the neoformation vessels bring pro-inflammatory cells and mediators, but also oxygen and nutrients to the inflamed tissues [10]. The inflammation of the gingiva, which is the main mechanism for periodontal lesions, is associated with the activation of pathological angiogenesis and the existence of a high number of newly formed blood vessels quantified as a microvessel density (MVD) [11].

The transition from gingivitis without bone loss to periodontitis is explained by the propagation of the inflammatory response, correlated with the failure of the innate inflammation resolving mechanisms. In the end, it results in the chronicity of the inflammatory lesion, which is histologically characterized by the present repair mechanisms signs (angiogenesis and fibrosis) occurring concurrently with inflammation [12]. It plays a significant role as well in bone regeneration, contributing to the inflammatory and regenerative phase of the alveolar bone. The microvessel density evaluation targets the acknowledgment of the angiogenesis level and its implication in multiple inflammatory conditions has been widely accepted.

Different markers (monoclonal antibodies) such as CD34, CD31, CD105, vascular endothelial growth factor (VEGF), and beta fibroblast growth factor (FGFβ) are used to measure microvessel density (MVD) in each microscopic field [13,14].

CD34 is a monomeric transmembrane glycoprotein with a molecular weight of 110–120 KD, which has a high sensitivity and moderate specificity. The anti-CD34 antibody, the QBEnd10 clone, is the most widely used immunohistochemical marker in the study of tumor angiogenesis and microvessel density, being positive on paraffin sections, ice, and Western blotting techniques. CD34 expression is frequently used to evaluate MVD, unlike CD31 which, in addition to being present in endothelial cells, is also localized in the macrophages [15,16].

In the scientific literature, existing studies regarding the angiogenesis evaluation in gingivitis are very limited, with the emphasis being on periodontitis and oral neoplasms. Starting from this aspect, in the present study, we aim to evaluate by immunohistochemical methods the morphology of blood vessels and microvessel density in inflammatory gingival lesions compared to normal, healthy gingiva. The quantification of MVD was established by the number of vessels in the inflammatory infiltrate, in the surrounding stroma, and also in the epithelium. Taking into consideration that gingivitis and its persistence influences the further development of periodontitis, the assessment of the microvessel density and heterogeneity in this stage could be an evolution marker in the possible progression of this disease. Our study brings a new point of view regarding the histologic aspects of gingivitis without bone loss and can promote further studies to establish the mechanism of clinical aggravation of gingivitis and transformation in periodontitis.

2. Materials and Methods

Our study was approved by the Ethics Committee of "Victor Babeș" University of Medicine and Pharmacy Timișoara (no.12/2021) and patients agreed and signed an informed consent form that followed the guidelines of the Declaration of Helsinki.

2.1. Patients' Data

In this study, we included patients based on the following inclusion and exclusion criteria. Inclusion criteria:

- Age: 18–60 years;
- Both males and females;
- Diagnosed gingivitis with no attachment loss;
- Periodontal and gingivitis-free patients (for the control group);
- No known general comorbidities;
- Non-smokers;
- Non-alcohol drinkers.

Exclusion criteria:

- Gingivitis modified by systemic factors, such as medication;
- Periodontitis;
- Patients with periodontal therapies;
- Patients with medication.

After the application of the inclusion and exclusion criteria, a total of 51 patients were included in the study, 28 females—54.9% and 23 males—45.09%. The Gingival Index (GI) used for the assessment of the gingivitis had the following values: $GI = 0$, $n = 12$; $GI = 1$, $n = 15$; $GI = 2$, $n = 16$; and $GI = 3$, $n = 8$, with a mean value of 1.82. The biopsy samples taken from healthy patients that were included in the control group were based on the following clinical criteria: the absence of gingival erythema, no bleeding while probing, no clinical visible plaque deposits, and a probing depth within 2 mm.

In Figure 1, the clinical assessment of gingivitis is presented in the three stages of inflammation.

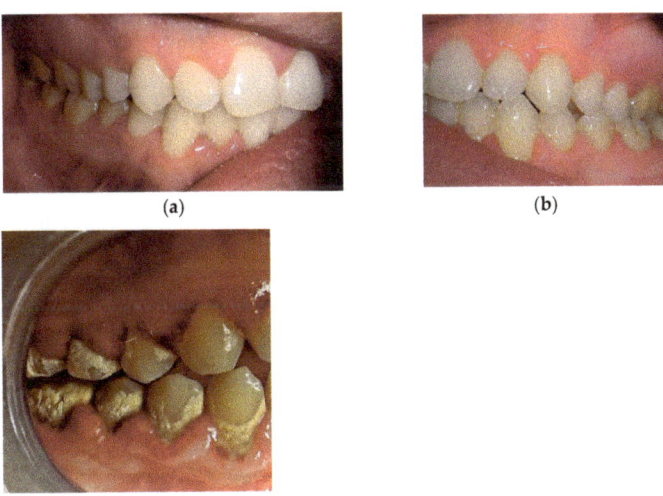

Figure 1. Clinical images of gingivitis: (**a**) mild inflammation-GI = 1; (**b**) moderate inflammation-GI = 2; and (**c**) severe inflammation-GI = 3.

The present study included a total of 51 gingival biopsies that were processed according to the standard histological technique. The gingival biopsies were obtained from the interdental papilla between the mandibular first and second premolar. A biopsy was taken from each patient and washed with buffer saline.

2.2. Primary Processing

Gingival biopsies were fixed in 10% buffered formalin for 48 h and then embedded in paraffin using the standard histological technique. The primary processing was completely standardized using the Shandon embedding center (Thermo-Shandon, Runcorn, Chershire, UK). Five micrometer-thick sections were prepared for each case and were stained with the routine hematoxylin–eosin method. These slides were used to analyze the morphological changes of the epithelium and to evaluate the density of the inflammatory infiltrate. Additional slides were prepared and selected for the immunohistochemical study.

Scoring

The inflammatory infiltrate was scored as 0 (absent), value 1 (isolated inflammatory cells, less than 10 inflammatory cells/microscopic field, and low inflammation), value 2 (aggregates of inflammatory cells in the lamina propria only and moderate inflammation), and value 3 (aggregates of inflammatory cells in the lamina propria associated with intraepithelial lymphocytes and severe inflammation).

2.3. Imunohistochimical Technique

Blood vessels were detected with anti-CD34 antibody—monoclonal mouse, clone QBEnd 10, ready to use, and Leica Bond (Leica Biosystem, Newcastle Ltd., Newcastle upon Tyne, UK). A heat-induced epitope retrieval with Bond Epitope Retrieval Solution 1 citrate buffer (pH 6.0) (Leica Biosystems, Newcastle Ltd., Newcastle upon Tyne, UK) for 30 min was applied. Endogenous peroxidase was blocked for five minutes with 3% hydrogen peroxide and followed by incubation with the primary antibody for 30 min. The Bond Polymer Refine Detection System (Leica Biosystems, Newcastle upon Tyne, UK) was used to develop the immunohistochemical reaction and the final product was visualized with 3,3′ diaminobenzidine dihydrochloride (DAB). The chromogen was applied for 10 min and the hematoxylin was used for 5 min for the counterstaining. The full immunohistochemical procedure was performed with a Leica Bond-Max (Leica Biosystems, Newcastle upon Tyne, UK) autostainer.

2.4. Staining Interpretation

All the sections were examined using a Nikon Eclipse 600 optical microscope. Initially, the examination was made using the ×100 lens in order to identify the most intensely positive areas for CD34. Vessel quantification was performed using the ×40 lens. The area of each field was approximately 0.2 mm^2. The endothelial cells colored with brown CD34 (CD34-positive) that formed a cluster of endothelial cells with a lumen were considered to be blood vessels. Single CD34-positive endothelial cells were also included in the count. The blood vessels with a muscle wall were excluded. The three fields with the largest number of blood vessels were chosen and then examined from left to right, avoiding counting the vessels from the same areas. The arithmetic mean of the total number of vessels encountered in the three examined fields was performed, representing the final result. The statistical evaluation was made by SPSS 17 software (IBM Analytics, Armonk, NY, USA) and a p-value of <0.05 was considered statistically significant.

3. Results

Microscopically, in normal healthy gingiva (n = 12) there were no inflammatory changes present. The normal histological structure of the gingival mucosa was preserved. It was noticed that a parakeratinized stratified squamous epithelium and lamina propria were composed of dense irregular connective tissue (Figure 2a).

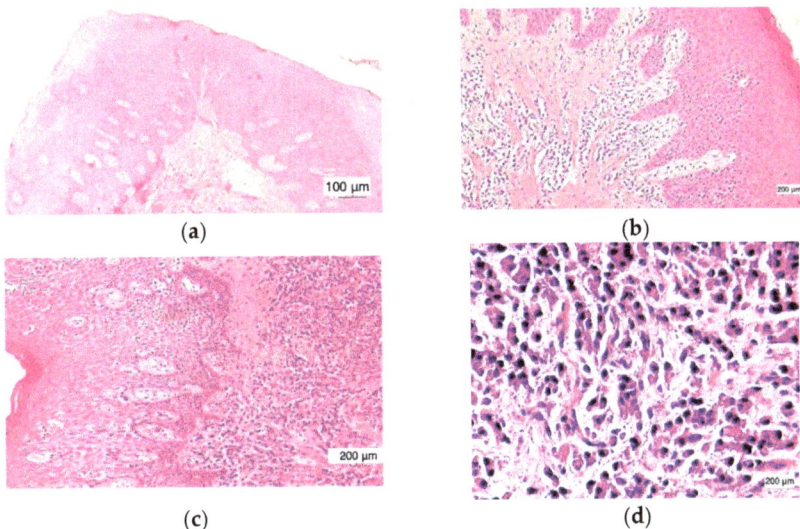

Figure 2. Different hematoxylin–eosin microscopic images for assessment of the morphological changes of the epithelium evaluation of the density of the inflammatory infiltrate: (**a**) gingiva without inflammatory changes GI = 0, ×200 magnification; (**b**) inflammatory infiltrate in the lamina propria with focal distribution, epithelium without modification GI = 1, ×200 magnification; (**c**) inflammatory infiltrate in the lamina propria, intraepithelial lymphocytes GI = 2, ×200 magnification; and (**d**) inflammatory infiltrate with polymorphic cellularity GI = 3, ×400 magnification.

In the cases evaluated with a score value of +1, low inflammation, the inflammatory infiltrate was found in the lamina propria with focal distribution, but also as isolated inflammatory cells. The covering epithelium had no changes and intraepithelial lymphocytes were very rare (Figure 2b).

In the cases evaluated with a score value of +2, moderate inflammation, the inflammatory infiltrate was noticed in the lamina propria over extended areas, reaching as far as the covering epithelium. Basal cell layer hyperplasia was found in the covering epithelium (Figure 2c).

The cases evaluated with a score value of +3 were characterized by severe inflammation. The aggregates of inflammatory cells in the lamina propria distributed over large areas associated with numerous intraepithelial lymphocytes were noticed. A tendency of inflammatory infiltrate distribution around the blood vessels was found. The presence of large amounts of lymphocytes in the covering epithelium induced an alteration of its structure. Thus, a hyperplasia of basal and parabasal cells was observed (Figure 2d).

Inflammatory changes were observed in 39 of the 51 cases included in our study. The inflammatory infiltrate consisted mainly of lymphocytes, macrophages, and neutrophilic granulocytes. Rarely contained eosinophilic granulocytes and plasma cells were also identified (Figure 2c).

Out of the 39 cases with inflammatory lesions, 15 cases showed mild inflammation (G I = 1, score value 1), 16 cases showed moderate inflammation (GI = 2, score value 2), and 8 cases had severe inflammatory lesions (GI = 3, score value 3), as found by clinical examination. The microscopic features of the normal gingiva, mild, moderate, and severe periodontal disease are shown in Figure 2. CD34 + vessels with a normal morphological appearance were observed in all 12 cases of healthy gingiva. The identified vessels are predominantly capillary and distributed throughout the gingival lamina, including the papillae to the proximity of the surface epithelium. In all of these cases, the blood vessels were small in diameter and all had a lumen. In cases of inflammatory lesions, the morphology of the blood vessels showed changes in accordance with the evolution of the periodontal lesions. Thus, both small-caliber vessels with a very narrow lumen delimited by proliferative endothelial cells and small vessels without a lumen were observed (Figure 3).

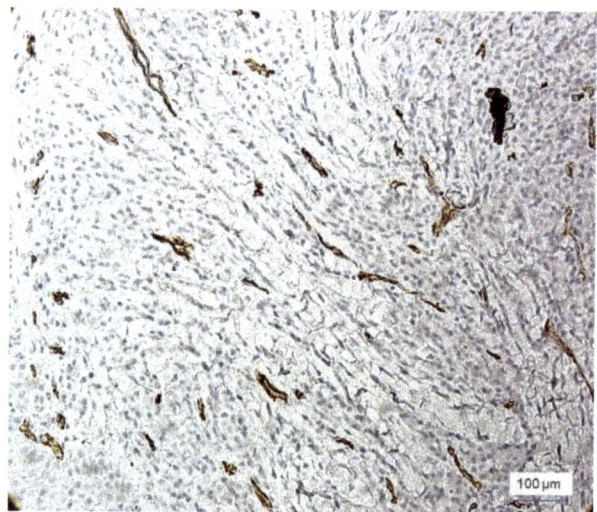

Figure 3. Severe inflammation marked vascular polymorphism, small vessels with or without lumen narrow, anti-CD34 immunohistochemical staining, and DAB chromogen, ×100 magnification.

Small narrow-lumen vessels have been observed in large amounts in gingival lesions with moderate and severe inflammation. In the cases of severe inflammation, vascular structures in the form of cords with a tendency to form a lumen were encountered.

Most cases with severe inflammation showed extensive areas of bleeding. In these cases, we identified large dilated vessels with dilated stasis and numerous branches, suggesting the activation of endothelial cells (Figure 4).

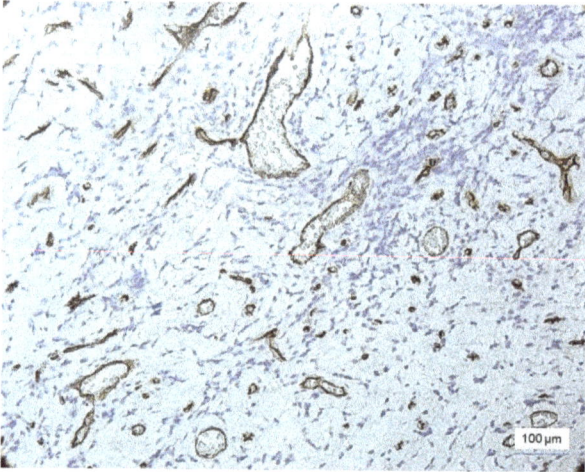

Figure 4. Large dilated and branched vessels, anti-CD34 immunohistochemical staining, and DAB chromogen, ×200 magnification.

In severe inflammation, a particular aspect was observed in the vessels: the presence of the phenomenon of intussusception, characterized by invagination of the vascular wall with the formation of intraluminal bridges that divided the initial vessel into two smaller vessels (Figure 5).

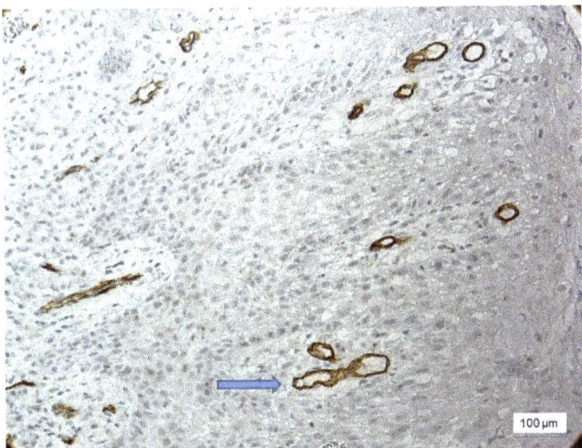

Figure 5. Severe inflammation, intussusception (arrow), intraluminal bridges dividing the blood vessel, anti-CD34 immunohistochemical staining, and DAB chromogen, ×200 magnification.

All these aspects related to the changes found in the morphology of the blood vessels in cases with inflammatory changes suggest that the initiation of angiogenesis in moderate and severe periodontal lesions was present.

Microvessel density (MVD) was quantified and the number of CD34 + vessels near the inflammatory infiltrate, in the surrounding stroma, and in the epithelium was observed. In all cases of inflammatory lesions, an increase in MVD was observed in proportion to the severity of the inflammation. Regardless of the severity of inflammation, the MVD was significantly increased in the stroma compared to the MVD in the infiltrate. Thus, in mild inflammation, the total number of vessels was between 12 and 35 vessels/microscopic field. Only two cases with mild inflammation showed a higher MVD (approximately 46 vessels/field).

In moderate inflammation, MVD was slightly increased compared to the cases with mild inflammation. The number of vessels was 15–49/field, with the majority being identified in the stroma around the inflammatory infiltrate (Figure 6).

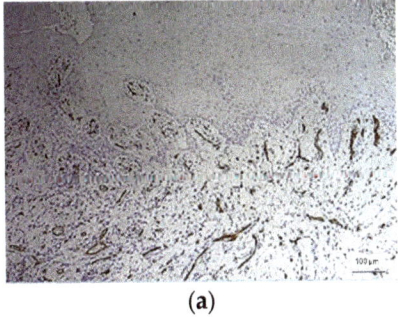
(a)

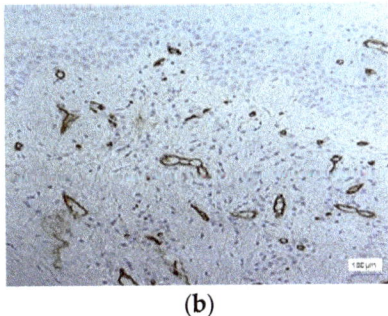
(b)

Figure 6. Moderate inflammation, GI = 2, and increased microvessel density at the stromal level, ×100: (**a**) stromal vascular polymorphism and intussusception, ×200, and (**b**) anti-CD34 immunohistochemical staining and DAB chromogen.

As expected, the highest values for MVD were observed in cases of severe inflammation, where the total number of vessels was between 35–89/field, most of them being observed in the stroma (Figure 7). Two cases with severe inflammation showed a lower MVD (20–25 vessels/field).

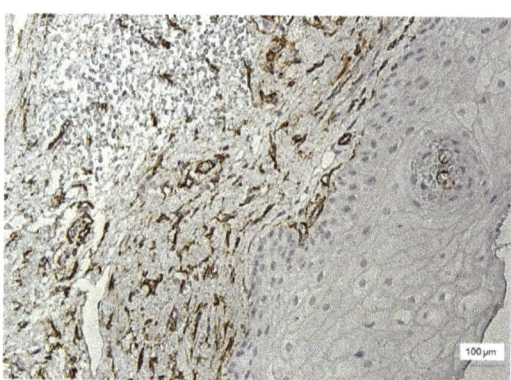

Figure 7. Severe inflammation, GI = 3, increased microvessel density at the stromal level, vascular polymorphism, anti-CD34 immunohistochemical staining, and DAB chromogen, ×100.

The presence of small capillary vessels was observed in the gingival epithelium, as well as in the cases with severe inflammation (Figure 8). Capillaries have been identified in the basal layer of the gingival epithelium.

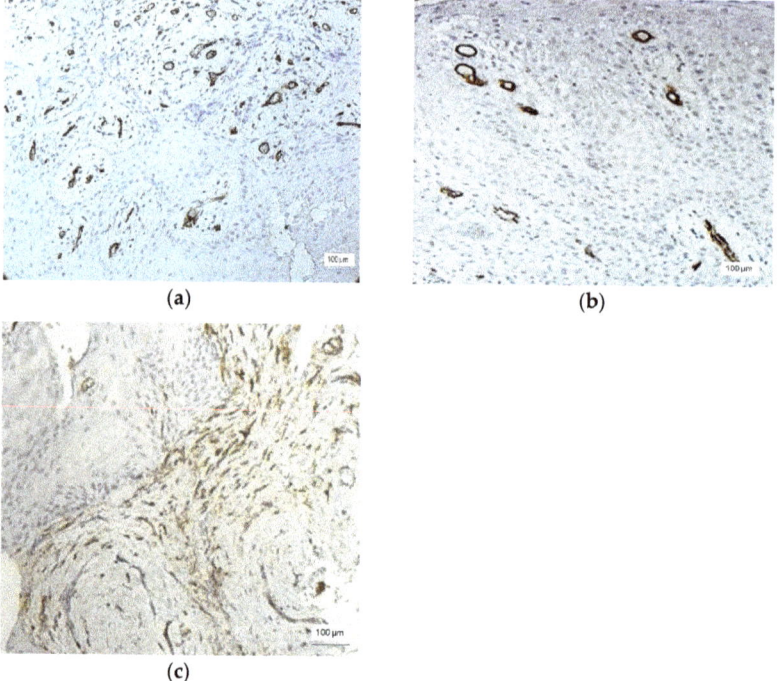

Figure 8. (a–c) Capillaries in the basal layer of the epithelium, anti-CD34 immunohistochemical staining, and DAB chromogen, ×200 magnification.

4. Discussion

According to the new classification scheme for periodontal and peri-implant diseases and conditions established at the World Workshop on the Classification of Periodontal and Peri-implant Diseases in 2017, gingivitis is defined as a site-specific inflammatory condition initiated by dental biofilm accumulation and characterized by edema and erythema of the gingival tissue with the absence of periodontal attachment loss [6,17]. Generally, it is a painless condition, which rarely leads to spontaneous bleeding. The tissue changes are completely reversible, once the dental biofilm is removed. Gingivitis is a precursor of periodontitis, which is characterized by gingival inflammation combined with connective tissue attachment and bone loss [17].

The development of new vessels from pre-existing vessels, called angiogenesis, is a complex process involving the remodeling of the extracellular matrix, the migration and proliferation of endothelial cells, and the morphogenesis of microvessels. Angiogenesis is often a significant and independent prognostic indicator for both overall survival rates and diseases [18]. Angiogenesis is one of the most well-known stromal factors involved in tumor progression as well as in inflammatory lesions, such as periodontal lesions. It has been extensively investigated in various tumors, such as breast carcinoma, hepatocellular carcinoma, astrocytoma, cervical carcinoma, and ovarian carcinoma, but also in several lesions and odontogenic tumors such as ameloblastoma [19].

As a result of the interaction between the gingival epithelium and the stromal compartment, angiogenesis is an early and constant process in gingivitis and periodontal diseases, occurring at all stages [20]. Angiogenesis and the dilation of capillaries appear to be characteristic of the vascular response in chronic inflammation, and apart from gingivitis and periodontitis, are also reported in rheumatoid arthritis, psoriasis, and other chronic inflammatory lesions [21].

Persistence of the gingival inflammation under the presence of various local and general risk factors progresses to the destruction of the underlying connective tissue and eventually to the destruction of the alveolar bone [22].

The proximity of this thick inflammatory infiltrate to the sulcular epithelium, which is in direct contact with the bacterial plaque irritant, demonstrates the importance of the bacterial plaque which plays a key role in the initiation and progression of gingivitis. A single kind of organism is not involved in the change from a healthy periodontium to an inflammatory periodontium. In periodontal diseases, the microbial communities are dysbiotic, with uncontrolled microbial species composition and abundance resulting in a pathogenic situation. Despite the fact that the Gram-negative organisms, "red complex" are associated with periodontal disease, they are also found at low levels in healthy patients without periodontal disease, suggesting that they are pathobionts rather than pathogens [21].

Periodontitis shares many of the same histological characteristics as gingivitis, with the exception that the connective tissues at the base of the gingival sulcus are destroyed, resulting in the formation of a deep periodontal pocket bordered by epithelium. In our findings, the inflammatory infiltrate consisted mainly of lymphocytes, macrophages, and neutrophilic granulocytes-PMN, and more rarely consisted of eosinophilic granulocytes and plasma cells. Vascular alterations appear to either assist or inhibit PMN activity, influencing the progress of the disease. In periodontitis, high endothelial cells are engaged with PMN rather than lymphocyte emigration, contrary to most circumstances [23].

The findings obtained in our study sustain the heterogeneity of the angiogenic process dependent on the level of gingiva inflammation. In tissues, the degree of angiogenesis can be evaluated by microvessel density (MVD) using an antibody against CD34, a glycosylated transmembrane protein present on progenitor endothelial cells [24]. Antibodies to the CD34 molecule are widely used for immunohistochemical staining of gingival microvessels MVD found in the early stages of gingivitis and may be considered the first step of a complex process with damages countable depending on the gingival index. MVD measurement is a widely known predictor of tumor growth, metastasis, and patient survival rate and correlates with tumor aggression [19]. In addition to this, MVD is also associated with the progression of gingivitis lesions as observed in our study. Increased MVD could cause a higher apport of different cytokines, adhesion molecules, and other inflammation factors. In gingivitis and periodontitis, the transport of inflammatory cells, nutrients, and oxygen caused by angiogenesis could enhance the severity of the inflammation [24].

Vascular changes are essential to the initiation of both acute and chronic inflammation, and blood flow is essential to its resolution. Inflammation begins with vasodilation, increasing circulation, and increased vascularization into the area. The progressive disorder of affected gingiva perfusion and oxygenation, the presence of increased vascular permeability, and functional failure of the microvascular system are the main processes involved in disease progression [25,26].

In the development of gingivitis, an important role is played by the vascular endothelial growth factor (VEGF), a 45-kd homodimeric proinflammatory glycoprotein that causes vascular permeability and angiogenesis. This protein seems to be involved in the onset and progression of gingivitis and periodontitis, mainly promoting the vascular network expansion generally observed in inflammation [27]. Endothelial cells produce proteases and plasminogen activators in response to VEGF, which break down the vascular basement membrane and allow endothelial cells to proliferate and migrate [28]. The double correlation of intraepithelial-increased MVD with VEGF may be considered a unique and specific feature of mild gingivitis lesions progressing to moderate lesions, indicating the initiation of the 'vascularization' phenomenon, which refers to the acquisition of new blood vessels by the affected gingival epithelium [11]. Lucarini et al. [29] in their study concluded the fact that the gingival mucosa affected by an inflammatory condition has significantly higher levels of VEGF and MVD compared to the healthy mucosa. VEGF has a direct implication in the vascular network, it increases the tissue edema, and influences the blood flow by decreasing it, suggesting a high implication in the etiology of gingivitis.

Acknowledging the heterogeneity of the blood vessels and the microvessel density in gingivitis is an important aspect of fully understanding the evolution of this disease and its possible progress towards periodontitis with high clinical relevance. The vascular changes encountered in gingivitis could represent a viable correlation in anticipating the incidence of periodontal involvement.

5. Conclusions

The modifications observed in patients presenting gingivitis indicate the presence of angiogenesis, an aspect suggested by increased vascular polymorphism, the phenomenon of intussusception, and finally, the acquisition of vessels in the gingival epithelium. MVD increases with the severity of gingival lesions, with the highest density being observed in severe inflammation.

Author Contributions: Conceptualization, C.R. and P.N.G.; methodology, P.N.G.; formal analysis, A.R.; investigation, M.R. and L.C.R.; resources, E.R.B., S.B., A.R. and R.E.L.; data curation, A.R. and M.R.; writing—original draft preparation, C.R., M.R. and L.C.R.; writing—review and editing, C.R., P.N.G. and R.A.C.; visualization, E.R.B., S.B., A.R. and R.E.L.; supervision, M.R. All authors have equal contributions. All authors have read and agreed to the published version of the manuscript.

Funding: This research received no external funding.

Institutional Review Board Statement: Our study was approved by the Ethics Committee of "Victor Babeș" University of Medicine and Pharmacy Timișoara, (no. 12/2021) and patients agreed and signed an informed consent form that followed the guidelines of the Declaration of Helsinki.

Informed Consent Statement: Informed consent was obtained from all subjects involved in the study.

Data Availability Statement: Data sharing is not applicable to this article.

Conflicts of Interest: The authors declare no conflict of interest.

References

1. Chapple, I.; Mealey, B.L.; Van Dyke, T.E.; Bartold, P.M.; Dommisch, H.; Eickholz, P.; Geisinger, M.L.; Genco, R.J.; Glogauer, M.; Goldstein, M.; et al. Periodontal health and gingival diseases and conditions on an intact and a reduced periodontium: Consensus report of workgroup 1 of the 2017 World Workshop on the Classification of Periodontal and Peri-Implant Diseases and Conditions. *J. Periodontol.* **2018**, *89*, S74–S84. [CrossRef] [PubMed]
2. Nagarajan, R.; Miller, C.S.; Dawson, D.; Al-Sabbagh, M.; Ebersole, J.L. Patient-Specific variations in biomarkers across gingivitis and periodontitis. *PLoS ONE* **2015**, *10*, e0136792. [CrossRef] [PubMed]
3. Lang, N.P.; Schätzle, M.A.; Löe, H. Gingivitis as a risk factor in periodontal disease. *J. Periodontol.* **2009**, *36*, 3–8. [CrossRef] [PubMed]
4. Schätzle, M.; Faddy, M.J.; Cullinan, M.P.; Seymour, G.J.; Lang, N.P.; Bürgin, W.; Anerud, A.; Boysen, H.; Löe, H. The clinical course of chronic periodontitis: V. Predictive factors in periodontal disease. *J. Periodontol.* **2009**, *36*, 365–371. [CrossRef] [PubMed]
5. Schätzle, M.; Löe, H.; Bürgin, W.; Anerud, A.; Boysen, H.; Lang, N.P. Clinical course of chronic periodontitis. I. Role of gingivitis. *J. Periodontol.* **2003**, *30*, 887–901. [CrossRef]
6. Caton, J.G.; Armitage, G.; Berglundh, T.; Chapple, I.; Jepsen, S.; Kornman, K.S.; Mealey, B.L.; Papapanou, P.N.; Sanz, M.; Tonetti, M.S. A new classification scheme for periodontal and peri-implant diseases and conditions-Introduction and key changes from the 1999 classification. *J. Periodontol.* **2018**, *89*, S1–S8. [CrossRef]
7. Armitage, G.C. Learned and unlearned concepts in periodontal diagnostics: A 50-year perspective. *Periodontology* **2013**, *62*, 20–36. [CrossRef]
8. Syndergaard, B.; Al-Sabbagh, M.; Kryscio, R.J.; Xi, J.; Ding, X.; Ebersole, J.L.; Miller, C.S. Salivary biomarkers associated with gingivitis and response to therapy. *J. Periodontol.* **2014**, *85*, e295–e303. [CrossRef]
9. Newman, M.G.; Takei, H.H.; Klokkevold, P.R.; Carranza, F.A. Classification of diseases and conditions affecting the periodontium. In *Newman and Carranza's Essentials of Clinical Periodontology*, 13th ed.; Elsevier: Philadelphia, PA, USA, 2019; p. 57.
10. Legorreta-Villegas, I.; Trejo-Remigio, D.A.; Ramírez-Martínez, C.M.; Portilla-Robertson, J.; Leyva-Huerta, E.R.; Jacinto-Alemán, L.F. Análisis de microdensidad vascular y factores de crecimiento en carcinoma oral de células escamosas. *Rev. ADM* **2020**, *77*, 287–294. [CrossRef]
11. Vladau, M.; Cimpean, A.M.; Balica, R.A.; Jitariu, A.A.; Popovici, R.A.; Raica, M. VEGF/VEGFR2 axis in periodontal disease progression and angiogenesis: Basic approach for a new therapeutic strategy. *In Vivo* **2016**, *30*, 53–60.
12. Meyle, J.; Chapple, I. Molecular aspects of the pathogenesis of periodontitis. *Periodontology* **2015**, *69*, 7–17. [CrossRef] [PubMed]
13. Kademani, D.; Lewis, J.T.; Lamb, D.H.; Rallis, D.J.; Harrington, J.R. Angiogenesis and CD34 expression as a predictor of recurrence in oral squamous cell carcinoma. *J. Oral Maxillofac. Surg.* **2009**, *67*, 1800–1805. [CrossRef] [PubMed]
14. Pereira, T.; Dodal, S.; Tamgadge, A.; Bhalerao, S.; Tamgadge, S. Quantitative evaluation of microvessel density using CD34 in clinical variants of ameloblastoma: An immunohistochemical study. *JOMFP* **2016**, *20*, 51–58. [CrossRef] [PubMed]
15. Natkunam, Y.; Rouse, R.V.; Zhu, S.; Fisher, C.; van De Rijn, M. Immunoblot analysis of CD34 expression in histologically diverse neoplasms. *Am. J. Clin. Pathol.* **2000**, *156*, 21–27. [CrossRef]
16. Vieira, S.C.; Silva, B.B.; Pinto, G.A.; Vassallo, J.; Moraes, N.G.; Santana, J.O.; Santos, L.G.; Carvasan, G.A.; Zeferino, L.C. CD34 as a marker for evaluating angiogenesis in cervical cancer. *Pathol. Res. Pract.* **2005**, *201*, 313–318. [CrossRef]
17. Trombelli, L.; Farina, R.; Silva, C.O.; Tatakis, D.N. Plaque-induced gingivitis: Case definition and diagnostic considerations. *J. Clin. Periodontol.* **2018**, *45*, S44–S67. [CrossRef]
18. Hande, A.H.; Gadbail, A.R.; Sonone, A.M.; Chaudhary, M.S.; Wadhwan, V.; Nikam, A. Comparative analysis of tumour angiogenesis in solid multicystic and unicystic ameloblastoma by using CD 105 (endoglin). *Arch. Oral Biol.* **2011**, *56*, 1635–1640. [CrossRef]
19. Segatelli, V.; de Oliveira, E.C.; Boin, I.F.; Ataide, E.C.; Escanhoela, C.A. Evaluation and comparison of microvessel density using the markers CD34 and CD105 in regenerative nodules, dysplastic nodules and hepatocellular carcinoma. *Hepatol. Int.* **2014**, *8*, 260–265. [CrossRef]
20. Kranti, K.; Mani, A.; Elizabeth, A. Immunoexpression of vascular endothelial growth factor and Ki-67 in human gingival samples: An observational study. *Indian J. Dent.* **2015**, *6*, 69–74. [CrossRef]
21. Zoellner, H.; Chapple, C.C.; Hunter, N. Microvasculature in gingivitis and chronic periodontitis: Disruption of vascular networks with protracted inflammation. *Microsc Res. Tech.* **2002**, *56*, 15–31. [CrossRef]
22. Kumar, S. Evidence-based update on diagnosis and management of gingivitis and periodontitis. *Dent. Clin. N. Am.* **2019**, *63*, 69–81. [CrossRef] [PubMed]
23. Jiang, Q.; Huang, X.; Yu, W.; Huang, R.; Zhao, X.; Chen, C. mTOR Signaling in the Regulation of CD4+ T Cell Subsets in Periodontal Diseases. *Front. Immunol.* **2022**, *13*, 827461. [CrossRef] [PubMed]
24. Aspriello, S.D.; Zizzi, A.; Spazzafumo, L.; Rubini, C.; Lorenzi, T.; Marzioni, D.; Bullon, P.; Piemontese, M. Effects of enamel matrix derivative on vascular endothelial growth factor expression and microvessel density in gingival tissues of periodontal pocket: A comparative study. *J. Periodontol.* **2011**, *82*, 606–612. [CrossRef] [PubMed]
25. Eldzharov, A.; Kabaloeva, D.; Nemeryuk, D.; Goncharenko, A.; Gatsalova, A.; Ivanova, E.; Kostritskiy, I.; Carrouel, F.; Bourgeois, D. Evaluation of Microcirculation, cytokine profile, and local antioxidant protection indices in periodontal health, and Stage II, Stage III Periodontitis. *J. Clin. Med.* **2021**, *10*, 1262. [CrossRef] [PubMed]

26. Kerdvongbundit, V.; Vongsavan, N.; Soo-Ampon, S.; Hasegawa, A. Microcirculation and micromorphology of healthy and inflamed gingivae. *Odontology* **2003**, *91*, 19–25. [CrossRef]
27. Aspriello, S.D.; Zizzi, A.; Lucarini, G.; Rubini, C.; Faloia, E.; Boscaro, M.; Tirabassi, G.; Piemontese, M. Vascular endothelial growth factor and microvessel density in periodontitis patients with and without diabetes. *J. Periodontol.* **2009**, *80*, 1783–1789. [CrossRef]
28. Cross, M.J.; Claesson-Welsh, L. FGF and VEGF function in angiogenesis: Signalling pathways, biological responses and therapeutic inhibition. *Trends Pharmacol. Sci.* **2001**, *22*, 201–207. [CrossRef]
29. Lucarini, G.; Zizzi, A.; Rubini, C.; Ciolino, F.; Aspriello, S.D. VEGF, Microvessel Density, and CD44 as Inflammation Markers in Peri-implant Healthy Mucosa, Peri-implant Mucositis, and Peri-implantitis: Impact of Age, Smoking, PPD, and Obesity. *Inflammation* **2019**, *42*, 682–689. [CrossRef]

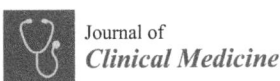

Case Report

Long-Term Results after Placing Dental Implants in Patients with Papillon-Lefèvre Syndrome: Results 2.5–20 Years after Implant Insertion

Katrin Nickles [1,*,†], Mischa Krebs [2,†], Beate Schacher [1], Hari Petsos [1] and Peter Eickholz [1]

1. Department of Periodontology, Center for Dentistry and Oral Medicine (Carolinum), Johann Wolfgang Goethe-University Frankfurt am Main, 60596 Frankfurt, Germany; schacher@em.uni-frankfurt.de (B.S.); petsos@med.uni-frankfurt.de (H.P.); eickholz@med.uni-frankfurt.de (P.E.)
2. Department of Oral Surgery and Implantology, Center for Dentistry and Oral Medicine (Carolinum), Johann Wolfgang Goethe-University Frankfurt am Main, 60596 Frankfurt, Germany; mischa@dr-krebs.net
* Correspondence: nickles@med.uni-frankfurt.de; Tel.: +49-69-6301-5642; Fax: +49-69-6301-3753
† These authors contributed equally to this work.

Abstract: Aim: A retrospective evaluation of patients with Papillon-Lefèvre syndrome (PLS) treated with dental implants to identify factors that may influence treatment outcomes. Methods: All PLS patients with dental implants currently registered at the Department of Periodontology, Goethe-University Frankfurt (20–38 years; mean: 29.6 years), were recruited. Five patients from three families (two pairs of siblings) with a total of 48 dental implants (inserted in different dental institutions) were included with a follow-up time of 2.5–20 years (mean: 10.4 years). Results: Implant failure occurred in three patients (at least 15 implants). Nearly all patients demonstrated peri-implantitis in more or less advanced stages; 60% of patients demonstrated bone loss ≥50% around the implants. Two patients did not follow any supportive therapy. Conclusions: Implants in PLS patients who did not follow any maintenance programme had a high risk of peri-implantitis and implant loss.

Keywords: dental implants; Papillon-Lefèvre syndrome; peri-implantitis; periodontitis; long-term results

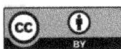

1. Introduction

Papillon-Lefèvre syndrome (PLS) is an infrequent genetic disorder characterised by palmoplantar hyperkeratosis combined with rapidly progressive severe periodontitis affecting both the deciduous and permanent dentitions [1]. The prevalence of PLS is 1–4 per million [2] with no sex or race predominance and is inherited as an autosomal-recessive trait. A loss-of-function mutation affecting the cathepsin C gene (CTSC) on chromosome 11q14.1-q14.3 has traditionally been related to the disorder [3,4], its main functions being protein degradation and proenzyme activation [5].

As periodontal therapy often fails in PLS patients [6–8], they typically lose their teeth early in life and eventually become edentulous with significant ridge resorption. For an increasing number of cases of PLS patients, it is reported that periodontitis may be arrested even in the long term. In those cases, therapy consists of treatment of the infection with the extraction of severely diseased teeth, combined mechanical and antibiotic periodontal treatment, oral hygiene instructions, intensive maintenance therapy, and microbiological monitoring [9–11].

However, PLS patients who have lost many or all teeth need prosthetic rehabilitation. Over the last few years, dental implants have become a common treatment alternative to replace missing teeth. The use of dental implants in young patients with rapidly progessing periodontitis (1999 classification: aggressive periodontitis; 2018 classification: periodontitis grade C) has already been reported [12,13]. Patients with periodontitis grade C (GAgP) had a five times greater risk of implant failure, a three times larger risk of mucositis, and 14 times higher risk of peri-implantitis [13]. Swierkot et al. concluded that patients with treated periodontitis grade C (GAgP) are more susceptible to mucositis and peri-implantitis and experience lower implant survival and success rates than periodontally healthy individuals [13].

Based on the fact that PLS is a rare disease, there are limited studies (mainly case reports) with small numbers of patients assessed in the literature. To the best of our knowledge, just eight articles report outcomes of dental implants in PLS patients [11,14–20]. Furthermore, long-term results are only occasionally reported.

Therefore, the aim of the present retrospective study was to analyse (long-term) outcomes of dental implants in five PLS patients and to identify factors that may influence treatment outcomes. As is presently best known, this is the largest group of PLS patients treated with dental implants reported thus far.

2. Materials and Methods

Patients and Data Collection

We studied all PLS patients with dental implants registered at the Department of Periodontology, Center for Dentistry and Oral Medicine, Johann Wolfgang Goethe-University Frankfurt (20–38 years; mean: 29.6 years). In all patients, the diagnosis of PLS was based on the clinical findings during the initial examination and confirmed by detecting mutations in the cathepsin C gene by analysing blood samples. The study was registered by the Institutional Review Board for Human Studies of the Medical Faculty Goethe-University under the number 31/05 in 2005.

Five patients (four female) were included. They belonged to three families and included two pairs of siblings. Implant therapy in two patients was performed exclusively at the Department of Oral Surgery and Implantology in Frankfurt, and in the three other patients, it was carried out at external dental clinics or by local dentists or oral surgeons. The initial periodontal therapy in Patients 1 and 2 had been described previously [21] as well as the periodontal development of Patients 1, 2, 3, and 4 [11]. All data were collected from the documents in the patients' files. The patients included in our study are listed in Table 1.

Table 1. The patients included and their dental implant characteristics.

Family	Patient	Implants In Situ (Number/Jaw/Type); Year Implants Were Placed; Follow-Up (Years)	Implants Lost (Number)	Bone Grafting (Yes/No/Material)	Prosthetic Restoration	Supportive Therapy (Yes/No/Main Contents)
A	1 (♀/*1988)	6× maxilla 4× mandible Ankylos® (Dentsply Friadent, York, PA, USA) (all Ø 3.5 mm, length 11 mm); Placed in 2007; 2.5 years	-	Yes (maxilla) Bio-Oss Block® (Geistlich, Wolhusen, Switzerland), autologous bone (zygomaticum), Bio-Gide® (Geistlich)	Removable telescopic crown-supported restoration (galvano)	no
A	2 (♀/*1991)	6× maxilla 4× mandible Ankylos® (Dentsply Friadent, York, PA, USA) (all Ø 3.5 mm, length 9.5 and 11 mm); Placed in 2010; 5 years	-	Yes (maxilla) Bio-Oss Block® (Geistlich), autologous bone (zygomaticum), Bio-Gide® (Geistlich)	Removable telescopic crown-supported restoration (galvano)	yes (but irregular): professional dental cleaning once a year; measuring of PPD (irregular), subgingival cleaning (glycine) in case of increased PPD + BOP

Table 1. Cont.

Family	Patient	Implants In Situ (Number/Jaw/Type); Year Implants Were Placed; Follow-Up (Years)	Implants Lost (Number)	Bone Grafting (Yes/No/Material)	Prosthetic Restoration	Supportive Therapy (Yes/No/Main Contents)
B	3 (♀/*1974)	4× maxilla 8× mandible maxilla: Astra® (Dentsply, York, PA, USA) mandible: Brånemark® (Nobel Biocare, Kloten, Switzerland) Placed in 1992; re-implantation maxilla in 2008 and 2010; 20 years (mandible), 4/2 years (maxilla)	4	Yes (maxilla) Autologous bone (iliac crest)	Removable bar-carried restoration	yes: professional dental cleaning every 3 months; no measuring of PPD, no subgingival cleaning; systemic amoxicillin + clavulanic acid and metronidazole for seven days twice a year; no professional supportive therapy
B	4 (♀/*1983)	1× maxilla 4× mandible 1 disc-shaped implant (unknown manufacturer); all others: Brånemark® (Nobel Biocare, Kloten, Switzerland) implants Placed in 1993; 19 years	11	Yes (maxilla) Autologous bone and bone substitute (unknown material)	Removable telescopic crown- and ball-shaped head-supported restoration	yes: professional dental cleaning every 3 months; no measurement of PPD, no subgingival cleaning; systemic amoxicillin + clavulanic acid and metronidazole for seven days twice a year; no professional supportive therapy
C	5 (♂/*1971)	5× maxilla 6× mandible 1 Biomet® 3i implant, all other: IMZ® implants (Dentsply, York, PA, USA); Placed in 1992; 20 years	Several implants were lost, number unknown	Yes (maxilla) (unknown material)	Removable bar-supported (maxilla) and removable telescopic crown-supported restoration (mandible)	no

♀female, ♂male, * born.

3. Results

3.1. Implant Therapy

Patients 1 and 2 were treated at the Department of Oral Surgery and Implantology, Center for Dentistry and Oral Medicine (Carolinum), Johann Wolfgang Goethe-University Frankfurt am Main with the same surgical technique (for details, see Table 1). Despite being provided with extensive information about the importance of supportive implant therapy (SIT), Patient 1 participated in just one maintenance visit. Supportive implant therapy (SIT) consisted of oral hygiene instructions, professional implant cleaning (professional mechanical plaque removal [PMPR] and stain removal), and—bi-annually—a comprehensive periodontal/peri-implant examination. In this way, a rapid intervention was possible whenever needed. In probing pocket depths of 4 mm that showed bleeding on probing (BOP) and/or pockets that were deeper than 4 mm, subgingival/mucosal instrumentation

(SI) with titan curettes and/or air-polishing with glycine powder, as well as instillation of 1% chlorhexidine gel, was performed. In the course of every maintenance visit, oral hygiene indices were assessed.

In patient 1, peri-implant mucositis and in two implants, peri-implantitis lesions could be detected already. In Patient 2, compliance improved over time. However, the patient participated in SIT only once a year. Peri-implant mucositis could also be clearly diagnosed in Patient 2 (Table 1).

In Patients 3 (see Figure 1), 4, and 5, implants were primarily inserted years before in different private practices (for details, see Table 1).

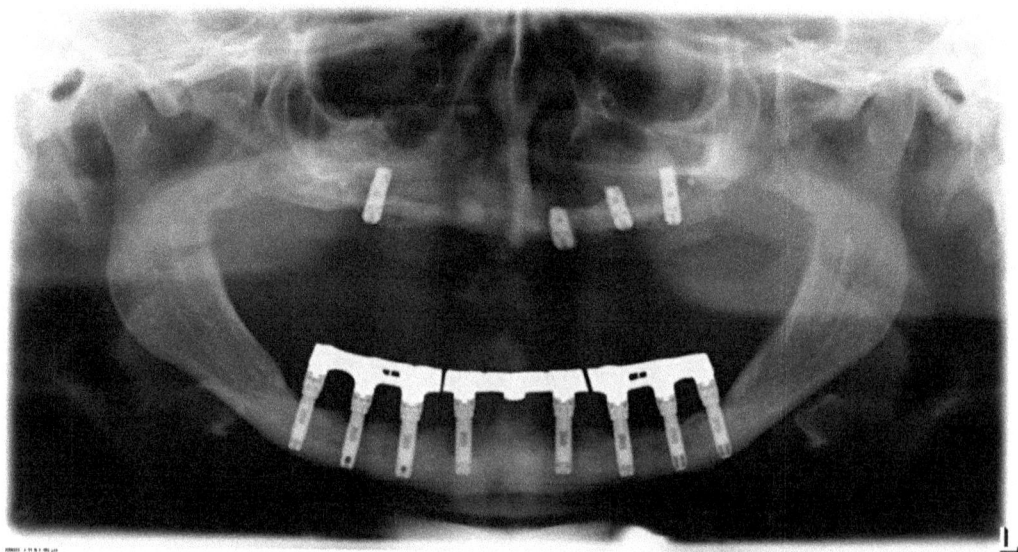

Figure 1. Patient 3 (panoramic radiograph performed in 2008): Eight hollow-screw implants (mandible) inserted in 1992 (16 years in situ); Four Astra® implants (maxilla) inserted in 2008 (six months in situ), two implants (maxilla) have already been lost.

3.2. Clinical, Microbiological and Radiological Findings

At six sites per implant (mesiobuccal, midbuccal, distobuccal, distooral, midoral, mesiooral), probing pocket depths (PPD) were measured using a manual rigid periodontal probe (PCP UNC15, Hu-Friedy, Chicago, IL, USA) to the nearest millimetre. Bleeding on probing (BOP) was recorded 30 s after probing. Suppuration was documented for each implant (see Table 2). Three patients were already exhibiting PPD $\geq$ 7 mm. All patients exhibited high BOP scores (>20%) except for Patient 4, who took systemic antibiotics at the time of scoring.

Table 2. Clinical data: probing pocket depths (PPD), bleeding on probing (BOP), suppuration, and microbiological findings at last visit.

Patient	PPD 1–3 mm (%)	PPD 4–6 mm (%)	PPD $\geq$ 7 mm (%)	BOP (%)	Suppuration (Yes/No)	AA +/−
1	55%	45%	0%	38%	no	AA −
2	58%	42%	0%	25%	no	AA −
3	71%	22%	7%	20%	yes	AA −
4	80%	20%	0%	9%	no	- *
5	32%	54%	14%	26%	Yes	AA −

* Patient was treated with systemic antibiotics at the time, - no microbiological examination.

Except for Patient 4, in each patient that was treated with systemic antibiotics, a microbiological examination was performed with sterile paper points from the deepest pocket of each quadrant. For analysis, a commercially available real-time PCR (Meridol Paro Diagnostik Test, Carpegen, Münster, Germany) for the quantitative determination of six periodontal pathogens (*Aggregatibacter actinomycetemcomitans*, *Porphyromonas gingivalis*, *Tannerella forsythia*, *Treponema denticola*, *Prevotella intermedia*, and *Fusobacterium nucleatum*) was employed. None of the patients showed subgingival presence of the periodontal key pathogen, *Aggregatibacter actinomycetemcomitans* (see Table 2).

Panoramic radiographs were either performed on the day of investigation in the university hospital or earlier by private practices and collected at the following appointment. The proportional bone loss was determined by use of a Schei-ruler [22] on the mesial and distal aspect of each implant (distance of implant shoulder to implant apex) and was classified into three categories (Bone loss 0– < 25%, 25– < 50%, ≥50%) (see Table 3). Three (60%) patients demonstrated bone loss ≥50% around the implants.

Table 3. Bone loss around implants (bone loss in % around implant [distance implant shoulder—implant apex], mesial and distal).

Patient	Bone Loss 0– < 25%	Bone Loss 25– < 50%	Bone Loss ≥ 50%
1	75%	25%	0%
2	95%	5%	0%
3	29%	46%	25%
4	60%	20%	20%
5	13%	55%	32%

4. Discussion

PLS is a rare genetic disease characterised by hyperkeratosis of the palms and soles. It also manifests in a rapidly progressive, severe periodontitis that leads to premature loss of the primary and secondary teeth if not treated early and consequently. A mutation affecting the CTSC gene on chromosome 11q14.1-q14.3 has been associated with the disorder [3]. The cathepsin C enzyme is expressed by epithelial and immune cells and mainly acts as a key enzyme in the activation of granule serine proteases, e.g., elastase. Several studies have studied the pathogenesis of periodontitis in PLS patients. Compromised neutrophil function, including phagocytosis, chemotaxis, and bacterial killing [23], as well as severely depressed natural killer cell cytotoxicity, have been described in patients with PLS [24,25]. Hence, it is plausible that patients with PLS are also very likely to develop disease around dental implants. For this reason, the use of dental implants in patients with severe forms of periodontitis secondary to systemic disorders was not a treatment option for a long time. As a result of young patients having a need for oral rehabilitation that would otherwise not be treated with fixed prosthetics, the question arises of whether dental implants could also elicit success in PLS patients. Swierkot et al. assessed the prevalence of peri-implant mucositis, peri-implantitis, implant success, and survival in patients with GAgP/periodontitis grade C and in periodontally healthy individuals [13]. They reported implant survival rates of 100% in periodontally healthy individuals versus 96% in patients with GAgP/periodontitis grade C. Further, the implant success rate was 33% in GAgP/periodontitis grade C patients and 50% in periodontally healthy patients. The implant success rate was defined by the following parameters: (1) no implant movement; (2) no discomfort (pain, foreign body sensation, paresthesia); (3) PD ≤ 5 mm without BOP; (4) no continuous radiologic translucency; and (5) annual peri-implant bone loss ≤ 0.2 mm 1 year after insertion of the superstructure. Implants that failed to meet ≥1 criteria were considered a failure. In the GAgP/periodontitis grade C group, peri-implant mucositis could be detected in 56% and peri-implantitis in 26% of the implants. In the periodontally healthy group, 40% of the implants exhibited mucositis and 10% peri-implantitis. In addition, GAgP/periodontitis grade C patients demonstrated a five times greater risk of implant failure, a three times higher risk of mucositis, and 14 times more obvious risk of developing peri-implantitis. Ultimately, the authors contended that patients with treated GAgP/periodontitis grade C are more susceptible to mucositis and peri-implantitis and had lower success rates and implant survival [13]. Actually, to the best of our knowledge, just eight articles have reported the outcomes of dental implants in PLS patients [11,14–20]. The exception is Nickles et al. [11]—all others only described the outcome in a single PLS patient with a follow-up period of up to 4.5 years. At first sight, the results are positive. Here, we present data from five PLS patients treated with dental implants. In two patients, dental implants were inserted at the Department of Oral Surgery and Implantology at the Johann Wolfgang Goethe-University Frankfurt am Main with state-of-the-art techniques. In one patient, peri-implantitis was already documented after 2.5 years (see Figure 2). Non-compliance to SIT seemed to be the most probable cause of peri-implant destruction in this patient.

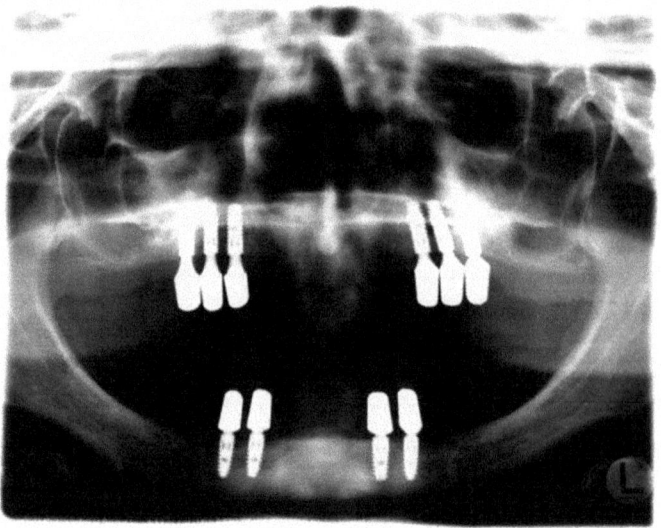

Figure 2. Patient 1 (panoramic radiograph performed in 2010): 10 Ankylos® implants (2.5 years in situ).

All patients treated with dental implants many years earlier (approximately 20 years in Patients 3, 4, and 5) exhibited advanced bone loss around the implants and suffered substantial implant loss. What could be the reasons for these failures? In two patients, Brånemark implants were utilised. The Brånemark system is a well-documented implant system—Ross-Jansåker et al. evaluated the long-term results of implant therapy with implant loss as the outcome variable. In 294 patients, Brånemark implants were inserted between 1988 and 1992 in Kristianstad (Sweden). One and five years after the placement of the suprastructure, the patients were scheduled to the clinic. Between 2000 and 2002 (9–14 years after implant insertion), the patients again underwent a clinical and radiographic examination. In total, 218 patients treated with 1057 implants were assessed and the overall implant survival rate was 95.7%. A significant connection could be noticed between implant loss and periodontal bone loss of the residual teeth. Overall, it appeared that a history of periodontitis was related to implant loss [26].

Documentation of long-term results with the IMZ® system is rare. Haas et al. presented a cumulative survival rate of 83.2% after 100 months in a study with 1920 IMZ® implants. The results demonstrated a statistically significant lower cumulative survival rate of maxillary (37.9%) versus mandibular implants (90.4%) [27]. In contrast to these findings, Willer et al. documented similar survival rates for upper and lower jaw implants in a prospective observation of 1250 IMZ dental implants. The cumulative survival rate after 10 years (82.4%) was very similar to the findings of Haas et al. [28] The cumulative survival rates associated with the IMZ system (83.2%/82.4%) seemed to be lower than those presented by a working group from Frankfurt University [29] with the Ankylos® Implant system with a survival rate of 93.3% after 204 months (17 years). Whether the implant system utilised in our three PLS cases had any influence on the outcomes remains questionable.

In 2014, a Cochrane review was published by Esposito et al. [30] concerning the success rates of different types of dental implants. Based on the available results of randomised clinical trials (RCTs), the authors felt there was limited evidence demonstrating that implants with relatively smooth (turned) surfaces were less prone to bone loss because of chronic infection (peri-implantitis) than those with rougher surfaces. On the other hand, there was no evidence indicating that any particular type of dental implant had superior long-term success. These results were based on a small number of RCTs, often at high risk of bias, with few participants and relatively short follow-up periods. More RCTs should be conducted with a follow-up of at least 5 years that also ascertain the inclusion of a sufficient number of patients in order to detect a true difference [30].

As tooth loss in PLS patients is usually accompanied by severe loss of alveolar bone structures in the mandible as well as in the maxilla, bone-grafting methods seem to be particularly necessary with respect to the maxilla. In the mandible, an inter-foraminal implant placement appears to be possible even in cases with severe resorption when short- and narrow-diameter implants are used. These implants seem to be similarly successful to longer implants [29,31].

In the maxilla, depending on the amount of bone loss and the desired form of prosthetic reconstructions, vertical grafting with autologous bone transplants and sinus grafting are apparently possible options for implant-retained reconstructions. Sinus graftings seem to be equally successful when performed with bovine substitutes or autologous materials [32–36]. Iliac bone was employed in at least one of the three PLS patients here with a follow-up period of approximately 20 years. Fretwurst et al. [37] examined the long-term results after onlay grafting with iliac bone. The authors could demonstrate that in patients with atrophic jaws, an adequately long-term reconstruction could be achieved with iliac onlay grafting in combination with dental implants.

Another issue common in the literature was the time at which the implants were placed. In Patients 3, 4, and 5, the first implants were placed by and next to remaining teeth, meaning there was no edentulous period for these patients.

The most important reason for peri-implant disease, however, was the lack of any professional supportive periodontal/peri-implant therapy. Rocuzzo et al. [38] compared the long-term outcomes of implants placed in patients treated for periodontitis (periodontally-compromised patients; PCPs) and in periodontally healthy patients (PHP) in relation to the adherence of SPT. It was observed that patients with a history of periodontitis had a lower survival rate and a statistically significantly higher number of sites with peri-implant bone loss. Furthermore, PCPs that did not faithfully adhere to SPT exhibited a higher implant failure rate. This underlines the value of SPT for enhancing the long-term outcomes of implant therapy, particularly in subjects affected by periodontitis, in order to control reinfection and limit biological complications [38].

Although in Patients 3 and 4, professional dental/implant cleanings (professional mechanical plaque removal [PMPR] and stain removal) were performed every three months, no measurement of probing depths, assessment of BOP/suppuration, or subgingival/-mucosal cleaning took place. Instead, systemic amoxicillin + clavulanic acid and metronidazole were prescribed for seven days twice a year, though no subgingival cleaning was performed concordantly. Altogether, no professional supportive therapy was conducted on these patients. In Patient 5, no supportive therapy took place at all.

Fazele et al. [39] assessed the success of dental implant placement in PLS patients in a systematic review: the authors studied 15 cases with 136 dental implants and they concluded that dental implants may be a viable treatment option for PLS patients and implantation can help preserve alveolar bone if the patients' immunological and growing conditions are well-considered and proper oral hygiene and compliance with the maintenance program are continued. Nevertheless, in 3 patients, 20 implants failed.

Some PLS patients receive systemic retinoid medication. In the literature, supposedly positive effects have been reported for a systemic medication with oral retinoids [40,41], but also not for others [42]. One of our patients (patient 2) is receiving a systemic retinoid (acitretin) for several years now—despite this, she has lost all of her teeth.

5. Conclusions

A history of periodontal disease is a risk factor for peri-implant disease in general and PLS periodontitis in particular. Thus, PLS patients are high-risk patients with regard to peri-implant disease. We report 5 PLS patients losing all teeth and being treated with dental implants. Only one patient receives proper (oral hygiene indices, PPD charting, PMPR, SI) SPT on a yearly basis. Patient 1 received just one proper SPT, Patients 3 and 4 received twice a year systemic antibiotics but only supramucosal PMPR, Patient 5 did not receive any maintenance treatment whatsoever. Thus, two main factors seem to drive bone loss: (1) time (which is trivial) and (2) lack of SPT (which is particularly evident in comparison to Patients 1 and 2).

In light of what we have presented in this work, it remains debatable whether implants should be used in patients with PLS-associated periodontitis. The impaired immune system in PLS patients represents a risk factor that cannot be controlled. These patients have to be classified as high-risk patients and informed of their circumstances. Many of these patients lose their teeth very early, yielding orthodontic and physiognomic, and, hence, psychosocial consequences. Implants often represent the only opportunity to insert fixed or at least stable prostheses in these patients. PLS patients—along with their treating dentist—should be aware of the risks associated with not complying with the prescribed regimen of supportive care, i.e., peri-implantitis and implant loss. Therefore it is of crucial importance that PLS patients are informed about the importance of supportive therapy.

The authors are aware of the fact that the number of patients included in the study was very small. Nevertheless, the manuscript clearly provides the prevalence, i.e., 1 to 4 under 1 million population. The authors are also aware of the fact that the treatment modalities (implant types, various bone grafts, etc.) are very heterogeneous and hard to compare.

In spite of everything, the present study represents the largest on implant treatment in PLS patients so far.

Author Contributions: All authors contributed substantially to the interpretation of the data for the work, they contributed to drafting and critically revising the manuscript, they agreed to be accountable for all aspects of the work. Additionally, P.E., M.K. and K.N. conceived the ideas for the concept and design of the study; K.N., M.K., B.S., H.P. and P.E. collected the data; B.S. and H.P. supervised methodical approaches; K.N. analysed the data and managed the group; P.E. and K.N. led the writing. All authors have read and agreed to the published version of the manuscript.

Funding: The microbiological examinations in four patients were partially funded by Carpegen GmbH, Münster.

Institutional Review Board Statement: The trial was approved by the Institutional Review Board for Human Studies of the Medical Faculty of the Johann Wolfgang Goethe-University Frankfurt/Main (31–05; 7 March 2005) with the 3rd Amendment (2015).

Informed Consent Statement: All participants were informed of the risks, benefits, and procedures of the study, and gave written informed consent.

Data Availability Statement: The data that support the findings of this study are not available due to data protection restrictions.

Acknowledgments: This study was kindly supported by Carpegen GmbH, Münster, Germany.

Conflicts of Interest: The authors declare that they have no conflict of interest. This study was self-funded by the authors and their institutions. The microbiological examinations in four patients were partially funded by Carpegen GmbH, Münster.

References

1. Papillon, M.M.; Lefèvre, P. Two cases of symmetrically familiary palmar and plantar hyperkeratosis (Meleda disease) within brother and sister combined with severe dental alterations in both cases (in French). *Soc. Franc. Dermat. Syph.* **1924**, *31*, 82–84.
2. Gorlin, R.J.; Sedano, H.; Anderson, V.E. The syndrome of palmar–plantar hyperkeratosis and premature periodontal destruction of the teeth. *J. Pediatr.* **1964**, *65*, 895–906. [CrossRef]
3. Hart, T.C.; Hart, P.S.; Bowden, D.W.; Michalec, M.D.; Callison, S.A.; Walker, S.J.; Zhang, Y.; Firatli, E. Mutations of the cathepsin C gene are responsible for Papillon-Lefèvre syndrome. *J. Med. Genet.* **1999**, *36*, 881–887. [PubMed]
4. Toomes, C.; James, J.; Wood, A.J.; Wu, C.L.; McCormick, D.; Lench, N.; Hewitt, C.; Moynihan, L.; Roberts, E.; Woods, C.G.; et al. Loss-of-function mutations in the cathepsin C gene result in periodontal disease and palmoplantar keratosis. *Nat. Genet.* **1999**, *23*, 421–424. [CrossRef] [PubMed]
5. Rao, N.V.; Rao, G.V.; Hoidal, J.R. Human Dipeptidyl-peptidase I. *J. Biol. Chem.* **1997**, *272*, 10260–10265. [CrossRef]
6. Bimstein, E.; Lustmann, J.; Sela, M.N.; Ben Neriah, Z.; Soskolne, W.A. Periodontitis Associated with Papillon-Lefèvre Syndrome. *J. Periodontol.* **1990**, *61*, 373–377. [CrossRef] [PubMed]
7. Bullon, P.; Pascual, A.; Fernandez-Novoa, M.C.; Borobio, M.V.; Muniain, M.A.; Camacho, F. Late onset Papillon–Lefèvre syndrome? A chromosomic, neutrophil function and microbiological study. *J. Clin. Periodontol.* **1993**, *20*, 662–667. [CrossRef]
8. de Vree, H.; Steenackers, K.; de Boever, J.A. Periodontal treatment of rapid progressive periodontitis in 2 siblings with Papillon–Lefèvre syndrome: 15-years follow-up. *J. Clin. Periodontol.* **2000**, *27*, 354–360. [CrossRef]
9. Schacher, B.; Baron, F.; Ludwig, B.; Valesky, E.; Noack, B.; Eickholz, P. Periodontal therapy in siblings with Papillon–Lefèvre syndrome and tinea capitis: A report of two cases. *J. Clin. Periodontol.* **2006**, *33*, 829–836. [CrossRef]
10. Nickles, K.; Schacher, B.; Schuster, G.; Valesky, E.; Eickholz, P. Evaluation of Two Siblings with Papillon-Lefèvre Syndrome 5 Years After Treatment of Periodontitis in Primary and Mixed Dentition. *J. Periodontol.* **2011**, *82*, 1536–1547. [CrossRef]
11. Nickles, K.; Schacher, B.; Ratka-Krüger, P.; Krebs, M.; Eickholz, P. Long-term results after treatment of periodontitis in patients with Papillon-Lefèvre syndrome: Success and failure. *J. Clin. Periodontol.* **2013**, *40*, 789–798. [CrossRef]
12. Mengel, R.; Stelzel, M.; Hasse, C.; Flores-de-Jacoby, L. Osseointegrated implants in patients treated for generalized severe adult periodontitis. An interim report. *J. Periodontol.* **1996**, *67*, 782–787. [CrossRef] [PubMed]
13. Swierkot, K.; Lottholz, P.; Flores-De-Jacoby, L.; Mengel, R. Mucositis, Peri-Implantitis, Implant Success, and Survival of Implants in Patients with Treated Generalized Aggressive Periodontitis: 3- to 16-Year Results of a Prospective Long-Term Cohort Study. *J. Periodontol.* **2012**, *83*, 1213–1225. [CrossRef]
14. Ullbro, C.; Crossner, C.G.; Lundgren, T.; Stålblad, P.A.; Renvert, S. Osseointegrated implants in a patient with Papillon–Lefèvre syndrome. A 4 1/2-year follow up. *J. Clin. Periodontol.* **2000**, *27*, 951–954. [CrossRef]
15. Woo, I.; Brunner, D.P.; Yamashita, D.-D.R.; Le, B.T. Dental Implants in a Young Patient with Papillon-Lefevre Syndrome: A Case Report. *Implant Dent.* **2003**, *12*, 140–144. [CrossRef] [PubMed]
16. Toygar, H.U.; Kircelli, C.; Firat, E.; Guzeldemir-Akcakanat, E. Combined Therapy in a Patient with Papillon-Lefèvre Syndrome: A 13-Year Follow-Up. *J. Periodontol.* **2007**, *78*, 1819–1824. [CrossRef] [PubMed]
17. Etöz, O.A.; Ulu, M.; Kesim, B. Treatment of Patient With Papillon-Lefevre Syndrome with Short Dental Implants: A Case Report. *Implant Dent.* **2010**, *19*, 394–399. [CrossRef] [PubMed]
18. Ahmadian, L.; Monzavi, A.; Arbabi, R.; Hashemi, H.M. Full-Mouth Rehabilitation of an Edentulous Patient with Papillon-Lefèvre Syndrome Using Dental Implants: A Clinical Report. *J. Prosthodont.* **2011**, *20*, 643–648. [CrossRef]
19. Senel, F.C.; Altintas, N.Y.; Bagis, B.; Cankaya, M.; Pampu, A.A.; Satıroglu, I.; Senel, A.C. A 3-Year Follow-Up of the Rehabilitation of Papillon-Lefèvre Syndrome by Dental Implants. *J. Oral Maxillofac. Surg.* **2012**, *70*, 163–167. [CrossRef]
20. Al Farraj, A.L.; Dosari, A. Oral rehabilitation of a case of Papillon-Lefevre syndrome with dental implants. *Saudi. Med. J.* **2013**, *34*, 424–427.
21. Rüdiger, S.; Petersilka, G.; Flemming, T.F. Combined systemic and local antimicrobial therapy of periodontal disease in Papillon–Lefèvre syndrome. *J. Clin. Periodontol.* **1999**, *26*, 847–854. [PubMed]
22. Schei, O.; Waerhaug, J.; Lovdal, A.; Arno, A. Alveolar Bone Loss as Related to Oral Hygiene and Age. *J. Periodontol.* **1959**, *30*, 7–16. [CrossRef]
23. Liu, R.; Cao, C.; Meng, H.; Tang, Z. Leukocyte functions in 2 cases of Papillon-Lefèvre syndrome. *J. Clin. Periodontol.* **2000**, *27*, 69–73. [CrossRef] [PubMed]
24. Lundgren, T.; Parhar, R.S.; Renvert, S.; Tatakis, D.N. Impaired cytotoxicity in Papillon–Lefèvre syndrome. *J. Dent. Res.* **2005**, *84*, 414–417. [CrossRef] [PubMed]
25. Khocht, A.; Albandar, J.M. Aggressive forms of periodontitis secondary to systemic disorders. *Periodontology* **2014**, *65*, 134–148. [CrossRef] [PubMed]
26. Roos-Jansaker, A.M.; Lindahl, C.; Renvert, H.; Renvert, S. Nine- to fourteen-year follow-up of implant treatment. Part I: Implant loss and associations to various factors. *J. Clin. Periodontol.* **2006**, *33*, 283–289. [CrossRef]

27. Haas, R.; Mensdorff-Pouilly, N.; Mailath, G.; Watzek, G. Survival of 1920 IMZ implants followed for up to 100 months. *Int. J. Oral Maxillofac. Implant.* **1996**, *11*, 581–588.
28. Willer, J.; Noack, N.; Hoffmann, J. Survival rate of IMZ implants: A prospective 10-year analysis. *J. Oral Maxillofac. Surg.* **2003**, *61*, 691–695. [CrossRef]
29. Krebs, M.; Schmenger, K.; Neumann, K.; Weigl, P.; Moser, W.; Nentwig, G.H. Long-term evaluation of ANKYLOS® dental implants, part i: 20-year life table analysis of a longitudinal study of more than 12,500 implants. *Clin. Impl. Dent. Rel. Res.* **2015**, *17*, e275–e286. [CrossRef]
30. Esposito, M.; Ardebili, Y.; Worthington, H. Interventions for replacing missing teeth: Different types of dental implants. *Cochrane Database Syst. Rev.* **2014**, *22*, CD003815. [CrossRef]
31. Pohl, V.; Thoma, D.S.; Sporniak-Tutak, K. Short dental implants (6 mm) versus long dental implants (11–15 mm) in combination with sinus floor elevation procedures: 3-year results from a multi-center, randomized, controlled clinical trial. *J. Clin. Periodontol.* **2017**, *44*, 438–445. [CrossRef] [PubMed]
32. Sbordone, C.; Sbordone, L.; Toti, P.; Martuscelli, R.; Califano, L.; Guidetti, F. Apical and marginal bone alterations around implants in maxillary sinus augmentation grafted with autogenous bone or bovine bone material and simultaneous or delayed dental implant positioning. *Clin. Oral Impl. Res.* **2011**, *22*, 485–491. [CrossRef]
33. Sbordone, C.; Toti, P.; Guidetti, F.; Califano, L.; Bufo, P.; Sbordone, L. Volume changes of autogenous bone after sinus lifting and grafting procedures: A 6-year computerized tomographic follow-up. *J. Cranio-Maxillofac. Surg.* **2013**, *41*, 235–241. [CrossRef] [PubMed]
34. Sbordone, C.; Toti, P.; Guidetti, F.; Califano, L.; Pannone, G.; Sbordone, L. Volumetric changes after sinus augmentation using blocks of autogenous iliac bone or freeze-dried allogeneic bone. A non-randomized study. *J. Craniomaxillofac. Surg.* **2014**, *42*, 113–118. [CrossRef] [PubMed]
35. Hatano, N.; Shimizu, Y.; Ooya, K. A clinical long-term radiographic evaluation of graft height changes after maxillary sinus floor augmentation with a 2:1 autogenous bone/xenograft mixture and simultaneous placement of dental implants. *Clin. Oral Implant. Res.* **2004**, *15*, 339–345. [CrossRef] [PubMed]
36. Zijderveld, S.A.; Schulten, E.A.J.M.; Aartman, I.H.A.; ten Bruggenkate, C.M. Long-term changes in graft height after maxillary sinus floor elevation with different grafting materials: Radiographic evaluation with a minimum follow-up of 4.5 years. *Clin. Oral Implant. Res.* **2009**, *20*, 691–700. [CrossRef]
37. Fretwurst, T.; Nack, C.; Al-Ghrairi, M.; Raguse, J.; Stricker, A.; Schmelzeisen, R.; Nelson, K.; Nahles, S. Long-term retrospective evaluation of the peri-implant bone level in onlay grafted patients with iliac bone from the anterior superior iliac crest. *J. Cranio-Maxillofac. Surg.* **2015**, *43*, 956–960. [CrossRef]
38. Roccuzzo, M.; De Angelis, N.; Bonino, L.; Aglietta, M. Ten-year results of a three-arm prospective cohort study on implants in periodontally compromised patients. Part 1: Implant loss and radiographic bone loss. *Clin. Oral Implant. Res.* **2010**, *21*, 490–496. [CrossRef]
39. Atarbashi-Moghadam, F.; Atarbashi-Moghadam, S.; Kazemifard, S.; Sijanivandi, S.; Namdari, M. Oral rehabilitation of Papillon–Lefèvre syndrome patients by dental implants: A systematic review. *J. Korean Assoc. Oral Maxillofac. Surg.* **2020**, *46*, 220–227. [CrossRef]
40. Nazzaro, V.; Blanchet-Bardon, C.; Mimoz, C.; Revuz, J.; Puissant, A. Papillon-Lefèvre Syndrome Ultrastructural Study and Successful Treatment with Acitretin. *Arch. Dermatol.* **1988**, *124*, 533–539. [CrossRef]
41. Gelmetti, C.; Nazzaro, V.; Cerri, D.; Fracasso, L. Long-Term Preservation of Permanent Teeth in a Patient with Papillon-Lefevre Syndrome Treated with Etretinate. *Pediatr. Dermatol.* **1989**, *6*, 222–225. [CrossRef] [PubMed]
42. Lundgren, T.; Renvert, S. Periodontal treatment of patients with Papillon-Lefevre syndrome: A 3-year follow-up. *J. Clin. Periodontol.* **2004**, *31*, 933–938. [CrossRef] [PubMed]

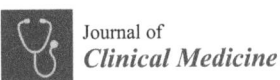

Article

Effect of Subgingival Instrumentation on Neutrophil Elastase and C-Reactive Protein in Grade B and C Periodontitis: Exploratory Analysis of a Prospective Cohort Study

Peter Eickholz [1,*], Anne Asendorf [1], Mario Schröder [1], Beate Schacher [1], Gerhard M. Oremek [2], Ralf Schubert [3], Martin Wohlfeil [1] and Otto Zuhr [1,4]

[1] Center for Dentistry and Oral Medicine (Carolinum), Department of Periodontology, Johann Wolfgang Goethe-University Frankfurt/Main, Theodor-Stern-Kai 7, 60596 Frankfurt, Germany; anne.asendorf@googlemail.com (A.A.); m.schroeder@med.uni-frankfurt.de (M.S.); schacher@em.uni-frankfurt.de (B.S.); martinwohlfeil@gmail.com (M.W.); o.zuhr@huerzelerzuhr.com (O.Z.)
[2] Centre for Internal Medicine, Department of Laboratory Medicine, Hospital of the Johann Wolfgang Goethe-University Frankfurt/Main, Theodor-Stern-Kai 7, 60590 Frankfurt, Germany; gerhardmaximilian.oremek@kgu.de
[3] Department for Children and Adolescence, Division for Allergy, Pneumology and Cystic Fibrosis, Goethe-University, 60590 Frankfurt, Germany; ralf.schubert@kgu.de
[4] Private Practice Hürzeler/Zuhr, Rosenkavalierplatz 18, 81925 Munich, Germany
* Correspondence: eickholz@med.uni-frankfurt.de; Tel.: +49-6301-5642; Fax: +49-6301-3753

Abstract: Background: Assessment of the effect of subgingival instrumentation (SI) on systemic inflammation in periodontitis grades B (BP) and C (CP). Methods: In this prospective cohort study, eight BP and 46 CP patients received SI. Data were collected prior to and 12 weeks after SI. Blood was sampled prior to, one day, 6, and 12 weeks after SI. Neutrophil elastase (NE), C-reactive protein (CRP), leukocyte count, lipopolysaccharide binding protein, interleukin 6 (IL-6) and IL-8 were assessed. Results: Both groups showed significant clinical improvement. NE was lower in BP than CP at baseline and 1 day after SI, while CRP was lower in BP than CP at baseline ($p < 0.05$). NE and CRP had a peak 1 day after SI ($p < 0.05$). Between-subjects effects due to CP ($p = 0.042$) and PISA ($p = 0.005$) occurred. Within-subjects NE change was confirmed and modulated by grade ($p = 0.017$), smoking ($p = 0.029$), number of teeth ($p = 0.033$), and PISA ($p = 0.002$). For CRP between-subjects effects due to BMI ($p = 0.008$) were seen. Within-subjects PISA modulated the change of CRP over time ($p = 0.017$). Conclusions: In untreated CP, NE and CRP were higher than in BP. SI results in better PPD and PISA reduction in BP than CP. Trial registration: Deutsches Register Klinischer Studien DRKS00026952 28 October 2021 registered retrospectively.

Keywords: neutrophil elastase; CRP; cytokine(s); non-surgical periodontal therapy; periodontal–systemic disease interactions; periodontitis

Citation: Eickholz, P.; Asendorf, A.; Schröder, M.; Schacher, B.; Oremek, G.M.; Schubert, R.; Wohlfeil, M.; Zuhr, O. Effect of Subgingival Instrumentation on Neutrophil Elastase and C-Reactive Protein in Grade B and C Periodontitis: Exploratory Analysis of a Prospective Cohort Study. *J. Clin. Med.* 2022, 11, 3189. https://doi.org/10.3390/jcm11113189

Academic Editor: Fa-Ming Chen

Received: 31 March 2022
Accepted: 1 June 2022
Published: 2 June 2022

Publisher's Note: MDPI stays neutral with regard to jurisdictional claims in published maps and institutional affiliations.

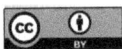

Copyright: © 2022 by the authors. Licensee MDPI, Basel, Switzerland. This article is an open access article distributed under the terms and conditions of the Creative Commons Attribution (CC BY) license (https://creativecommons.org/licenses/by/4.0/).

1. Introduction

The 1999 Classification of Periodontal Diseases distinguished between chronic (ChP) and aggressive periodontitis (AgP) with regard to onset of the disease at different ages and progressions at different speeds in different patients [1]. Individual predisposition and modifying factors explain these differences. The 2018 classification assigns different grades to different rates of progression (slow progression: (A); moderate progression: (B); rapid progression: (C)). Molar–incisor pattern and case phenotype are elements of the actual classification that recollect AgP [2].

Tooth brushing, flossing, and even chewing may frequently cause bacteraemia in patients with severe untreated periodontitis [3]. AgP and periodontitis grade C exhibit more rapid progression. This may be due to a hyperinflammatory phenotype that also may result in a higher systemic inflammatory burden (i.e., serum C-reactive protein (CRP) and neutrophil elastase (NE)), as shown for AgP [4–7]. Frequent bacteraemia and the systemic spill of proinflammatory cytokines [4] from periodontal pockets result in the release of NE and acute-phase proteins (e.g., CRP). NE and CRP are markers of systemic inflammatory burden and may be part of the link that connects the oral inflammation periodontitis with other parts of the body. Non-surgical periodontal therapy (subgingival instrumentation: SI) resulted in a serum NE reduction in AgP but not in ChP [5]. Is this difference still detectable if patients are reclassified according to the 2018 classification?

This is an exploratory analysis of a prospective cohort study that originally observed serum NE, CRP, and LPS binding protein to be significantly higher in AgP than ChP and a significant difference regarding the change of serum NE 12 weeks after SI between AgP and ChP [4,5]. Therefore, the primary aim of this exploratory analysis was to compare these inflammatory serum parameters at baseline and after non-surgical subgingival instrumentation (SI) in the same patients after reclassification according to the 2018 classification into grade B (BP) and C (CP) periodontitis.

2. Material and Methods

This is the exploratory analysis of data of a prospective cohort study on the effect of SI on serum inflammatory parameters. An exploratory analysis of haematological parameters and heat shock protein 27 has been published recently [7]. Clinical examinations and therapy have been described in detail before [5,7]. Thus, only a brief description is provided in the following. Sixty-six patients with untreated severe periodontal disease (31 generalised severe ChP; 35 AgP) were recruited at the Department of Periodontology of the Center for Dentistry and Oral Medicine (Carolinum), Johann Wolfgang Goethe-University Frankfurt/Main, Germany.

The following inclusion criteria had to be fulfilled: (1) at least 16 years of age, (2) at least 20 remaining teeth and (3) written informed consent.

Patients were diagnosed as aggressive periodontitis if the following criteria were present: (1) clinically healthy patients, i.e., he or she does not suffer from systemic diseases predisposing to periodontitis (e.g., diabetes mellitus); (2) probing pocket depths (PPD) $\geq$ 3.6 mm at more than 30% of sites [5] (according to the Periodontal Screening and Recording (PSR) index [8] and the directives for treatment of statutorily insured patients in Germany [9], a PPD of 3.5 mm was the threshold for periodontal disease and thus requirement of therapy. However, Florida probes provide measurements to the nearest 0.2 mm. Thus, the threshold for treatment requirement was PPD $\geq$ 3.6 mm); (3) radiographic bone loss of at least 50% at a minimum of 2 separate teeth; (4) age at time of diagnosis up to 35 years (severe periodontitis below age up to 35 years is a rough threshold to identify rapid destruction in AgP) [4,10]; (5) age at time of recruitment up to 37 years of age [4].

Patients were diagnosed as generalised severe chronic periodontitis if the following criteria were fulfilled: (1) PPD at least 3.6 mm and probing vertical attachment loss (PAL-V) at least 5 mm at more than 30% of sites, (2) PPD at least 7 mm at a minimum of 4 sites (to provide a minimum of deep pockets in each patient); (2) older than 35 years of age.

The following inclusion criteria led to exclusion: (1) requirement of preventive use of systemic antibiotics for measurements that may cause transitory bacteraemia (e.g., pocket probing); (2) self-reported chronic disease influencing the serum CRP level (e.g., rheumatoid arthritis, Crohn's disease or ulcerative colitis); (3) self-reported infectious disease within the last 8 weeks before examination (history of fever); (4) any clinically assessed chronic dermal or mucosal inflammatory condition (e.g., lichen planus); (5) non-surgical or surgical periodontal treatment within the last 24 months before examination; (6) systemic or topical subgingival antibiotics within the last 8 weeks before examination.

The following parameters were assessed as self-report: (1) current body weight and height, (2) current and past cigarette smoking habits. Patients currently smoking or having quit smoking for less than five years were classified as smokers [11]. Additionally, ethnic origin was recorded [4]. The study protocol fulfilled the rules of the Declaration of Helsinki. The Institutional Review Board for Human Studies of the Medical Faculty of the Goethe-

University Frankfurt/Main approved the protocol (Application# 188/06). Information on the risks and benefits as well as the procedures of the study was provided to all participants.

2.1. Clinical Examination

An earlier publication of our group reports clinical examinations in detail [4].

One experienced examiner (MW) performed all measurements. He assessed the following parameters at 6 sites per tooth (mesiobuccal, buccal, distobuccal, mesiooral, oral, distooral) at baseline (T0), 6 (T2), and 12 weeks (T3) after SI: (1) Gingival Bleeding Index (GBI) [12], (2) Plaque Control Record (PCR) [13]. MW scored probing parameters immediately prior to the first session of SI and at T3. With an electronic probe (Florida Probe, Version 3.2, Gainesville, FL, USA), he assessed PPD (standard probe) and relative vertical probing attachment level (RAL-V) (disk probe) to the nearest 0.2 mm. Thirty seconds after probing, he scored bleeding on probing (BOP). MW assessed recession to the nearest 0.5 mm using a manual periodontal probe (PCPUNC 15, Hu-Friedy, Chicago, IL, USA) from the cemento-enamel junction (CEJ) to the gingival margin and calculated PAL-V as the sum of PPD and recession. If CEJ was located apical to the gingival margin, PAL-V was calculated as PPD minus the distance from the gingival margin to the CEJ.

2.2. Reclassification

Assignment of stage for each patient was performed using the baseline interproximal PAL scores and number of teeth lost [2]. Due to the fact that only patients suffering from AgP or generalised severe ChP had been included originally, it was assumed that all missing teeth had been lost due to periodontitis with the exception of missing 3rd molars that were never considered as lost due to periodontal reasons. For each patient, the percentage of teeth indicating stage III (CAL-V $\geq$ 5 mm, PPD $\geq$ 6 mm, furcation involvement class II and III) was documented [7].

Each patient was assigned to a grade using radiographs obtained at baseline (primary criteria) as well as modifying factors (smoking, diabetes mellitus). An experienced periodontologist (PE) viewed the radiographs on a screen (Universal Viewer, Dentsply Rinn®, New York, NY, USA) in a darkened room. At the tooth with most severe bone loss, the distances from the CEJ to the most apical extension of bone loss (BD) and to the tip of the root were measured to the next 1.0 mm with a periodontal probe (PCPUNC15, HuFriedy, Chicago, IL, USA). The distance from CEJ to BD was divided by the distance CEJ to root tip to calculate bone loss relative to root length. The division of relative bone loss by patients' age provided the bone loss age coefficient [7]. Patients with bone loss age coefficient >1 were assigned to grade C [2].

2.3. Blood Samples

Twenty millilitres of blood was sampled from an arm vein (T0; T1: one day later immediately prior to the 2nd session of SI; T2, T3). Serum levels of CRP, NE and leukocyte count were analysed at the Department of Laboratory Medicine of the Centre for Internal Medicine, Hospital of the Johann Wolfgang Goethe-University Frankfurt/Main.

Serum IL-6, IL-8, and lipopolysaccharide-binding protein (LBP) concentrations were analysed in duplicates by the ELISA technique according to the manufacturers' instructions at the Department for Children and Adolescence, Division for Allergy, Pneumology and Cystic Fibrosis, Goethe-University, Frankfurt, Germany. All laboratory methods have been described in detail before [5].

2.4. Anti-Infective Therapy

All patients underwent oral hygiene instructions and professional prophylaxis until the full mouth plaque score (PCR) was $\leq$50% (1st step of therapy) [14]. SI was performed in 2 visits on 2 consecutive days under local anaesthesia (UDS, Sanofi-Aventis Deutschland GmbH, Frankfurt/Main, Germany) according to a modification of the full-mouth disinfection protocol [5,15] (2nd step of therapy). All teeth exhibiting PPD $\geq$ 3.5 mm underwent

SI using sonic scalers (Sonicsys, KaVo, Biberach, Germany) and hand instruments. If *A. actinomycetemcomitans* had been detected from subgingival plaque, 500 mg amoxicillin and 400 mg metronidazole were prescribed 3 times daily for 7 days. In case of sensitivity to penicillin, 250 mg ciprofloxacin and 500 mg metronidazole were prescribed 2 times daily for 7 days [16–18]. For 14 days after start of SI for all patients, oral home care included rinsing 2 times daily for 60 s with 10 mL of 0.12% chlorhexidine mouth wash (ParoEx, Sunstar, Schönau, Germany), which was followed by tooth brushing and brushing the back of the tongue with 1% CHX gel. At T2 and T3, all patients received oral hygiene instructions and professional prophylaxis [7].

2.5. Statistical Analysis

Statistical analysis was performed using a PC program (Systat™ for Windows Version 13, Systat Inc., Evanston, IL, USA). The sample size had originally been calculated for the main outcome variables NE and CRP for a comparison between ChP and AgP [6,8]. Inferential statistics were intended to be exploratory, not confirmatory. *p*-values represent a metric measure of evidence against the respective null hypothesis and were used only to generate new hypotheses. Therefore, no adjustment for multiple testing was applied. *p*-values < 0.05 were considered as significant. For a description of demographic and clinical parameters, standard univariate statistical analyses were performed. Numbers and percentages describe categorical variables. Continuous variables are reported as means and standard deviations for clinical parameters and as medians (lower/upper quartile) for serum parameters. Patients' characteristics were compared between BP and CP patients as well as between patients treated with adjunctive systemic antibiotics or not using Fisher's exact tests for categorical variables and Mann–Whitney U tests for continuous data.

For all individuals, the body mass index (BMI) and cigarette pack years were calculated. Group frequencies (BP, CP) were expressed for sex and current smoking. Group means and standard deviations were calculated for the following parameters: age, number of remaining teeth, pack years, BMI, GBI, PCR and BOP at baseline and 12 weeks as well as for the changes between baseline and 12 weeks. For all site-based periodontal parameters (PPD, PAL-V, RAL-V), means per individual were calculated at T0 and T3 as well as for changes from T0 to T3. Furthermore, using these numbers, group means and standard deviations were calculated. Additionally, the periodontal inflamed surface area (PISA) was calculated per individual to describe the size of the interface between the periodontal pocket and vascular system [19].

For comparisons, repeated measures analysis of variance (MANOVA) was used for log-transformed NE and CRP with the following independent variables: time point of examination (T0, 1, 2, 3), diagnosis (BP = 0, CP = 1), African origin, female sex, smoking (never and former smoker = 0, current smoker = 1), adjunctive systemic antibiotics (no = 0, yes = 1), number of teeth, BOP, BMI and baseline PISA. An effect with a probability of $p < 0.05$ was accepted as significant.

3. Results

Between October 2006 and December 2009, 31 ChP and 29 AgP patients were enrolled. Of originally 56 patients three had been recruited but were not enrolled because they violated the inclusion criteria. Furthermore, three patients did not attend the baseline examination and were also not enrolled. The results on these 60 patients' NE, CRP, leukocyte counts, IL-6 and IL-8, as well as LBP regarding ChP and AgP had already been published [5]. Because the respective radiographs were not available anymore, the assignment of new diagnoses according to the 2018 classification was not possible in six of 60 patients. Thus, the data of 54 patients were analysed [7]. Of those patients assigned to grade B according to interproximal bone loss (%) divided by age, neither was a current heavy smoker ($\geq$10 cigarettes per day) nor suffered from diabetes mellitus. Thus, modifying factors did not affect grade. A total of originally 24 AgP were reclassified to 19 generalised stage III (all CP), none in stage IV and 5 molar incisor pattern (all CP). A total of originally 30 ChP were reclassified to 25 generalised stage III (5 BP, 20 CP), 5 stage IV (3 BP, 2 CP) and no molar incisor patterns [7]. One BP (12.5%) and 24 CP (52.2%) were female ($p = 0.056$), all BP and 39 CP (84.8%) were of European ethnicity, two CP (4.3%) were of African and 5 (10.9%) of Asian ethnicity ($p = 0.497$). The BP group consisted of one current (12.5%) and two (25%) former smokers (CP: current: 15/31% ($p = 0.411$); former: 9/20% ($p = 0.659$)). Four BP (50%) and 17 CP (37%) received SI with adjunctive systemic antibiotics ($p = 0.697$). Table 1 provides further patient characteristics.

Table 1. Individuals' characteristics.

Parameters Mean ± Standard Deviation	Periodontitis Grade B ($n = 8$)	Periodontitis Grade C ($n = 46$)	Grade B/C p
Age (years)	61.0 ± 6.7	40.5 ± 11.5	<0.001
Remaining teeth (n)	26.6 ± 3.2	27.4 ± 2.9	0.492
Pack years	6.8 ± 11.6	8.4 ± 15.0	0.665
Body mass index (kg/m^2)	24.4 ± 2.8	26.2 ± 4.7	0.324

After SI, clinical parameters (GBI, BOP, PPD, RAL-V, PISA) improved in general significantly ($p < 0.05$). Only PCR improvement at T3 in BP was not significant. At T3, PPD ($p = 0.006$) and PISA ($p = 0.046$) were significantly better in BP than in CP (Table 2) [7]. Adjunctive systemic antibiotics (AB) failed to make a difference with regard to PPD reduction (AB: $-1.3 ± 0.5$ mm; no AB: $-1.0 ± 0.4$ mm; $p = 0.186$) and CAL gain (AB: 0.6 ± 0.4 mm; no AB: 0.4 ± 0.3 mm; $p = 0.059$).

Table 2. Individuals' periodontal variables and change of periodontal variables after therapy (PAL-V: clinical vertical attachment level; RAL-V: relative vertical attachment level).

Parameters Mean ± Standard Deviation		Periodontitis Grade B ($n = 8$)	Periodontitis Grade C ($n = 46$)	Grade B/C p
Gingival Bleeding Index (%)	Baseline	15.0 ± 7.9	13.4 ± 10.8	0.526
	6 weeks	6.3 ± 5.3 [a]	3.7 ± 4.7 [b]	0.113
	12 weeks	6.4 ± 6.5 [a]	5.9 ± 4.8 [b,c]	0.981
Plaque Control Record (%)	Baseline	40.1 ± 26.2	35.8 ± 14.1	0.856
	6 weeks	22.0 ± 14.5 [a]	31.5 ± 18.6 [a]	0.169
	12 weeks	32.8 ± 11.7	28.2 ± 16.8 [a]	0.233
Bleeding on probing (%)	Baseline	49.4 ± 15.9	52.0 ± 13.7	0.575
	12 weeks	20.3 ± 7.6 [a]	26.7 ± 10.4 [b]	0.092
Probing pocket depth (PPD) (mm)	Baseline	3.4 ± 0.3	3.8 ± 0.7	0.242
	12 weeks	2.2 ± 0.3 [a]	2.6 ± 0.4 [b]	0.006
PPD reduction (mm)		1.2 ± 0.3	1.1 ± 0.5	0.342
Attachment level (mm) (PAL-V)	Baseline	4.3 ± 1.0	3.6 ± 1.8	0.093
(RAL-V)	Baseline	11.1 ± 1.2	10.8 ± 1.5	0.715
(RAL-V)	12 weeks	10.6 ± 1.2 [a]	10.4 + 1.4 [b]	0.715
Attachment gain (mm) (ΔRAL-V)		0.4 ± 0.3	0.5 ± 0.4	0.789
PISA (mm^2)	Baseline	1169 ± 201	1372 ± 543	0.273
	12 weeks	288 ± 112 [a]	460 ± 303 [b]	0.046

Significantly different to baseline [a] ($p < 0.05$); [b] ($p < 0.001$). Significantly different to 6 weeks [c] ($p < 0.05$).

CP exhibited higher serum NE than BP at all time points. However, this difference was significant only at T0 and T1. Furthermore, NE was significantly increased at T1 ($p < 0.05$) (Table 3). Repeated measures analysis of variance identified between subjects significant effects due to CP ($p = 0.042$) and PISA ($p = 0.005$). Within subjects, the change of serum NE over time was confirmed and modulated by grade (p = 0.017), smoking (p = 0.029), number of teeth (p = 0.033), and PISA (p = 0.002). Adjunctive systemic antibiotics failed to modulate change of serum NE (Table 4).

Table 3. Individuals' neutrophil elastase and C-reactive protein (median (lower/upper quartile)).

Parameters		Periodontitis Grade B (n = 8)	Periodontitis Grade C (n = 46)	Grade B/C p
Neutrophil elastase (ng/mL) (NE)	Baseline	8.75 (7/13.25)	30.55 (12.4/37.2)	0.008
	1 day	19.3 (14.5/25.1) [b]	33.05 (21.8/40.1) [a]	0.036
	6 weeks	9.4 (8.01/17.55)	32 (13.1/37.68)	0.059
	12 weeks	17.65 (10.75/34.65)	28 (11.3/36.2)	0.422
Change baseline to 12 weeks		3.75 (−0.14/0.05)	−1.15 (−4.2/1.4)	0.051
C-reactive protein (mg/dL) (CRP)	Baseline	0.09 (0.08/0.13)	0.17 (0.10/0.34)	0.033
	1 day	0.75 (0.23/1.41) [a]	0.54 (0.29/1.16) [a]	0.990
	6 weeks	0.15 (0.05/0.27)	0.17 (0.11/0.34)	0.336
	12 weeks	0.14 (0.07/0.21)	0.23 (0.10/0.34)	0.278
Change baseline to 12 weeks		0.01 (−0.05/0.14)	0 (−0.06/0.05)	0.542
CRP reduction ≥ 0.3 mg/dL (n/%) baseline to 12 weeks		0 (0)	4 (9)	1.000
CRP < 0.1 mg/dL (n) (%)	Baseline	5 (63)	8 (17)	0.015
	12 weeks	3 (37)	11 (24)	0.413
CRP 0.1 to 0.3 mg/dL (n) (%)	Baseline	3 (37)	26 (57)	0.449
	12 weeks	4 (50)	20 (43)	1.000
CRP > 0.3 mg/dL (n) (%)	Baseline	0 (0)	12 (26)	0.176
	12 weeks	1 (13)	15 (33)	0.411

Significantly different to all other time points [a] ($p < 0.001$), [b] ($p < 0.05$).

Table 4. Repeated measures analysis of variance of log-transformed neutrophil elastase (NE).

	Degrees of Freedom	F-Ratio	p-Value
Between subjects			
Grade C	1	4.397	0.042
African origin	1	2.589	0.115
Female	1	0.464	0.499
Bleeding on probing (T0)	1	1.669	0.203
Smoker	1	1.359	0.250
Systemic antibiotics	1	0.001	0.973
Number of teeth	1	1.079	0.305
Body mass index (T0)	1	2.716	0.107
PISA (T0)	1	8.858	0.005
Error	43		
Within subjects			
NE	3	3.406	0.020
NE × grade C	3	3.533	0.017
NE × African origin	3	0.666	0.574
NE × female	3	0.107	0.956

Table 4. *Cont.*

	Degrees of Freedom	F-Ratio	p-Value
NE × bleeding on probing (T0)	3	0.481	0.696
NE × smoker	3	3.091	0.029
NE × systemic antibiotics	3	1.203	0.312
NE × number of teeth	3	3.005	0.033
NE × body mass index	3	0.524	0.666
NE × PISA (T0)	3	5.218	0.002
Error	129		

Serum CRP was only significantly higher in CP than in BP at T0 ($p = 0.033$). Furthermore, the percentage of patients with serum CRP < 0.1 mg/dl was significantly lower in CP than in BP ($p = 0.015$) (Table 3). Repeated measures analysis of variance identified between subjects significant effects due to BMI ($p = 0.008$). Within subjects, the change of serum CRP over time was modulated by PISA ($p = 0.017$). Adjunctive systemic antibiotics failed to modulate the change of serum CRP (Table 5).

Table 5. Repeated measures analysis of variance of log-transformed C-reactive protein (CRP).

	Degrees of Freedom	F-Ratio	p-Value
Between subjects			
Grade C	1	0.254	0.617
African origin	1	1.385	0.246
Female	1	0.047	0.830
Bleeding on probing (T0)	1	0.358	0.553
Smoker	1	0.004	0.950
Systemic antibiotics	1	1.284	0.263
Number of teeth	1	0.178	0.675
Body mass index (T0)	1	7.691	0.008
PISA (T0)	1	1.129	0.294
Error	44		
Within subjects			
CRP	3	0.539	0.657
CRP × grade C	3	1.311	0.274
CRP × African origin	3	0.581	0.628
CRP × female	3	0.248	0.863
CRP × bleeding on probing (T0)	3	0.818	0.486
CRP × smoker	3	0.294	0.829
CRP × systemic antibiotics	3	2.238	0.087
CRP × number of teeth	3	0.243	0.866
CRP × body mass index	3	0.467	0.706
CRP × PISA (T0)	3	3.539	0.017
Error	132		

Univariate analysis failed to find any significant difference between BP and CP for leucocyte count, serum LBP, IL-6, and IL-8. However, LBP was significantly increased at T1 for CP ($p < 0.001$) and IL-6 for BP and CP ($p < 0.05$) (Table 6).

Table 6. Leukocyte counts LPS binding protein, interleukin 6 and 8 (median (lower/upper quartile)).

Parameters		Periodontitis Grade B (n = 8)	Periodontitis Grade C (n = 46)	Grade B/C p
Leukocyte count (nL^{-1})	Baseline	5.86 (3.95/7.62)	6.37 (5.12/7.47)	0.559
	1 day	5.05 (4.51/6.66)	6.34 (4.98/7.34)	0.330
	6 weeks	5.01 (4.56/5.79)	6.02 (4.9/7.49) [b]	0.189
	12 weeks	4.92 (4.29/5.30)	5.97 (4.85/7.5)	0.056
LPS binding protein (µg/mL) (LBP)	Baseline	22.2 (15.3/27.9)	30.4 (22.3/45) [a]	0.108
	1 day	40.4 (25.5/49.7)	44.3 (31.7/57.6)	0.488
	6 weeks	32 (20.5/43.1)	26.6 (19.5/42.9) [a]	0.961
	12 weeks	34 (18/44)	24.7 (19.2/36.8) [a]	0.618
Interleukin 6 (pg/mL) (IL-6)	Baseline	1.55 (1.25/2.5) [b]	1.5 (0.9/2) [a]	0.510
	1 day	2.95 (2.25/3.65)	2.8 (2/5.1)	0.855
	6 weeks	1.25 (1/3) [b]	1.25 (0.8/1.7) [a,c]	0.626
	12 weeks	1.2 (0.85/2.55) [a]	1.5 (1.1/2.2) [a,d]	0.502
Interleukin 8 (pg/mL) (IL-8)	Baseline	21.5 (17/29)	17 (11/25)	0.223
	1 day	27 (24/35.5)	20.5 (13/29)	0.125
	6 weeks	36 (20/58.5)	17 (13/28)	0.108
	12 weeks	24.5 (19.5/29)	22.5 (15/37) [c]	0.884

Significantly different to 1 day [a] ($p < 0.001$); [b] ($p < 0.05$); significantly different to baseline [c] ($p < 0.05$); significantly different to 6 weeks [d] ($p < 0.05$).

4. Discussion

This is an exploratory analysis of a prospective cohort study that originally observed serum NE, CRP, and LPS binding protein to be significantly higher in AgP than ChP and observed a significant difference regarding change of serum NE 12 weeks after SI (T3) between AgP and ChP [4,5]. The primary aim of this exploratory analysis therefore was to compare these inflammatory serum parameters at T0 and after step 2 periodontal therapy (SI) [14] in the same patients after reclassification according to the 2018 classification into eight patients with untreated grade B (BP) and 46 with grade C (CP) periodontitis (6 patients were lost due to missing data). In both groups, significant clinical improvement was achieved ($p < 0.05$). NE was significantly lower in BP than in CP at T0 and T1, while CRP was significantly lower in BP than CP only at T0. NE and CP were significantly higher at T1 than at T0, 2 and 3. Between-subjects significant effects due to CP and PISA were observed. Change of NE over time was modulated by grade, smoking, number of teeth, and PISA, and significant effects due to BMI were seen. Change of serum CRP over time was modulated by PISA. In untreated CP, serum NE and CRP are higher than in BP. SI results in better PPD and PISA 12 weeks after SI in BP than CP. Adjunctive systemic antibiotics modulated neither change of serum NE nor of CRP.

Oral microbiota may enter internal tissues and circulation via the parakeratinised and ulcerated pocket epithelium of established gingivitis and periodontitis. Summing up the pocket walls of all periodontally compromised teeth in an untreated patient, the periodontal wound surface is estimated to be as large as 8 to 20 cm^2 [20]. The size of this wound surface was assessed in this analysis as PISA which ranged in this study from 9 to 15 cm^2 in BP and from 3 to 25 cm^2 in CP at T0.

Bacteraemia from periodontal pockets and the resulting systemic spill of proinflammatory cytokines cause an acute inflammatory host response [21–23]. The cohort studied in this analysis exhibited in AgP significantly higher serum NE and CRP at baseline and 12 weeks after treatment than in ChP [5]. This significant difference persisted even 5 years after treatment, indicating a stronger inflammatory response in AgP than in ChP [6]. In the 1999 classification, AgP represents periodontitis with rapid progression, whereas in the 2018 classification, rapid progression is classified by grade C. With serum NE being significantly higher in CP than BP at baseline and 1 day after SI and CRP at baseline, this exploratory analysis confirms the observation made in AgP for CP. One day after SI, an inflammatory host response was observed in the patients of this study as elevated levels of NE, CRP, LBP, and IL-6 in both ChP and AgP [5]. In this exploratory analysis, the same was observed. Elevation of NE, CRP, and IL-6 was significant for CP and BP. However, for LBP, this was observed only for CP. This difference may be due to the small size of the BP group ($n = 8$).

This study failed to provide any significant differences between BP and CP with regard to leukocyte count, LBP, IL-6 and IL-8. This confirms the results comparing ChP and AgP for leukocyte counts, IL-6 and IL-8. However, for LBP, higher serum LBP was observed in AgP at baseline and 1 day after SI than ChP. This difference may also be due to the small size of the BP group ($n = 8$).

Untreated periodontitis associated with elevated serum NE and CRP may thereby contribute to the risk for CVD and COPD. For AgP, serum CRP was reduced by 0.23 mg/dL at T3 [5]. This was far more than the weighted mean (0.067 mg/dL) calculated by a structured review over two studies which included a total of 40 patients with generalised severe periodontitis [24]. However, neither difference reached statistical significance. Interestingly, in contrast to the analysis of ChP versus AgP, this exploratory analysis failed to show SI reducing any of the investigated systemic inflammatory parameters. In part, this may be due to the loss of patients and rearrangement of groups.

Non-surgical periodontal therapy in this study was effective. It resulted in significant mean PPD reduction (BP: 1.2 mm; CP: 1.0 mm) and attachment gain (BP: 0.4 mm; CP: 0.5 mm), confirming results reported by other groups [25–27].

What are the limitations of this analysis? First of all, this is an exploratory analysis of a cohort originally aiming at serum NE and CRP in comparison of ChP and AgP [5]. Since this distinction has been abandoned in the 2018 classification of periodontal diseases, this is an attempt to use the new diagnoses (BP/CP). The exploratory analyses were not adjusted for multiple testing. Thus, there is a high risk to detect differences that are due to chance. Furthermore, the sample size is quite small with a high risk of being underpowered. Another weakness is connected to staging according to tooth loss due to periodontitis. Most patients cannot name the exact reason why teeth have been extracted in particular if tooth loss is a while ago. If extractions have not been performed in one's own clinic, it is quite difficult to estimate the reason. This is a general difficulty of this parameter in the 2018 classification. Due to the fact that only patients suffering from AgP or generalised severe ChP had been included originally, it was assumed that all missing teeth had been lost due to periodontitis with the exception of missing 3rd molars that were never considered as lost due to periodontal reasons. This may be a pragmatic approach to stage periodontitis due to tooth loss in this analysis. However, to the best of our knowledge, this is the first analysis to compare BP and CP regarding systemic inflammatory host responses.

5. Conclusions

Within the limitations of the present study, the following conclusion may be drawn: In untreated grade C periodontitis (CP), serum NE and CRP are higher than in grade B periodontitis (BP). SI results in better PPD and PISA reduction in BP than CP.

Author Contributions: Conceptualisation: P.E., B.S. and O.Z.; methodology: O.Z.; formal analysis: P.E.; funding acquisition: P.E.; investigation: M.W., G.M.O., R.S., P.E.; data curation: A.A., M.S.; writing—original draft preparation: O.Z.; writing—review and editing: P.E., B.S., A.A., M.S., G.M.O., R.S., M.W.; supervision: P.E. All authors have read and agreed to the published version of the manuscript.

Funding: This study was in part funded by the authors and their institutions and in part by grants of the German Society of Periodontology (DG PARO), the German Society of Dental, Oral, and Maxillofacial Medicine (DGZMK), the New Working Group for Periodontology (NAgP) (3 months examination), and the Freiherr Carl von Rothschild'sche Stiftung Carolinum, Frankfurt, Germany (statistical analysis for NE, CRP, leukocyte count, LPS, IL-6, IL-8).

Institutional Review Board Statement: Approval for the study was obtained from the Institutional Review Board for Human Studies of the Medical Faculty of Goethe-University Frankfurt/Main (Application# 188/06). Informed consent was obtained from all subjects involved in the study.

Informed Consent Statement: Informed consent was obtained from all subjects involved in the study.

Data Availability Statement: The datasets used and/or analysed during the current study are available from the corresponding author on reasonable request.

Conflicts of Interest: The authors declare no conflict of interest.

Abbreviations

AgP	aggressive periodontitis
BD	most apical extension of bone loss
BMI	body mass index
BOP	bleeding on probing
BP	grade B periodontitis
CEJ	cemento-enamel junction
ChP	chronic periodontitis
COPD	chronic obstructive pulmonary disease
CP	grade C periodontitis
CRP	C-reactive protein
CVD	cardiovascular disease
GBI	gingival bleeding index
IL	interleukin
LBP	lipopolysaccharide-binding protein
MANOVA	repeated measures analysis of variance
NE	neutrophil elastase
PAL-V	vertical probing attachment loss
PCR	plaque control record
PISA	periodontal inflamed surface area
PMN	polymorphonuclear leukocytes
PPD	probing pocket depth
RAL-V	vertical relative attachment level
SI	subgingival instrumentation

References

1. Armitage, G.C. Development of a classification system for periodontal diseases and conditions. *Ann. Periodontol.* **1999**, *4*, 1–6. [CrossRef] [PubMed]
2. Tonetti, M.S.; Greenwell, H.; Kornman, K.S. Staging and grading of periodontitis: Framework and proposal of a new classification and case definition. *J. Clin. Periodontol.* **2018**, *45* (Suppl. 20), S149–S161. [CrossRef] [PubMed]
3. Wilson, W.; Taubert, K.A.; Gewitz, M.; Lockhart, P.B.; Baddour, L.M.; Levison, M.; Durack, D.T. Prevention of infective endocarditis: Guidelines from the American Heart Association: A guideline from the American Heart Association Rheumatic Fever, Endocarditis and Kawasaki Disease Committee, Council on Cardiovascular Disease in the Young, and the Council on Clinical Cardiology, Council on Cardiovascular Surgery and Anesthesia, and the Quality of Care and Outcomes Research Interdisciplinary Working Group. *J. Am. Dent. Assoc.* **2007**, *138*, 739–745, 747–760. [PubMed]
4. Wohlfeil, M.; Scharf, S.; Siegelin, Y.; Schacher, B.; Oremek, G.M.; Sauer-Eppel, H.; Eickholz, P. Increased systemic elastase and C-reactive protein in aggressive periodontitis (CLOI-D-00160R2). *Clin. Oral Investig.* **2012**, *16*, 1199–1207. [CrossRef] [PubMed]
5. Eickholz, P.; Siegelin, Y.; Scharf, S.; Schacher, B.; Oremek, G.M.; Sauer-Eppel, H.; Schubert, R.; Wohlfeil, M. Non-surgical periodontal therapy decreases serum elastase levels in aggressive but not in chronic periodontitis. *J. Clin. Periodontol.* **2013**, *40*, 327–333. [CrossRef] [PubMed]

6. Ramich, T.; Asendorf, A.; Nickles, K.; Oremek, G.M.; Schubert, R.; Nibali, L.; Wohlfeil, M.; Eickholz, P. Inflammatory serum markers up to 5 years after comprehensive periodontal therapy of aggressive and chronic periodontitis. *Clin. Oral Investig.* **2018**, *22*, 3079–3089. [CrossRef] [PubMed]
7. Eickholz, P.; Schroder, M.; Asendorf, A.; Schacher, B.; Oremek, G.M.; Kaiser, F.; Wohlfeil, M.; Nibali, L. Effect of nonsurgical periodontal therapy on haematological parameters in grades B and C periodontitis: An exploratory analysis. *Clin. Oral Investig.* **2020**, *24*, 4291–4299. [CrossRef]
8. Covington, L.L.; Breault, L.G.; Hokett, S.D. The application of Periodontal Screening and Recording (PSR) in a military population. *J. Contemp. Dent. Pract.* **2003**, *4*, 36–51.
9. Krankenkassen, B.Z. (Ed.) *Richtlinien des Bundesausschusses der Zahnärzte und Krankenkassen für eine Ausreichende, Zweckmäßige und Wirtschaftliche Vertragszahnärztliche Versorgung (Behandlungsrichtlinien)*; Bundesanzeiger: Köln, Germany, 2006.
10. Pretzl, B.; Salzer, S.; Ehmke, B.; Schlagenhauf, U.; Dannewitz, B.; Dommisch, H.; Eickholz, P.; Jockel-Schneider, Y. Administration of systemic antibiotics during non-surgical periodontal therapy-a consensus report. *Clin. Oral Investig.* **2019**, *23*, 3073–3085. [CrossRef]
11. Lang, N.P.; Tonetti, M.S. Periodontal risk assessment (PRA) for patients in supportive periodontal therapy (SPT). *Oral Health Prev. Dent.* **2003**, *1*, 7–16.
12. Ainamo, J.; Bay, I. Problems and proposals for recording gingivitis and plaque. *Int. Dent. J.* **1975**, *25*, 229–235.
13. O'Leary, T.J.; Drake, R.B.; Naylor, J.E. The plaque control record. *J. Periodontol.* **1972**, *43*, 38. [CrossRef]
14. Sanz, M.; Herrera, D.; Kebschull, M.; Chapple, I.; Jepsen, S.; Beglundh, T.; Sculean, A.; Tonetti, M.S.; EFP Workshop Participants and Methodological Consultants. Treatment of stage I-III periodontitis-The EFP S3 level clinical practice guideline. *J. Clin. Periodontol.* **2020**, *47* (Suppl. 22), 4–60. [CrossRef]
15. Quirynen, M.; Bollen, C.M.; Vandekerckhove, B.N.; Dekeyser, C.; Papaioannou, W.; Eyssen, H. Full- vs. partial-mouth disinfection in the treatment of periodontal infections: Short-term clinical and microbiological observations. *J. Dent. Res.* **1995**, *74*, 1459–1467. [CrossRef]
16. Harks, I.; Koch, R.; Eickholz, P.; Hoffmann, T.; Kim, T.S.; Kocher, T.; Meyle, J.; Kaner, D.; Schlagenhauf, U.; Doering, S.; et al. Is progression of periodontitis relevantly influenced by systemic antibiotics? A clinical randomized trial. *J. Clin. Periodontol.* **2015**, *42*, 832–842. [CrossRef]
17. Griffiths, G.S.; Ayob, R.; Guerrero, A.; Nibali, L.; Suvan, J.; Moles, D.R.; Tonetti, M.S. Amoxicillin and metronidazole as an adjunctive treatment in generalized aggressive periodontitis at initial therapy or re-treatment: A randomized controlled clinical trial. *J. Clin. Periodontol.* **2011**, *38*, 43–49. [CrossRef]
18. Feres, M.; Soares, G.M.; Mendes, J.A.; Silva, M.P.; Faveri, M.; Teles, R.; Socransky, S.S.; Figueiredo, L.C. Metronidazole alone or with amoxicillin as adjuncts to non-surgical treatment of chronic periodontitis: A 1-year double-blinded, placebo-controlled, randomized clinical trial. *J. Clin. Periodontol.* **2012**, *39*, 1149–1158. [CrossRef]
19. Nesse, W.; Abbas, F.; van der Ploeg, I.; Spijkervet, F.K.; Dijkstra, P.U.; Vissink, A. Periodontal inflamed surface area: Quantifying inflammatory burden. *J. Clin. Periodontol.* **2008**, *35*, 668–673. [CrossRef]
20. Loos, B.G. Systemic markers of inflammation in periodontitis. *J. Periodontol.* **2005**, *76*, 2106–2115. [CrossRef]
21. Tonetti, M.S.; D'Aiuto, F.; Nibali, L.; Donald, A.; Storry, C.; Parkar, M.; Suvan, J.; Hingorani, A.D.; Vallance, P.; Deanfield, J. Treatment of periodontitis and endothelial function. *N. Engl. J. Med.* **2007**, *356*, 911–920. [CrossRef]
22. D'Aiuto, F.; Nibali, L.; Parkar, M.; Suvan, J.; Tonetti, M.S. Short-term effects of intensive periodontal therapy on serum inflammatory markers and cholesterol. *J. Dent. Res.* **2005**, *84*, 269–273. [CrossRef]
23. D'Aiuto, F.; Parkar, M.; Andreou, G.; Suvan, J.; Brett, P.M.; Ready, D.; Tonetti, M.S. Periodontitis and systemic inflammation: Control of the local infection is associated with a reduction in serum inflammatory markers. *J. Dent. Res.* **2004**, *83*, 156–160. [CrossRef]
24. Paraskevas, S.; Huizinga, J.D.; Loos, B.G. A systematic review and meta-analyses on C-reactive protein in relation to periodontitis. *J. Clin. Periodontol.* **2008**, *35*, 277–290. [CrossRef]
25. Guerrero, A.; Griffiths, G.S.; Nibali, L.; Suvan, J.; Moles, D.R.; Laurell, L.; Tonetti, M.S. Adjunctive benefits of systemic amoxicillin and metronidazole in non-surgical treatment of generalized aggressive periodontitis: A randomized placebo-controlled clinical trial. *J. Clin. Periodontol.* **2005**, *32*, 1096–1107. [CrossRef]
26. Kim, T.S.; Schenk, A.; Lungeanu, D.; Reitmeir, P.; Eickholz, P. Nonsurgical and surgical periodontal therapy in single-rooted teeth. *Clin. Oral Investig.* **2007**, *11*, 391–399. [CrossRef]
27. Cionca, N.; Giannopoulou, C.; Ugolotti, G.; Mombelli, A. Amoxicillin and metronidazole as an adjunct to full-mouth scaling and root planing of chronic periodontitis. *J. Periodontol.* **2009**, *80*, 364–371. [CrossRef]

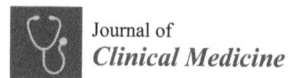

Article

Phenotypic and Functional Alterations of Immune Effectors in Periodontitis; A Multifactorial and Complex Oral Disease

Kawaljit Kaur [1], Shahram Vaziri [1], Marcela Romero-Reyes [2], Avina Paranjpe [3] and Anahid Jewett [1,4,*]

[1] Division of Oral Biology and Oral Medicine, School of Dentistry and Medicine, Los Angeles, CA 90095, USA; drkawalmann@g.ucla.edu (K.K.); ajewett@dentistry.ucla.edu (S.V.)
[2] Department of Neural and Pain Sciences, University of Maryland, Baltimore, MD 21201, USA; mromero@umaryland.edu
[3] Department of Endodontics, University of Washington, Seattle, DC 98195, USA; avina@u.washington.edu
[4] The Jonsson Comprehensive Cancer Center, UCLA School of Dentistry and Medicine, Los Angeles, CA 90095, USA
* Correspondence: ajewett@ucla.edu; Tel.: +1-310-206-3970; Fax: +1-310-794-7109

Abstract: Survival and function of immune subsets in the oral blood, peripheral blood and gingival tissues of patients with periodontal disease and healthy controls were assessed. NK and CD8 + T cells within the oral blood mononuclear cells (OBMCs) expressed significantly higher levels of CD69 in patients with periodontal disease compared to those from healthy controls. Similarly, TNF-α release was higher from oral blood of patients with periodontal disease when compared to healthy controls. Increased activation induced cell death of peripheral blood mononuclear cells (PBMCs) but not OBMCs from patients with periodontal disease was observed when compared to those from healthy individuals. Unlike those from healthy individuals, OBMC-derived supernatants from periodontitis patients exhibited decreased ability to induce secretion of IFN-γ by allogeneic healthy PBMCs treated with IL-2, while they triggered significant levels of TNF-α, IL-1β and IL-6 by untreated PBMCs. Interaction of PBMCs, or NK cells with intact or NFκB knock down oral epithelial cells in the presence of a periodontal pathogen, *F. nucleatum*, significantly induced a number of pro-inflammatory cytokines including IFN-γ. These studies indicated that the relative numbers of immune subsets obtained from peripheral blood may not represent the composition of the immune cells in the oral environment, and that orally-derived immune effectors may differ in survival and function from those of peripheral blood.

Keywords: cell death; periodontitis; CD69; oral blood; *F. nucleatum*; NFκB; IFN-γ

1. Introduction

Periodontitis is an inflammatory disease affecting the supporting tissues of the tooth, and is characterized by a wide range of clinical, microbiological and immunological manifestations [1]. The hallmark of periodontitis is the gradual destruction of supporting tissues, which are composed of gingival and periodontal connective tissue, cementum and alveolar bone [2,3]. Several established causes of periodontitis relate to the imbalance in microbial organisms, heightened host's inflammatory and immune responses and a series of environmental and genetic factors [1,4,5]. Limited knowledge is available about the function, biology and phenotypic properties of oral blood and immune cells infiltrating the gingival tissues, and their comparison with immune cells within the peripheral blood; however, it is clear that pathogenesis of periodontitis is complex and involves both innate and adaptive immune responses [6,7]. In gingiva local inflammatory responses induced by the interaction of stromal cells with the immune effectors in the presence of oral bacteria activate innate immune responses resulting in the release of an array of cytokines and chemokines responsible for continuous recruitment of inflammatory cells to the gingival tissues, and the establishment of chronic inflammation [8]. In addition, many NF-kB-induced pathways are also known to be involved in periodontal diseases [9,10].

Citation: Kaur, K.; Vaziri, S.; Romero-Reyes, M.; Paranjpe, A.; Jewett, A. Phenotypic and Functional Alterations of Immune Effectors in Periodontitis; A Multifactorial and Complex Oral Disease. *J. Clin. Med.* 2021, 10, 875. https://doi.org/10.3390/jcm10040875

Academic Editor: Susanne Schulz

Received: 11 January 2021
Accepted: 17 February 2021
Published: 20 February 2021

Publisher's Note: MDPI stays neutral with regard to jurisdictional claims in published maps and institutional affiliations.

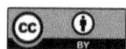

Copyright: © 2021 by the authors. Licensee MDPI, Basel, Switzerland. This article is an open access article distributed under the terms and conditions of the Creative Commons Attribution (CC BY) license (https://creativecommons.org/licenses/by/4.0/).

It has been reported that both T and B cells are present in periodontal tissues, and both gingival tissue-derived T and B cells were shown to be at a more advanced stage of the cell cycle than peripheral blood T and B cells, indicative of activation within the tissues [2]. Much less is known regarding the NK cells in periodontal diseases, which are known to be the regulators of adaptive immunity [11,12]. The adaptive immune responses in particular, CD4+ T cells and the proinflammatory cytokines IFN-γ and TNF-α are important effectors of bone loss in periodontal disease [13–15]. TNF-α was found to be higher in periodontal tissues in comparison to those from healthy individuals [16]. IFN-γ is primarily produced by activated T and NK cells and plays an important role in host defense. IFN-γ knock-out mice were shown to have a decreased bone loss in periodontal disease; however, due to the significance of this cytokine in bacterial defense, the function of this cytokine is very complex and is not clearly known in periodontal disease [17]. T cells from periodontitis patients also express higher secretion of IFN-γ compared to T cells from healthy individuals [18].

Oral microorganisms can induce activation of NK and T cells resulting in the secretion of pro-inflammatory cytokines IL-1β and TNF-α by these cells [19]. IL-1β and TNF-α can also induce the endothelial cells in the blood vessels to express higher ICAM-1 (CD54) and other adhesion molecules [20], allowing more leukocytes to migrate into the periodontal tissues. Previously, in the established lesions of periodontitis, massive accumulations of leukocytes primarily T and B cells were observed [2]. Despite the presence of immune cells, the disease fails to resolve if bacteria remain in the gingival sulcus. The potent activation and induction of cell death by bacteria in epithelial cells may also recruit more immune effectors to the sites of infection, thereby activating immune cells to prevent access of pathogenic oral microorganisms to deeper tissues. Indeed, we and other laboratories reported that F. *nucleatum* is capable of inducing cell death of immune effectors as well as oral keratinocytes in in vitro culture conditions [21]. Persistent recruitment and activation of immune effectors due to continuous activation and death of oral epithelial cells by the oral organisms may result in the increased survival of immune effectors and further the contribution of activated lymphocytes to increased tissue damage and inflammation.

In this paper we investigated the cell surface receptor expression, activation markers, cytokine secretion and cell death profiles of mononuclear cells obtained from peripheral blood, oral blood and gingival tissues of healthy individuals and patients with periodontitis when they were left untreated or treated with interleukin 2 (IL-2), interferon-gamma (IFN-γ) and phorbol myristate acetate (PMA)/ionomycin (I). Since genetic factors, primarily contributed by mutations seen in the pro-inflammatory cytokines such as IL-1β, TNF-α and many others, have been identified to be associated with periodontal disease, we studied NFkB signaling pathway in keratinocytes involved in the regulation of many pro-inflammatory cytokines in order to understand the complex interaction between the immune cells, keratinocytes and oral bacteria.

2. Materials and Methods

2.1. Cell Lines, Reagents and Antibodies

Mononuclear cells isolated from healthy individuals' and periodontitis patients' peripheral and oral blood were cultured in RPMI 1640 supplemented with 1% sodium pyruvate, 1% non-essential amino acids, 1% glutamine, 1% penicillin-streptomycin (Life Technologies, Carlsbad, CA, USA) and 10% fetal bovine serum (FBS) (Gemini Bio-Product, West Sacramento, CA, USA). HEp2 tumor cell lines were obtained from ATCC and maintained on DMEM media (Life Technologies, CA, USA) supplemented with 10% FBS. Oral squamous carcinoma cells (OSCCs) were maintained in RPMI 1640 supplemented with 10% FBS. Human oral keratinocytes (HOK-16B) were cultured in keratinocyte growth medium (KGM) supplemented with 4% bovine pituitary extract, 1% hydrocortisone, 1% gentamycin-sulfate, 1% bovine insulin and 1% epidermal growth factor obtained from Cambrex-Bio (Walkersville, MD, USA). Propidium iodide (PI), phorbol 12-myristate 13-acetate (PMA) and ionomycin were purchased from Sigma (St Louis, MO, USA). *Fusobacterium nucleatum*

(PK1594) was obtained from Paul Kolenbrander, National Institutes of Health. Recombinant human IL-2 and IFN-γ were obtained from NIH-BRB. IFN-γ was obtained from Peprotech (Piscataway, NJ, USA). Anti-CD16 mAb, as well as all of the human ELISA kits and flow cytometric antibodies were purchased from Biolegend (CA, USA). Multiplex assay kits were purchased from Millipore (Billerica, MA, USA). pRcCMV-IκB(S32AS36A) and pRcCMV vector alone were generated in our laboratory.

2.2. Donor Selection and Diagnostic Criteria

Oral blood and gingival tissues were obtained from consenting donors who were undergoing periodontal surgery at the UCLA school of dentistry, Los Angeles, CA, USA. Patients were classified as having periodontal disease on the basis of bleeding index, attachment loss, probing depth (6 sites/tooth) and radiographic examinations. Those classified as having periodontal disease had each of the following; probing depth of greater than 5 mm, spontaneous bleeding on probing, clinical attachment loss and radiographic evidence of severe alveolar bone loss. Donors were diagnosed as healthy individuals if they demonstrated a probing depth of equal or less than 4 mm, no clinical attachment loss and no radiographic evidence of alveolar bone loss. Periodontal surgery was performed either to remove diseased tissue (granulation tissue from alveolar defects) in patients with periodontal disease or to remove healthy tissue for cosmetic purposes such as crown lengthening, gingival thinning and cosmetic grafting in healthy individuals.

2.3. Isolation of Peripheral and Oral Blood Mononuclear Cells

Written informed consent approved by the UCLA Institutional Review Board (IRB# 11-000781-CR00010; Study ID#11-00781; Committee: UCLA Medical IRB 2) was obtained from healthy individuals and periodontitis patients, and all procedures were approved by the UCLA-IRB. Peripheral blood mononuclear cells (PBMCs) were isolated from peripheral blood as described before [22]. To obtain oral-gingival mononuclear cells approximately 3–6 mL of oral blood was drawn using 6 mL syringe with 16 G needle containing 0.5 mL of heparin. Oral blood was obtained during flap surgery and from granulation tissue (diseased tissue) around alveolar defects or from supra-periosteal tissue (healthy tissue). Collected oral blood was then added to 1:1 ratio of 1 $\times$ PBS and layered slowly on a ficoll gradient solution. The samples were then centrifuged for 20 min at 2000 rpm. The collected mononuclear cells (oral blood mononuclear cells, OBMCs) were washed twice with 1 $\times$ PBS and re-suspended in RPMI with 10% FBS. The cells were then counted using a hemocytometer and the viability was determined using trypan blue and propidium iodide staining and subsequent analysis by microscopy and flow-cytometry, respectively. Peripheral blood was obtained immediately after the recovery of oral blood from the same individuals. Blood and gingival samples were obtained from both male and female donors. The age range for patients with periodontal disease was 29–68 years, and for healthy individuals it was 27–46 years.

2.4. Mononuclear Cells Purified from Gingival Tissues

Gingival biopsies were thoroughly washed with 1 $\times$ PBS twice and cut into approximately 1 mm pieces. The cut tissues were placed in RPMI supplemented with DNAse (0.15 mg/mL) and collagenase type II (0.59 mg/mL) and incubated on a shaker for 1 h in °C. After that, the released cells in the supernatants were filtered through a 45–60-micron nylon mesh and the cells were collected in a 50 mL conical tube. The remaining undigested tissue was retreated with RPMI in the presence of DNAse and collagenase type II for a second digestion and incubated for an additional hour. The collected cells were layered on a ficoll gradient to separate the lymphocytes. The lymphocytes were then washed twice with 1 $\times$ PBS and re-suspended in RPMI with 10% FBS. The cells were then counted and the viability were determined as described above by trypan blue and propidium iodide staining immediately after purification, and after an overnight incubation at 37 °C.

2.5. Enzyme-Linked Immunosorbent Assays (ELISAs) and Multiplex Assays

Single ELISAs were performed as previously described [22]. To analyze and obtain the cytokine and chemokine concentration, a standard curve was generated by either two- or three-fold dilutions of recombinant cytokines provided by the manufacturer. For multiple cytokine array, the levels of cytokines and chemokines were examined by multiplex assay, which was conducted as described in the manufacturer's protocol for each specified kit. Analysis was performed using a Luminex multiplex instrument (MAGPIX, Millipore, Billerica, MA, USA), and data were analyzed using the proprietary software (xPONENT 4.2, Millipore, Billerica, MA, USA).

2.6. Cytotoxicity Assays

The ^{51}Cr release assay was performed as described previously [23]. Briefly, different numbers of effector cells were incubated with ^{51}Cr–labeled target cells. After a 4-h incubation period, the supernatants were harvested from each sample and the released radioactivity was counted using the gamma counter. The percentage specific cytotoxicity was calculated as follows:

$$\text{cytotoxicity} = \frac{\text{Experimental cpm} - \text{spontaneous cpm}}{\text{Total cpm} - \text{spontaneous cpm}}$$

LU $30/10^6$ is calculated by using the inverse of the number of effector cells needed to lyse 30% of tumor target cells $\times$ 100.

Cytotoxicity was also performed using xCELLigence Real Time Cell Analysis (RTCA). Tumor cells were added to microplates (E-Plates) overnight, before the addition of effector cells at 1:1 effector to target ratios, and the impedance was read by the instrument at different time intervals. Procedure was conducted as described in the manufacturer's protocol for xCELLigence immunotherapy kit.

2.7. Surface Staining and Cell Death Assays

Staining was performed by labeling the cells with antibodies or propidium iodide (PI), as described previously [22,24,25]. For surface staining, the cells were washed twice using ice-cold PBS + 1%BSA. Predetermined optimal concentrations of specific human monoclonal antibodies were added to 1×10^4 cells in 50 µL of cold PBS + 1%BSA, and were incubated on ice for 30 min. Thereafter cells were washed in cold PBS + 1%BSA and brought to 500 µL with PBS + 1%BSA. Flow cytometric analysis was performed using Beckman Coulter Epics XL cytometer (Brea, CA, USA).

2.8. Purification of Human NK Cells

Briefly, PBMCs were obtained after Ficoll-hypaque centrifugation and were used to isolate NK cells using the EasySep® Human NK cell purchased from Stem Cell Technologies (Vancouver, BC, Canada). Isolated NK cells stained with anti-CD16 to measure the cell purity using flow cytometric analysis.

2.9. Retroviral Transduction, Transfection and the Generation of Tumor Cell Transfectants

Cells were infected with culture supernatants of NIH 3T3 packaging cells infected with either GFP expressing a transdominant negative allele of IκB [26] or GFP alone. The mutant IκB-alpha (IκBαM) cDNA was excised from pCMX by digesting with *Bam*HI and EcoRV, and cloned into the pMX-IRES-EGFP retroviral vector and cut with *Not*I (Klenow-filled) and *Bam*HI. Forty-eight hours after infection the cells were sorted and high GFP expressing cells were grown and used in the experiments. The generation of tumor cell transfectants was described previously [23,27]. The stability of IκB(S32AS36A) super suppressor transfected cells in blocking NFκB function were regularly checked by western blot analysis and EMSA using nuclear extracts prepared from the cell transfectants, and a luciferase reporter assay described below.

2.10. Luciferase Reporter Assay

Cells were plated and maintained in RPMI supplemented with 10% FBS and 1% penicillin/streptomycin before transfection. Transfections were done using an NF-κB Luciferase reporter vector [28] and Lipofectamine 2000 reagent (Invitrogen, Carlsbad, CA, USA) in Opti-MEM media (Invitrogen, CA) for 18 h after which they were treated with TNF-α. The cells were then lysed with lysis buffer and the relative Luciferase activity was measured using the Luciferase assay reagent kit obtained from Promega (Madison, WI, USA).

2.11. Fusobacterium nucleatum Preparation

Viable or 1% paraformaldehyde fixed *F. nucleatum* were used for co-cultures with the immune cells and epithelial tumors at 30:2:1; bacteria: PBMCs: HEp2 tumor ratios. Similar results were obtained with either viable or paraformaldehyde fixed bacterial co-cultures with immune cells and epithelial tumors.

2.12. Statistical Analysis

An unpaired or paired, two-tailed Student's *t*-test was performed for experiments with two groups. One-way ANOVA with a Bonferroni post-test was used to compare different groups for experiments with more than two groups. Duplicate or triplicate samples were used in the in vitro studies for assessment. The following symbols represent the levels of statistical significance within each analysis: *** (p value < 0.001), ** (p value 0.001–0.01), * (p value 0.01–0.05).

3. Results

3.1. Periodontitis Patients' Oral Blood Exhibited Higher Percentages of NK Cells and Lower Percentages of B Cells in Comparison to Their Peripheral Blood

We first investigated the percentages of different immune cell subsets in oral and peripheral blood of healthy individuals and periodontitis patients. Similar percentages of NK, T and B cells in peripheral and oral blood were found for healthy individuals (Table 1 (upper two rows)). In contrast, decreased percentages of B cells, increased percentages of NK cells, and similar percentages of T cells were observed in oral blood compared to peripheral blood of periodontitis patients (Table 1 (lower two rows) and Figure S1). Overall, these results indicated that oral blood obtained from periodontitis patients contained higher numbers of NK cells when compared to those obtained from their peripheral blood. The percentages of NK cells within the oral blood were similar between heathy and periodontitis patients.

Table 1. Percentages of lymphocyte cell subsets in peripheral and oral blood of healthy individuals and periodontitis patients.

		CD16+	CD3+	CD19+	CD3 + CD4+	CD3 + CD8+
Healthy	Peripheral blood	15.5 ± 3.5 **	74 ± 7	10.5 ± 3.5 *	55 ± 7	19 ± 9
	Oral blood	15.8 ± 9.7	74 ± 6.9	7.8 ± 7.4	52 ± 6	22 ± 10
Patients	Peripheral blood	3.5 ± 0.7 **	71 ± 9.9	24.5 ± 9 *	51 ± 3	20 ± 1
	Oral blood	16 ± 10	73 ± 15	6.7 ± 4	53 ± 2	20 ± 7

Mononuclear cells were isolated from peripheral and oral blood of healthy individuals and periodontitis patients using Ficoll-Hypaque density gradient. The percentages of lymphocyte subsets were determined immediately after purification using specific antibody staining followed by flow cytometric analysis. The IgG2 isotype was used as a control. Significant differences were obtained between the levels of CD16 + NK (** p value of 0.001–0.01) and CD19 + B cells (* p value 0.01–0.05) in the peripheral blood between healthy individuals and those of the periodontitis patients, and for CD16+ NK cells (** p value of 0.001–0.01) and CD19 + B cells (* p value 0.01–0.05) between peripheral and oral blood in periodontitis patients. No significant differences (p = 0.8) were observed in peripheral and oral blood between healthy individuals and periodontitis patients for the levels of CD3, CD4 and CD8 lymphocyte subpopulations. The numbers for each immune subset reflect the mean percentages derived from six donors ± standard deviation.

3.2. Oral Gingival-Derived Immune Cells from Periodontitis Patients Exhibited Higher Percentages of B Cells and Lower Percentages of T Cells as Compared to Those from Healthy Individuals

We determined the percentages of immune cell subsets in the oral gingival cells using flow cytometric analysis. Higher percentages of CD19 expressing B cells, and lower percentages of CD3 and CD3 + CD4+ expressing T cells were observed in immune cells derived from gingival tissue of periodontitis patients when compared to those of healthy individuals (Table 2). No significant differences were seen for the percentages of CD16 expressing NK cells or CD3 + CD8+ expressing T cells (Table 2). The majority of CD45+ immune cells in gingival tissues were at an activated state as indicated by higher expression of CD69 surface receptor (Figure S2A). Gingival tissue derived immune cells from patients also expressed CD28 and CD95 (Fas) surface receptors (Figure S2B).

Table 2. Percentages of lymphocyte cell subsets in gingival tissues obtained from healthy individuals and periodontitis patients.

	CD16+	CD3+	CD19+	CD3 + CD4+	CD3 + CD8+
Healthy	4.7 ± 5.0	80 ± 19	6.7 ± 5.9	62 ± 8	18 ± 10
Patients	5.05 ± 3.9	68 ± 23	27 ± 23	47 ± 10	21 ± 4

Gingival tissue-associated mononuclear cells from healthy individuals and periodontitis patients were obtained as described in the Materials and Methods section. The percentages of lymphocyte subsets in mononuclear cells were determined using specific antibody staining followed by flow cytometric analysis. IgG2 isotype was used as controls. $p = 0.14$ was obtained for the difference between the levels of CD19 + B cells obtained from the healthy individuals and periodontitis patients. No significant differences ($p = 0.7$) were observed for CD16, CD3, CD4 and CD8 lymphocyte subpopulations between healthy individuals and periodontitis patients. The numbers for each immune subset reflect the mean percentages derived from six donors ± standard deviation.

3.3. NK Cells and CD8 + T Cells in Oral Blood of Periodontitis Patients Exhibited Significant Levels of Activation

Oral blood mononuclear cells (OBMCs), and peripheral blood mononuclear cells (PBMCs) of periodontitis patients and healthy individuals were left untreated, or treated with IL-2 or PMA plus ionomycin (PMA/I) overnight. To determine the levels of activation, the early activation antigen expression, CD69 was analyzed on the surfaces of CD16 + NK and CD8 + T cells. The surface expression levels of CD69 activation antigens were found to be elevated on the CD16 + NK cells and CD8 + T cells in OBMCs when compared to PBMCs of periodontitis patients (Figure 1). Moreover, increased surface expression levels of CD69 on NK cells were only observed on cells obtained from periodontitis patients and not form the healthy individuals (unpublished material). When CD16 + NK and CD8+ T cells were treated with IL-2 and PMA/I, higher intensity of CD69 was detected both in OBMCs and PBMCs of periodontitis patients, although the intensity remained higher in OBMCs (Figure 1 and Figure S3). PMA/I treatment resulted in a similar or slightly higher intensity of CD69 surface expression on CD16 + NK and CD8 + T cells in OBMCs as compared to PBMCs (Figure S3). Overall, these results indicated that OBMCs obtained from periodontitis patients exhibited higher activation levels.

3.4. PBMCs but Not OBMCs Obtained from Periodontitis Patients Demonstrated Significantly Higher Levels of Cell Death When Compared to Those from Healthy Individuals

Activation by PMA/I resulted in an increased level of cell death both in healthy individuals' and periodontitis patients' PBMCs but not in OBMCs (Figure 2). Approximately two-fold more cell deaths could be seen in PMA/I-treated PBMCs of periodontitis patients when compared to those from healthy individuals (Figure 2). In contrast, treatment with PMA/I did not exhibit significant cell death in OBMCs either from patients or healthy individuals (Figure 2).

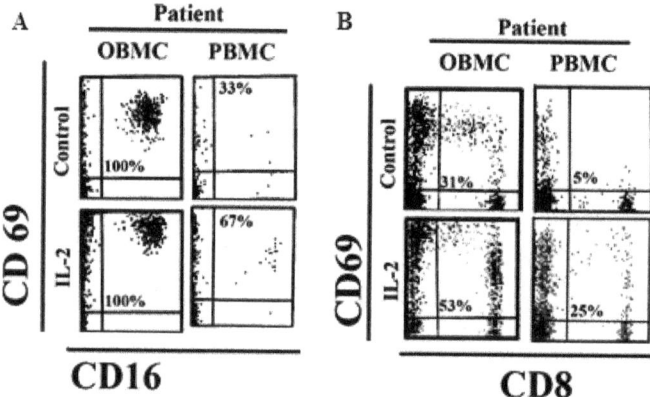

Figure 1. Increased activation of NK and CD8 + T cells in oral blood when compared to peripheral blood of periodontitis patients. Mononuclear cells (1×10^6/mL) obtained from oral and peripheral blood of periodontitis patients left untreated and treated with IL-2 (500 U/mL) for 18–24 h after which they were washed twice. The surface expression levels of CD16 and CD69 (**A**), and CD8 and CD69 (**B**) were determined using flow cytometry. IgG2 isotype was used as controls. Numbers in each quadrant represent the percentages of stained sub-population for the specific antigen. The oral and peripheral blood was obtained from the same donors. One of four representative experiments is shown in this figure.

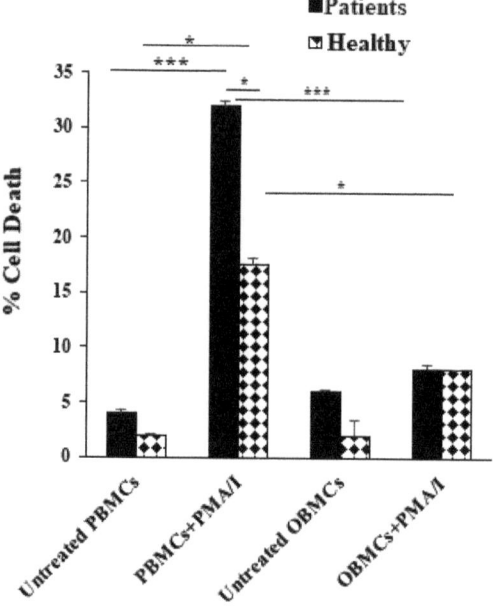

Figure 2. Higher levels of cell death were observed in periodontitis patients' PBMCs when compared to those from healthy individuals. Mononuclear cells obtained from peripheral and oral blood of healthy individuals and periodontitis patients were treated with PMA (10 ng/mL) + ionomycin (10 ng/mL) for 10–14 h. The samples were then washed and propidium iodide (30 μg/mL) was added to each sample. The percentages of dead cells were determined by flow cytometric analysis. PBMCs and OBMCs were obtained from the same donors. One of four representative experiments is shown in this figure. *** (p value <0.001), * (p value 0.01–0.05).

3.5. Increased TNF-α Secretion Was Observed from OBMCs of Periodontitis Patients When Compared to Those from Healthy Individuals

OBMCs and PBMCs of periodontitis patients were left untreated or treated with IL-2 or IFN-γ or PMA/I, and the levels of TNF-α secretion were determined after 12 to 18 h. Higher secretion of TNF-α was observed from OBMCs when compared to PBMCs of periodontitis patients (Figure 3A). IFN-γ treatment increased TNF-α secretion moderately by patient OBMCs whereas it induced significant levels of secretion by the patient PBMCs (Figure 3A). Although there was a moderate increase in TNF-α release by IFN-γ treated OBMCs obtained from patient and healthy donors, the increase was not statistically significant (Figure 3A). The lack of increase in TNF-α by IFN-γ could be due to higher basal activation of OBMCs in patients. The levels of TNF-α secretion between PMA/I-treated PBMCs and OBMCs plateaued since PMA/I activates lymphocytes in both cell populations maximally (Figure 3A). Next, we compared the TNF-α secretion in OBMCs obtained from healthy individuals and periodontitis patients. We observed increased secretion of TNF-α in OBMCs from periodontitis patients with and without IL-2 or IFN-γ treatment (Figure 3B). These results demonstrated the increased functional activities of mononuclear cells in oral blood as compared to peripheral blood of periodontitis patients. Furthermore, periodontal disease found to be associated with increased TNF-α secretion in oral blood immune cells.

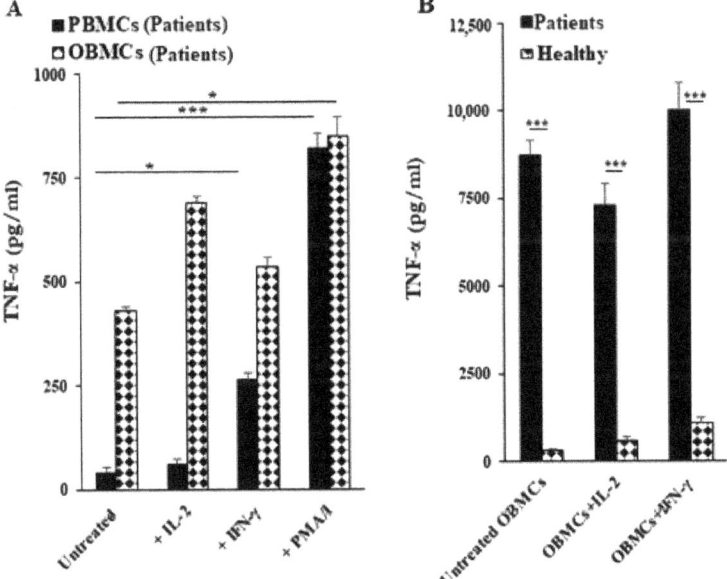

Figure 3. Periodontitis patients' OBMCs secreted higher levels of TNF-α secretion in comparison to their PBMCs; Periodontitis patients' OBMCs secreted higher levels of TNF-α when compared to those from healthy individuals. PBMCs and OBMCs of periodontitis patients were treated with IL-2 (500 U/mL), IFN-γ (500 U/mL) and PMA (10 ng/mL) + ionomycin (10 ng/mL). After 12–18 h of incubation, supernatants were harvested and the levels of TNF-α secretion were determined using single ELISA. *** (p value < 0.001), * (p value 0.01–0.05), p values were obtained for differences between untreated or IL-2 or IFN-γ treated PBMCs and OBMCs obtained from the periodontitis patients (**A**). OBMCs obtained from healthy individuals and periodontitis patients were left untreated, treated with IL-2 (500 U/mL) or treated with IFN-γ (500 U/mL). After an overnight incubation the supernatants were harvested and subjected to a single ELISA to determine TNF-α secretion levels. *** (p value < 0.001), p value was obtained for the difference between TNF-α secretion by OBMCs obtained from healthy individuals and periodontitis patients; control, IL-2 and IFN-γ treated OBMCs (**B**). One of four representative experiments is shown in this figure.

3.6. OBMC-Derived Supernatants from Periodontitis Patients Regulate Secretion of Cytokines by Allogeneic Healthy PBMCs

Since chronic periodontitis was shown to be associated with an altered balance between anti-inflammatory and pro-inflammatory cytokines, we tested the ability of OBMCs-derived supernatants from periodontitis patients and healthy individuals to modulate IFN-γ, IL-6, TNF-α and IL-1β secretions in untreated and IL-2-treated allogeneic PBMCs isolated from healthy individuals. When compared to OBMC-derived supernatants from healthy individuals, addition of those derived from OBMCs of periodontitis patients to IL-2 activated PBMCs had lower priming/activating capability of PBMCs to secrete IFN-γ and TNF-α, whereas IL-6 induction was similar between the two, likely due to the plateauing effect (Figure 4A–C). IL-1β induction was also lower in the presence of OBMC-derived supernatants from periodontitis patients, but with no statistical differences (Figure 4D). When adding to untreated PBMCs, OBMC-derived supernatants from patients or healthy individuals exhibited no change in IFN-γ induction whereas much higher levels of IL-6, TNF-α and IL-1β were induced in those treated with OBMC-derived supernatants from patients compared to those from healthy individuals (Figure 4A–D).

3.7. NFkB Deletion in Oral Epithelial Cells Increases IFN-γ Secretion by PBMCs and NK Cells in the Presence or Absence of Fusobacterium nucleatum

Since immune effectors in the periodontal tissues interact with a number of stromal cells as well as with the epithelial cells to induce cytokine secretion, we determined the induction of cytokines in the presence of a number of either non modified or genetically modified oral epithelial cell lines as shown below in the presence and absence of *F. nucleatum*. First, we determined NK cell-mediated cytotoxicity against the pRcCMV vector alone (HEp2-pRcCMV), or IκB(S32AS36A) transfected HEp2 (HEp2-IκB(S32AS36A)) cells as targets. The NK cell-mediated cytotoxicity was higher against HEp2-IκB(S32AS36A) cells in comparison to HEp2-pRcCMV cells by untreated, IL-2-treated or anti-CD16 mAbs treated NK cells (Figure 5A–C). Similar results were seen in oral squamous carcinoma cells (OSCCs) and human oral keratinocytes (HOK) cells. Inhibition of NFkB by the IkB(S32AS36A) super-repressor retroviral vector was confirmed by measuring NFkB activity using a luciferase reporter assay (Figure S4A,B). Overall, the NK cell-mediated cytotoxicity was higher against NFkB knock-down OSCCs and HOK cells when compared to EGFP transfected cells (Figure S4C,D).

To determine the effect of immune cells' interaction with epithelial cells in the presence and absence of *F. nucleatum*, we left PBMCs and NK cells untreated or treated them with IL-2 before they were co-cultured with HEp2-IκB(S32AS36A) and HEp2-pRcCMV in the presence or absence of *F. nucleatum*. We observed increased secretion of IFN-γ in co-cultures of PBMCs with HEp2-IκB(S32AS36A) tumors compared to those with HEp2-pRcCMV in the presence or absence of *F. nucleatum* (Figure 6A). Although similar results to IFN-γ were seen for TNF-α, GM-CSF, IL-13, MCP-1, and RANTES, the secretion of IL-6 was higher in immune cell cultures with HEp2-pRcCMV in comparison to those with HEp2-IκB(S32AS36A) tumors (Figure S5). Increased IFN-γ secretion was also observed when untreated and IL-2-treated NK cells were co-cultured with HEp2-IκB(S32AS36A) tumors compared to HEp2-pRcCMV in the absence or presence of *F. nucleatum* (Figure 6B). Similar results were seen when IL-2 treated NK cells were co-cultured with NFkB knock-down OSCCs and HOK cells in comparison to those cultured with EGFP transfected cells (Figure S4E,F). The treatment with *F. nucleatum* increased IFN-γ in all culture conditions and, the highest was seen in IL-2-treated PBMCs or NK cells co-cultured with HEp2-IκB(S32AS36A) tumors (Figure 6A,B). Increased secretion of TNF-α, IL-8, GM-CSF, and IL-13 was also seen when NK cells were co-cultured with HEp2-IκB(S32AS36A) in comparison to HEp2-pRcCMV tumors in the absence of *F. nucleatum* (Figure S6). The secretion of IL-6 was higher in HEp2-pRcCMV in comparison to HEp2-IκB(S32AS36A) tumors (Figure S6). Furthermore, IL-6 secretion was lower when NK cells were co-cultured with NFkB knock-down OSCCs and HOK cells in comparison to those cultured with EGFP transfected cells (Figure S4G,H). Interestingly, IL-13 and GM-CSF secretions were inhibited by *F. nucleatum* in IL-2-treated

NK cells co-cultured with HEp2-IκB(S32AS36A) and HEp2-pRcCMV cells (Figure S6). Overall, these results demonstrated that NFκB knock-down cells in comparison to their non-knock-down counterparts are more active inducers of PBMCs and NK cells to secrete IFN-γ, and presence of F. *nucleatum* enhances this functional activation.

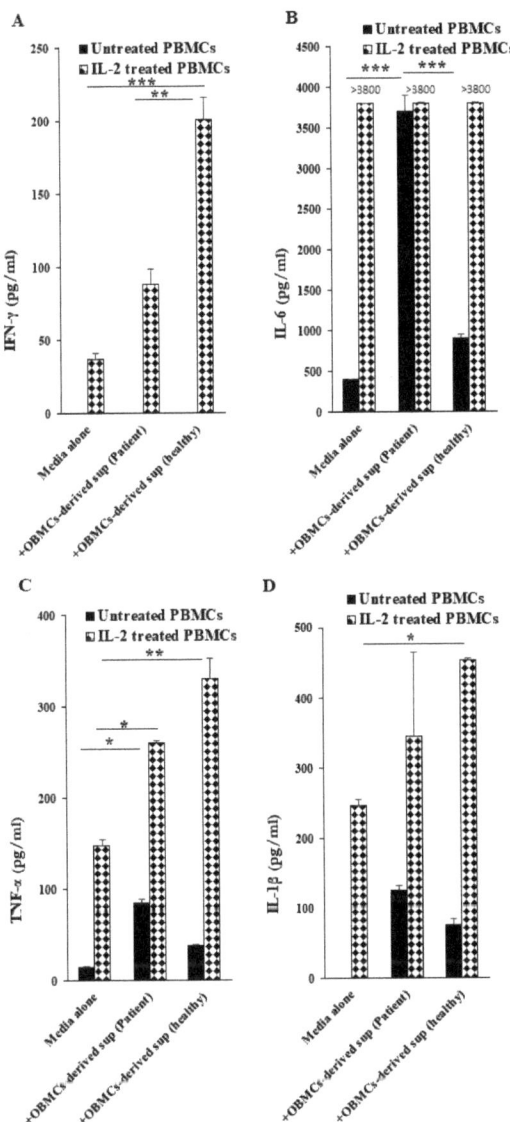

Figure 4. Periodontitis patients' OBMCs-derived supernatant had decreased ability to activate allogeneic healthy PBMCs in comparison to healthy individuals' OBMC-derived supernatant. Untreated OBMCs (1×10^6/mL) of healthy individuals and periodontitis patients were incubated at 37 °C for 6–12 h before supernatants were harvested. Allogeneic healthy PBMCs (1×10^6/mL) were left untreated or treated with IL-2 (500 U/mL) for 12–18 h, after which, OBMCs-derived supernatants were added to PBMCs, and 18–20 h later the supernatants were harvested to determine IFN-γ (**A**), IL-6 (**B**), TNF-α (**C**), IL-1β (**D**) secretion using single ELISAs. One of four representative experiments is shown in this figure. *** (p value < 0.001), ** (p value 0.001–0.01), * (p value 0.01–0.05).

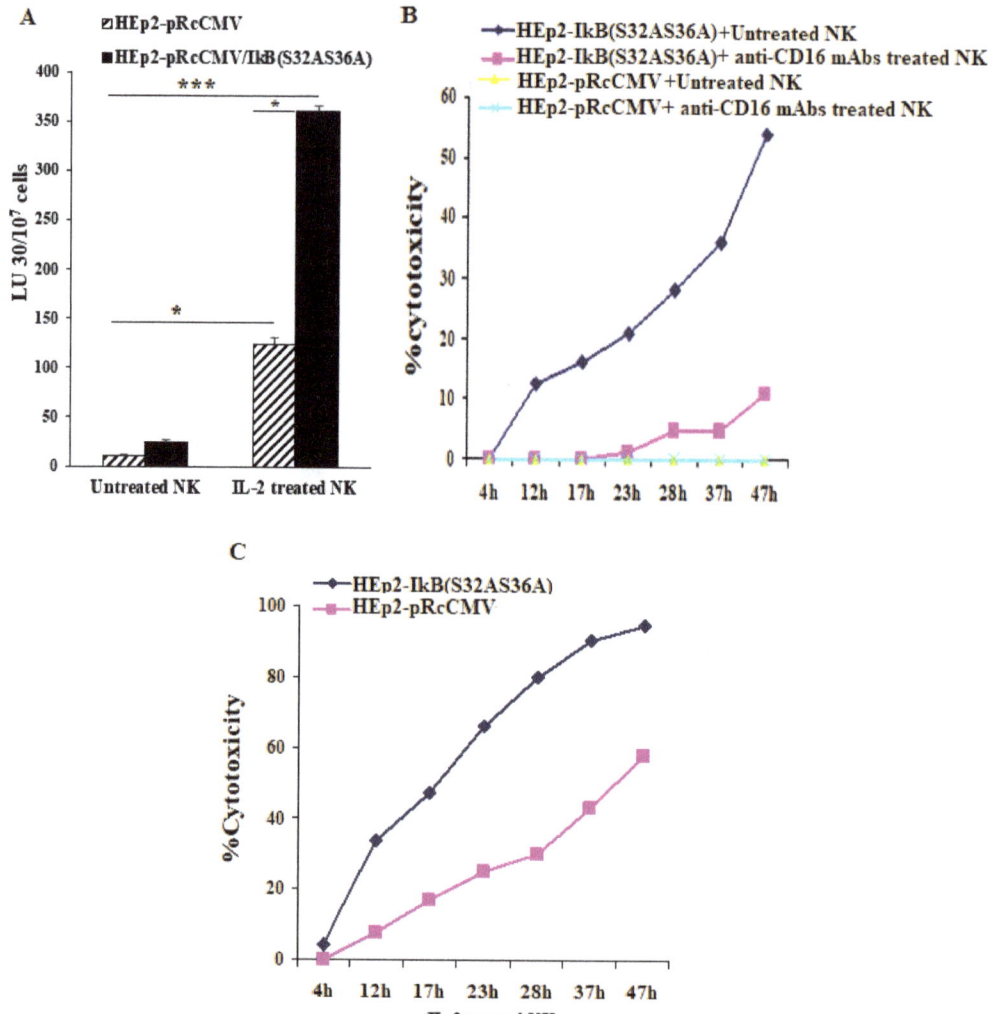

Figure 5. NFκB blocking in HEp2 tumors increased their susceptibility to NK cell-mediated cytotoxicity. NK cells were left untreated and treated with IL-2 (500 U/mL) overnight before they were added to ^{51}Cr-labeled pRcCMV vector alone or IκB(S32AS36A) transfected HEp2 cells at various effector-to-target ratios. NK cell-mediated cytotoxicity was measured using a standard 4-h ^{51}Cr release assay. The lytic units (LU) 30/10^7 cells were determined using the inverse number of NK cells required to lyse 30% of target cells × 100 (**A**). *** (p value < 0.001), * (p value 0.01–0.05). NK cells were left untreated and treated with anti-CD16 mAbs (3 μg/mL) overnight before they were added to ^{51}Cr-labeled pRcCMV vector alone or IκB(S32AS36A) transfected HEp2 cells at various effector-to-target ratios. NK cell-mediated cytotoxicity was measured using xCELLigence Real Time Cell Analysis (RTCA) (**B**). NK cells were treated with IL-2 (500 U/mL) overnight before they were added to ^{51}Cr-labeled pRcCMV vector or and IκB(S32AS36A) transfected HEp2 cells at various effector-to-target ratios. NK cell-mediated cytotoxicity was measured using xCELLigence Real Time Cell Analysis (RTCA) (**C**). One of four representative experiments is shown in this figure.

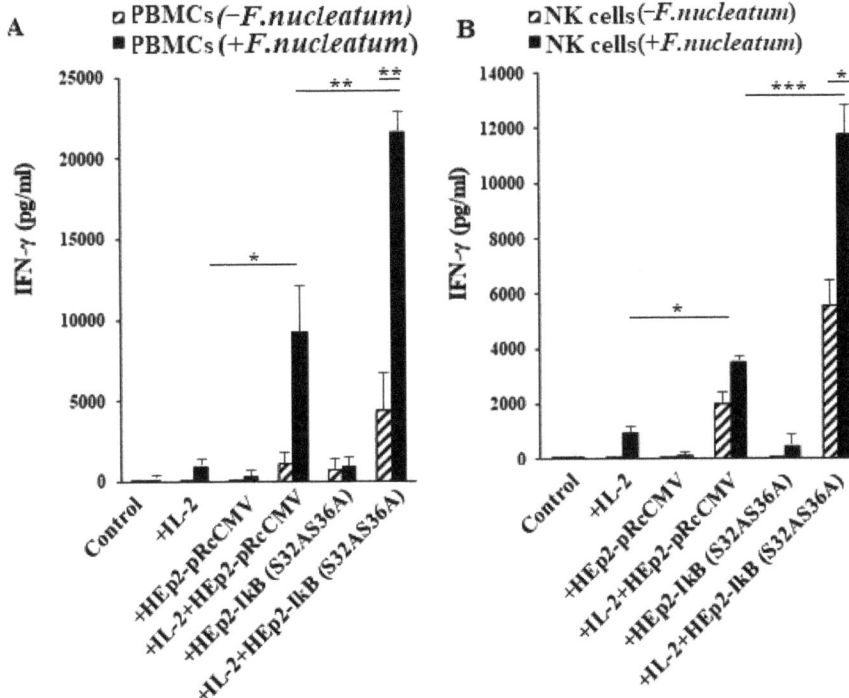

Figure 6. Increased IFN-γ secretion levels were observed in *F. nucleatum* treated PBMCs and NK cells; highest secretion levels were seen in the presence of NFκB blocked HEp2 tumors. PBMCs were left untreated or treated with IL-2 (2000 U/mL) overnight before their co-culture with HEp2-pRcCMV or HEp2-IκB(S32AS36A) cells in the presence or absence of *F. nucleatum* (bacteria: PBMCs: Hep2 tumors at 30:2:1 ratios). After an overnight incubation, the supernatants were harvested to determine IFN-γ secretion using multiplex cytokine array assay, one of four representative experiments are shown in the figure (**A**). NK cells were left untreated or treated with IL-2 (2000 U/mL) overnight before their co-culture with HEp2-pRcCMV or HEp2-IκB(S32AS36A) cells in the presence or absence of *F. nucleatum* at (bacteria: PBMCs: Hep2 tumors at 30:2:1 ratios). After an overnight incubation, the supernatants were harvested to determine IFN-γ secretion using multiplex cytokine array assay (**B**). One of four representative experiments is shown in this figure *** (p value < 0.001), ** (p value 0.001–0.01), * (p value 0.01–0.05).

4. Discussion

Although ample progress has previously been made regarding periodontal disease, a clear understanding of immune interaction with neighboring stromal cells with probable genetic and epigenetic modifications in the presence of complex oral microorganisms is still limited. In previous studies disease-relevant assumptions or interpretations were usually made based on the interaction of periodontal pathogens with peripheral blood immune effectors. In addition, the use of tissue-associated immune effectors from the infected sites also provided limited information regarding the disease pathogenesis since these cells were isolated largely at a non-functional state due to the harsh recovery methods. Indeed, in our experience the majority of the immune effectors isolated from the gingival tissues underwent cell death when the cells were incubated greater than 3–4 h. Furthermore, they were unable to secrete cytokines or mediate cytotoxicity even though they exhibited increased levels of activation markers on their surface. Thus, such experiments are great to assess the phenotype of the immune effectors at the time of isolation, but lack ability to provide functional readouts. These observations, therefore, prompted us to design strategies to obtain immune cells from the oral site using oral blood which remained functional and had the capacity to respond when exposed to self-bacterial and viral microflora.

Therefore, to understand potential similarities and differences between peripheral, oral and tissue-derived immune effectors, initially we obtained and characterized immune subsets from each of these sites in healthy individuals and from the patients with periodontal disease (Tables 1 and 2).

The rationale for using orally-derived blood to compare with the peripheral blood and tissue-derived immune effectors is; (1) to observe whether there were quantitative differences between the immune subsets from different compartments, and (2) to determine and compare the levels of their functional competency. It is likely that orally-derived immune effectors contain elements of saliva in addition to oral microorganisms, and thus exhibit phenotypic and functional properties that are distinct from those obtained from peripheral blood or even those found in the gingival tissues. Nevertheless, the analysis could shed light on their differences and help identify important questions regarding the pathogenesis of periodontal disease. For example, are there any phenotypic similarities between the oral blood immune effectors and those recovered from the gingival tissues? When comparing CD69 expression we observed similar increase in CD69 surface expression in oral blood mononuclear cells compared to those extracted from gingival tissues. It is interesting to note that lymphocytes obtained from healthy gingival tissues also expressed higher levels of CD69 expression when compared to the patients with periodontitis. However, the numbers of immune effectors obtained from healthy gingival tissues were far less than those obtained from patients with periodontitis.

The increased activation of orally-derived mononuclear cells from patients could be due to their exposure to periodontal pathogens during the recovery method. In this regard the oral mononuclear cells from patients may recognize and become strongly activated to their oral flora and/or they may be at a stage of maturation which is more susceptible to activation signals delivered by the oral pathogens. Indeed, it is believed that the nature of host immune cells is the determining factor for the response to periodontal pathogens [29,30]. In addition, patients with periodontal disease are shown to have genetic predisposition for increased cytokine secretion, particularly IL-1β and TNF-α [31]. Therefore, the studies reported here are likely to shed some light on the mechanisms of immune cell activation in patients since both the immune effectors and the combination of pathogenic oral bacterial and viral flora are derived from the same oral niche.

Orally-derived immune cells from patients with periodontal disease exhibited an increase in the activation of NK and CD8+ T cell fractions after an overnight incubation, and secreted higher levels of TNF-α, whereas those obtained from healthy donors exhibited a profile closer to those obtained from naïve peripheral blood immune cells. In this regard we have recently reported that activated NK cells are able to activate CD8+ T cells [32]. As indicated, the difference could be due to either higher innate capacity of the immune effectors to become activated and/or the increased activating capacity of periodontal pathogens in patients compared to healthy controls. Our results also indicated that mononuclear cells obtained from the oral blood did not undergo significant activation induced cell death after treatment with PMA/I when compared to peripheral blood, even though OBMCs demonstrated increased levels of activation when compared to PBMCs. No significant differences could be observed in cell death between OBMCs obtained from healthy individuals and those with periodontitis in the presence and absence of PMA/I treatment. The resistance of oral mononuclear cells to apoptotic cell death has been documented previously in chronic periodontal lesions [33,34]. Both IL-4 and Fas Ligand were found to be decreased or not expressed within the gingival tissues even though the IL-4 and Fas receptors were expressed on the immune cells, suggesting a lack of ligand for decreased cell death [33,34]. However, since PMA/I treatment bypasses the receptor mediated effects, this implies other underlying mechanisms for the lack of cell death in OBMCs. Whether there are pressures for selecting longer surviving immune cells in OBMCs requires further investigations. Therefore, continued inflammation and tissue damage in periodontal disease may partly be mediated by longer surviving oral mononuclear cells.

Activation-induced cell death in immune effectors is a well characterized cellular outcome which occurs upon potent activation of immune cells. As indicated above, PBMCs treated with PMA/I underwent significant cell death, whereas OBMCs demonstrated considerably lower levels of cell death upon activation with PMA/I. No significant correlation could be seen between levels of activation (using CD69 expression) and the extent of cell death in immune effectors isolated from peripheral and oral blood. Indeed, more cell death was observed in PBMCs that had a slightly lower CD69 expression when compared to OBMCs after treatment with PMA/I (Figure 2 and Figure S3). Therefore, other factors in addition to the extent of activation may be responsible for continued survival of these cells in an oral microenvironment. Whether components of saliva in addition to signals delivered by bacterial and viral flora provide a survival advantage for mononuclear cells awaits future investigation.

Higher numbers of CD16+ NK cells were observed in the oral blood of patients with periodontal disease when compared to the peripheral blood and gingival tissues. NK cells are a subset of lymphocytes which mediate first line defense against a variety of tumors and microorganisms. Indeed, NK cells are one of the primary sources of secreted IFN-γ. Thus, activation of NK cell function and elaboration of cytokines such as IFN-γ is essential for the expansion and amplification of immune responses mediated by the effectors of both an innate and adaptive immune system. In addition, IFN-γ is important in differentiation of stromal cells and subsequent cessation of NK cell function since NK cells are known to become activated by the stem cells and not by the well-differentiated cells [35,36]. Thus, IFN-γ can regulate its own production negatively and limit the levels of inflammation [35–38].

The rationale for a lower percentage of peripheral blood NK cells compared to oral blood NK cells in patients with periodontal disease is not clearly known yet. One can speculate regarding the increased homing of these cells to oral tissues from the peripheral blood in which a higher gradient of chemokines is secreted by epithelial cells upon activation by pathogenic organisms. In addition, it is also possible that lower percentages of NK cells seen in the gingiva of patients compared to those in the oral blood could be due to the higher induction of activation-induced cell death in NK cells in the gingiva where higher activation signals are given to the NK cells by the gingival microenvironment, a phenomenon that we and others have established previously in NK cells [39]. As for the differences in percentages of B cells in the peripheral and oral blood and gingival tissue, the decrease in the oral blood seems to be compensated for by the increase in the percentages of B cells in the gingival tissues of patients with periodontal disease. Such differences in the quantity of B cells could not be seen in different tissue compartments in healthy individuals. The percentages of T cells remained high in all compartments in healthy individuals as well as in patients with periodontal disease.

When added to IL-2-activated allogeneic PBMCs, supernatants obtained from OBMCs of periodontitis patients were only able to increase IFN-γ secretion by about 2.4-fold, whereas those obtained from healthy individuals increased by 5.4-fold. Since supernatants obtained from OBMCs of periodontitis patients contain significant levels of pro-inflammatory cytokines such as TNF-α, IL-6 and IL-1β, these cytokines may be inhibitory for the induction of IFN-γ. Indeed, we have previously shown that both TNF-α and IL-6 inhibit secretion of IFN-γ by the NK cells [24,27]. Higher induction of pro and anti-inflammatory cytokines in the presence of decreased IFN-γ secretion may, therefore, tilt the balance towards the establishment of chronic inflammation in periodontal infections. Indeed, we have shown in a series of studies that IFN-γ is important in the differentiation of stromal cells and the limitation of inflammation [36,40,41]. In addition, healthy stem cells or stem-like cancer stem cells, but not differentiated cells, are able to activate NK cells due to a lack of or decreased surface expression of MHC-class I [36,42,43]. Therefore, it is possible that due to a lower release of IFN-γ during chronic inflammation, adequate induction of MHC-class I expression does not occur in the stromal cells, thereby leading to a decreased activation and release of IFN-γ by the NK cells which maintains the stromal cells at a lower level of differentiation resulting in the chronicity of inflammation. These possibilities are currently under investigation in our laboratory.

Since both bacterial and viral agents have been implicated in the pathogenesis of periodontal disease [44–47], it is likely that suboptimal induction of IFN-γ will have profound effects on the clearance of both types of organism and the resolution of inflammation [48–50]. Therefore, the increase in the numbers and activation of NK cells in periodontal infection may have a direct relationship to the increase in colonization with the viral and bacterial infections since NK cells are the primary effectors that mediate lysis of virally infected cells. In addition, by secreting IFN-γ, NK cells will be able to increase lysis of bacteria by augmenting the activation of monocyte-macrophages and dendritic cells [51].

It is known that the number of bacteria in the periodontal tissues of the patients does not correlate with the severity of periodontal disease, and that it is likely that other factors are involved in the pathogenesis of disease [1,52]. Thus, periodontal disease is multifactorial. Since periodontal disease has been shown to have genetic as well as environmental components, it is likely that mutations either in the stromal cells or in the immune cells could likely exacerbate the disease [52–56]. We have shown previously that many genetic alterations in particular deletions of important genes in stromal cells or in the immune cells can directly activate NK cells which could lead to the expansion and differentiation of T cells [32,57,58]. In order to determine whether such interactions may have a significant activating effect on PBMCs and NK cells in the presence of an oral pathogenic bacteria *F. nucleatum* (known to be associated with periodontal disease), we determined the effect of NFkB knock-down epithelial cells in the activation of PBMCs and NK cells in the presence of *F. nucleatum*. Significant activation of PBMCs and NK cells and the augmented release of different cytokines and chemokines were observed under such conditions (Figure 6, Figure S5 and Figure S6). Indeed, Jung et al. and Raje et al. reported previously how Nuclear factor-kappa B Essential Modulator (NEMO) deficiency might lead to a genetic predisposition named "Mendelian Susceptibility to Mycobacterial Disease (MSMD)", which increases susceptibility to mycobacterial infections [59,60]. In addition, Javali et al. indicated that periodontal disease was the initial oral manifestations of abdominal tuberculosis that was caused by mycobacteria infections, implicating this organism in periodontal disease [61]. Therefore, since NEMO deficiency may lead to an overall manifestation of immune deficiency through poor response to bacterial and fungal infections from NK, B and T-cells, as well as neutrophils, macrophages and dendritic cells, the bacterial infections from Gram-negative anaerobic bacteria, which are implicated in the periodontal diseases, are also likely. It is of interest to note that NFkB deletion in epithelial tumors increased IFN-γ secretion in the presence of decreased IL-6 in the co-cultures of these tumors with immune cells (Figure 6 and Figures S4–S6). Such observation is likely due to the significantly decreased secretion of IL-6 in NFkB knock-down tumors as well as decreased synergistic induction of IL-6 in the co-cultures of immune cells with NFkB knock-down tumors (Figures S5 and S6). Increased activation of NK cells and higher lysis of the tumors by the NK cells might also contribute to the decreased IL-6 secretion seen in the co-cultures of NFkB tumors with the NK cells. These findings indicate that cellular alternations in those that interact with the immune cells and/or in immune cells can exacerbate the immune function in the presence of periodontal pathogens, and could be the likely cause of the destruction which is seen in periodontitis patients. Although NFkB deficiency in epithelial cells or in other stromal cells has not been reported to be one of the major causes of periodontal disease, nevertheless, such findings may implicate the potential for genetic alterations in the exacerbation of periodontal disease.

Overall, our studies have identified a number of characteristics of immune effectors from different tissue compartments, which may have relevance to the pathogenesis of periodontal infections.

Supplementary Materials: The following are available online at https://www.mdpi.com/2077-0383/10/4/875/s1, Figure S1: Increased NK cells in oral blood in comparison to peripheral blood in periodontitis patients; Figure S2: Characteristics of lymphocytes obtained from gingival tissues; Figure S3: Increased activation of NK and CD8+ T cells in oral blood as compared to peripheral blood of periodontitis patients; Figure S4: Increased cytotoxicity, IFN-γ secretion, and decreased IL-6 in co-culture of NK cells with NFκB knockdown OSCCs and HOK-16B cells; Figure S5: Cytokine secretion levels in *F. nucleatum* treated PBMCs co-cultured with HEp2-pRcCMV, and HEp2-IκB(S32AS36A) cells; Figure S6: Determined cytokine secretion levels in *F. nucleatum*-treated NK cells co-cultured with Hep2-pRcCMV, and Hep2-IκB(S32AS36A) cells.

Author Contributions: K.K. performed experiments, data analysis, figures preparation, manuscript writing/editing. S.V., M.R.-R., and A.P. performed the experiments. A.J. arranged funding, prepared study design, and worked with K.K. for data analysis, figures preparation, manuscript writing/editing. All authors have read and agreed to the published version of the manuscript.

Funding: This research was funded by NIH-NIDCR RO1-DE022552; RO1 DE12880; UCLA Academic senate grant and School of Dentistry Seed grant.

Institutional Review Board Statement: This study was conducted according to UCLA Institutional Review Board (IRB). #11-000781), and declaration of Helsinki Informed Consent Statement: Written informed consents approved by the UCLA Institutional Review Board (IRB) were obtained from healthy donors and patients with periodontal diseases, and all procedures were approved by the UCLA-IRB.

Informed Consent Statement: Written informed consent approved by the UCLA Institutional Review Board was obtained from healthy individuals and periodontitis patients, and all procedures were approved by the UCLA-IRB.

Data Availability Statement: The data presented in this study are available in the article or Supplementary Materials of "Phenotypic and functional alterations of immune effectors in periodontitis; a multifactorial and complex disease of oral gingival tissues".

Conflicts of Interest: The authors declare that the research was conducted in the absence of any commercial or financial relationships that could be construed as a potential conflict of interest.

Abbreviations

NK cells	Natural killer cells
OSCCs	Oral squamous carcinoma cells
IFN-γ	Interferon-gamma
TNF-α	Tumor necrosis factor-α
OBMCs	Oral blood mononuclear cells
PBMCs	Peripheral blood mononuclear cells
NFκB	Nuclear factor kappa B
IL	Interleukin
GM-CSF	Granulocyte macrophage colony-stimulating factor

References

1. Slots, J. Periodontology: Past, present, perspectives. *Periodontol 2000* **2013**, *62*, 7–19. [CrossRef]
2. Gemmell, E.; Yamazaki, K.; Seymour, G.J. Destructive periodontitis lesions are determined by the nature of the lymphocytic response. *Crit. Rev. Oral Biol. Med.* **2002**, *13*, 17–34. [CrossRef]
3. Teng, Y.T. The role of acquired immunity and periodontal disease progression. *Crit. Rev. Oral Biol. Med.* **2003**, *14*, 237–252. [CrossRef]
4. Page, R.C.; Kornman, K.S. The pathogenesis of human periodontitis: An introduction. *Periodontol 2000* **1997**, *14*, 9–11. [CrossRef] [PubMed]
5. Kinane, D.F. Causation and pathogenesis of periodontal disease. *Periodontol 2000* **2001**, *25*, 8–20. [CrossRef]
6. Kornman, K.S.; Page, R.C.; Tonetti, M.S. The host response to the microbial challenge in periodontitis: Assembling the players. *Periodontol 2000* **1997**, *14*, 33–53. [CrossRef] [PubMed]
7. Page, R.C. The role of inflammatory mediators in the pathogenesis of periodontal disease. *J. Periodontal Res.* **1991**, *26*, 230–242. [CrossRef]

8. Graves, D.T. The potential role of chemokines and inflammatory cytokines in periodontal disease progression. *Clin. Infect. Dis.* **1999**, *28*, 482–490. [CrossRef] [PubMed]
9. Peters, U.; Solominidou, E.; Korkmaz, Y.; Rüttermann, S.; Klocke, A.; Flemmig, T.F.; Beikler, T. Regulator of Calcineurin 1 in Periodontal Disease. *Mediat. Inflamm.* **2016**, *2016*, 5475821. [CrossRef]
10. Venugopal, P.; Koshy, T.; Lavu, V.; Rao, S.R.; Ramasamy, S.; Hariharan, S.; Venkatesan, V. Differential expression of microRNAs let-7a, miR-125b, miR-100, and miR-21 and interaction with NF-kB pathway genes in periodontitis pathogenesis. *J. Cell Physiol.* **2018**, *233*, 5877–5884. [CrossRef] [PubMed]
11. Fujita, S.; Takahashi, H.; Okabe, H.; Ozaki, Y.; Hara, Y.; Kato, I. Distribution of natural killer cells in periodontal diseases: An immunohistochemical study. *J. Periodontol.* **1992**, *63*, 686–689. [CrossRef]
12. Kamoda, Y.; Uematsu, H.; Yoshihara, A.; Miyazaki, H.; Senpuku, H. Role of activated natural killer cells in oral diseases. *JPN J. Infect. Dis.* **2008**, *61*, 469–474.
13. Kawai, T.; Eisen-Lev, R.; Seki, M.; Eastcott, J.W.; Wilson, M.E.; Taubman, M.A. Requirement of B7 costimulation for Th1-mediated inflammatory bone resorption in experimental periodontal disease. *J. Immunol.* **2000**, *164*, 2102–2109. [CrossRef]
14. Teng YT, A.; Nguyen, H.; Gao, X.; Kong, Y.Y.; Gorczynski, R.M.; Singh, B.; Ellen, R.P.; Penninger, J. M Functional human T-cell immunity and osteoprotegerin ligand control alveolar bone destruction in periodontal infection. *J. Clin. Investig.* **2000**, *106*, R59–R67. [CrossRef] [PubMed]
15. Salvi, G.E.; Brown, C.E.; Fujihashi, K.; Kiyono, H.; Smith, F.W.; Beck, J.D.; Offenbacher, S. Inflammatory mediators of the terminal dentition in adult and early onset periodontitis. *J. Periodontal Res.* **1998**, *33*, 212–225. [CrossRef]
16. Stashenko, P.; Jandinski, J.J.; Fujiyoshi, P.; Rynar, J.; Socransky, S.S. Tissue levels of bone resorptive cytokines in periodontal disease. *J. Periodontol.* **1991**, *62*, 504–509. [CrossRef] [PubMed]
17. Baker, P.J.; Dixon, M.; Evans, R.T.; Dufour, L.; Johnson, E.; Roopenian, D.C. CD4(+) T cells and the proinflammatory cytokines gamma interferon and interleukin-6 contribute to alveolar bone loss in mice. *Infect. Immun.* **1999**, *67*, 2804–2809. [CrossRef] [PubMed]
18. Takeichi, O.; Haber, J.; Kawai, T.; Smith, D.J.; Moro, I.; Taubman, M.A. Cytokine profiles of T-lymphocytes from gingival tissues with pathological pocketing. *J. Dent. Res.* **2000**, *79*, 1548–1555. [CrossRef]
19. Page, R.C. Periodontal diseases: A new paradigm. *J. Dent. Educ.* **1998**, *62*, 812–821. [CrossRef]
20. Page, R.C. The pathobiology of periodontal diseases may affect systemic diseases: Inversion of a paradigm. *Ann. Periodontol.* **1998**, *3*, 108–120. [CrossRef] [PubMed]
21. Jewett, A.; Hume, W.R.; Le, H.; Huynh, T.N.; Han, Y.W.; Cheng, G.; Shi, W. Induction of apoptotic cell death in peripheral blood mononuclear and polymorphonuclear cells by an oral bacterium, Fusobacterium nucleatum. *Infect. Immun.* **2000**, *68*, 1893–1898. [CrossRef]
22. Jewett, A.; Bonavida, B. Target-induced inactivation and cell death by apoptosis in a subset of human NK cells. *J. Immunol.* **1996**, *156*, 907–915.
23. Jewett, A.; Wang, M.Y.; Teruel, A.; Poupak, Z.; Bostanian, Z.; Park, N.H. Cytokine dependent inverse regulation of CD54 (ICAM1) and major histocompatibility complex class I antigens by nuclear factor kappaB in HEp2 tumor cell line: Effect on the function of natural killer cells. *Hum. Immunol.* **2003**, *64*, 505–520. [CrossRef]
24. Jewett, A.; Cavalcanti, M.; Bonavida, B. Pivotal role of endogenous TNF-alpha in the induction of functional inactivation and apoptosis in NK cells. *J. Immunol.* **1997**, *159*, 4815–4822. [PubMed]
25. Jewett, A.; Bonavida, B. Interferon-alpha activates cytotoxic function but inhibits interleukin-2-mediated proliferation and tumor necrosis factor-alpha secretion by immature human natural killer cells. *J. Clin. Immunol.* **1995**, *15*, 35–44. [CrossRef]
26. Van Antwerp, D.J.; Martin, S.J.; Kafri, T.; Green, D.R.; Verma, I.M. Suppression of TNF-alpha-induced apoptosis by NF-kappaB. *Science* **1996**, *274*, 787–789. [CrossRef]
27. Jewett, A.; Cacalano, N.A.; Teruel, A.; Romero, M.; Rashedi, M.; Wang, M.; Nakamura, H. Inhibition of nuclear factor kappa B (NFkappaB) activity in oral tumor cells prevents depletion of NK cells and increases their functional activation. *Cancer Immunol. Immunother.* **2006**, *55*, 1052–1063. [CrossRef] [PubMed]
28. Doyle, S.E.; Vaidya, S.A.; O'Connell, R.; Dadgostar, H.; Dempsey, P.W.; Wu, T.T.; Rao, G.; Sun, R.; Haberland, M.E.; Modlin, R.L.; et al. IRF3 mediates a TLR3/TLR4-specific antiviral gene program. *Immunity* **2002**, *17*, 251–263. [CrossRef]
29. Bartold, P.M.; Clayden, A.M.; Gao, J.; Haase, H.; Li, H.; Stevens, M.; Symsons, A.; Young, W.G.; Zhang, C.Z. The role of growth factors in periodontal and pulpal regeneration. *JNZ Soc. Periodontol.* **1998**, *83*, 7–14.
30. Jotwani, R.; Cutler, C.W. Adult periodontitis–specific bacterial infection or chronic inflammation? *J. Med. Microbiol.* **1998**, *47*, 187–188. [PubMed]
31. Graves, D.T.; Cochran, D. The contribution of interleukin-1 and tumor necrosis factor to periodontal tissue destruction. *J. Periodontol.* **2003**, *74*, 391–401. [CrossRef]
32. Kaur, K.; Ko, M.W.; Ohanian, N.; Cook, J.; Jewett, A. Osteoclast-expanded super-charged NK-cells preferentially select and expand CD8+ T cells. *Sci. Rep.* **2020**, *10*, 20363. [CrossRef]
33. Sawa, T.; Nishimura, F.; Ohyama, H.; Takahashi, K.; Takashiba, S.; Murayama, Y. In vitro induction of activation-induced cell death in lymphocytes from chronic periodontal lesions by exogenous Fas ligand. *Infect Immun.* **1999**, *67*, 1450–1454. [CrossRef]

34. Yamamoto, M.; Kawabata, K.; Fujihashi, K.; McGhee, J.R.; Van Dyke, T.E.; Bamberg, T.V.; Hiroi, T.; Kiyono, H. Absence of exogenous interleukin-4-induced apoptosis of gingival macrophages may contribute to chronic inflammation in periodontal diseases. *Am. J. Pathol.* **1996**, *148*, 331–339.
35. Tseng, H.C.; Cacalano, N.; Jewett, A. Split anergized Natural Killer cells halt inflammation by inducing stem cell differentiation, resistance to NK cell cytotoxicity and prevention of cytokine and chemokine secretion. *Oncotarget* **2015**, *6*, 8947–8959. [CrossRef]
36. Jewett, A.; Arasteh, A.; Tseng, H.C.; Behel, A.; Arasteh, H.; Yang, W.; Nicholas, A.; Paranjpe, A. Strategies to rescue mesenchymal stem cells (MSCs) and dental pulp stem cells (DPSCs) from NK cell mediated cytotoxicity. *PLoS ONE* **2010**, *5*, e9874. [CrossRef] [PubMed]
37. Jorgovanovic, D.; Song, M.; Wang, L.; Zhang, Y. Roles of IFN-γ in tumor progression and regression: A review. *Biomark. Res.* **2020**, *8*, 49. [CrossRef]
38. Ottsjö, L.S.; Flach, C.F.; Nilsson, S.; de Waal Malefyt, R.; Walduck, A.K.; Raghavan, S. Defining the Roles of IFN-γ and IL-17A in Inflammation and Protection against Helicobacter pylori Infection. *PLoS ONE* **2015**, *10*, e0131444.
39. Jewett, A.; Cacalano, N.A.; Head, C.; Teruel, A. Coengagement of CD16 and CD94 receptors mediates secretion of chemokines and induces apoptotic death of naive natural killer cells. *Clin. Cancer Res.* **2006**, *12*, 1994–2003. [CrossRef]
40. Tseng, H.-C.; Bui, V.; Man, Y.-G.; Cacalano, N.; Jewett, A. Induction of Split Anergy Conditions Natural Killer Cells to Promote Differentiation of Stem Cells through Cell-Cell Contact and Secreted Factors. *Front. Immunol.* **2014**, *5*, 269. [CrossRef] [PubMed]
41. Jewett, A.; Kos, J.; Kaur, K.; Safaei, T.; Sutanto, C.; Chen, W.; Wang, P.; Namagerdi, A.K.; Fang, C.; Ko, M.-W.; et al. Natural Killer Cells: Diverse Functions in Tumor Immunity and Defects in Pre-neoplastic and Neoplastic Stages of Tumorigenesis. *Mol. Ther. Oncolytics* **2020**, *16*, 41–52. [CrossRef]
42. Jewett, A.; Tseng, H.C.; Arasteh, A.; Saadat, S.; Christensen, R.E.; Cacalano, N.A. Natural killer cells preferentially target cancer stem cells; role of monocytes in protection against NK cell mediated lysis of cancer stem cells. *Curr. Drug Deliv.* **2012**, *9*, 5–16. [CrossRef]
43. Jewett, A.; Man, Y.G.; Tseng, H.C. Dual functions of natural killer cells in selection and differentiation of stem cells; role in regulation of inflammation and regeneration of tissues. *J. Cancer* **2013**, *4*, 12–24. [CrossRef]
44. Cappuyns, I.; Gugerli, P.; Mombelli, A. Viruses in periodontal disease—a review. *Oral Dis.* **2005**, *11*, 219–229. [CrossRef]
45. Kubar, A.; Saygun, I.; Ozdemir, A.; Yapar, M.; Slots, J. Real-time polymerase chain reaction quantification of human cytomegalovirus and Epstein-Barr virus in periodontal pockets and the adjacent gingiva of periodontitis lesions. *J. Periodontal Res.* **2005**, *40*, 97–104. [CrossRef] [PubMed]
46. Ling, L.J.; Ho, C.C.; Wu, C.Y.; Chen, Y.T.; Hung, S.L. Association between human herpesviruses and the severity of periodontitis. *J. Periodontol.* **2004**, *75*, 1479–1485. [CrossRef] [PubMed]
47. Slots, J.; Kamma, J.J.; Sugar, C. The herpesvirus-Porphyromonas gingivalis-periodontitis axis. *J. Periodontal Res.* **2003**, *38*, 318–323. [CrossRef]
48. Dybing, J.K.; Walters, N.; Pascual, D.W. Role of endogenous interleukin-18 in resolving wild-type and attenuated Salmonella typhimurium infections. *Infect. Immun.* **1999**, *67*, 6242–6248. [CrossRef]
49. Pontarini, E.; Lucchesi, D.; Fossati-Jimack, L.; Coleby, R.; Tentorio, P.; Croia, C.; Bombardieri, M.; Mavilio, D. NK cell recruitment in salivary glands provides early viral control but is dispensable for tertiary lymphoid structure formation. *J. Leukoc. Biol.* **2019**, *105*, 589–602. [CrossRef]
50. Owen, K.A.; Anderson, C.J.; Casanova, J.E. Salmonella Suppresses the TRIF-Dependent Type I Interferon Response in Macrophages. *Mbio* **2016**, *7*. [CrossRef] [PubMed]
51. Greenlee-Wacker, M.C.; Nauseef, W.M. IFN-gamma targets macrophage-mediated immune responses toward Staphylococcus aureus. *J. Leukoc. Biol.* **2017**, *101*, 751–758. [CrossRef] [PubMed]
52. Loos, B.G.; Van Dyke, T.E. The role of inflammation and genetics in periodontal disease. *Periodontol 2000* **2020**, *83*, 26–39. [CrossRef]
53. Hassell, T.M.; Harris, E.L. Genetic influences in caries and periodontal diseases. *Crit. Rev. Oral Biol. Med.* **1995**, *6*, 319–342. [CrossRef] [PubMed]
54. Irfan, U.M.; Dawson, D.V.; Bissada, N.F. Epidemiology of periodontal disease: A review and clinical perspectives. *J. Int. Acad. Periodontol.* **2001**, *3*, 14–21.
55. Kantaputra, P.N.; Bongkochwilawan, C.; Lubinsky, M.; Pata, S.; Kaewgahya, M.; Tong, H.J.; Cairns, J.R.K.; Guven, Y.; Chaisrisookumporn, N. Periodontal disease and FAM20A mutations. *J. Hum. Genet.* **2017**, *62*, 679–686. [CrossRef] [PubMed]
56. Kocher, T.; Sawaf, H.; Fanghänel, J.; Timm, R.; Meisel, P. Association between bone loss in periodontal disease and polymorphism of N-acetyltransferase (NAT2). *J. Clin. Periodontol.* **2002**, *29*, 21–27. [CrossRef] [PubMed]
57. Tseng, H.C.; Arasteh, A.; Kaur, K.; Kozlowska, A.; Topchyan, P.; Jewett, A. Differential Cytotoxicity but Augmented IFN-γ Secretion by NK Cells after Interaction with Monocytes from Humans, and Those from Wild Type and Myeloid-Specific COX-2 Knockout Mice. *Front. Immunol.* **2015**, *6*, 259. [CrossRef] [PubMed]
58. Kaur, K.; Cook, J.; Park, S.H.; Topchyan, P.; Kozlowska, A.; Ohanian, N.; Fang, C.; Nishimura, I.; Jewett, A. Novel Strategy to Expand Super-Charged NK Cells with Significant Potential to Lyse and Differentiate Cancer Stem Cells: Differences in NK Expansion and Function between Healthy and Cancer Patients. *Front. Immunol.* **2017**, *8*, 297. [CrossRef]
59. Jung, S.; Gies, V.; Korganow, A.S.; Guffroy, A. Primary Immunodeficiencies With Defects in Innate Immunity: Focus on Orofacial Manifestations. *Front. Immunol.* **2020**, *11*, 1065. [CrossRef]

60. Raje, N.; Dinakar, C. Overview of Immunodeficiency Disorders. *Immunol. Allergy Clin.* **2015**, *35*, 599–623. [CrossRef]
61. Javali, M.A.; Patil, V.; Ayesha, H. Periodontal disease as the initial oral manifestation of abdominal tuberculosis. *Dent. Res. J.* **2012**, *9*, 634–637. [CrossRef] [PubMed]

MDPI
St. Alban-Anlage 66
4052 Basel
Switzerland
www.mdpi.com

Journal of Clinical Medicine Editorial Office
E-mail: jcm@mdpi.com
www.mdpi.com/journal/jcm

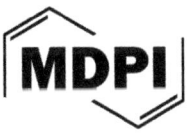

Disclaimer/Publisher's Note: The statements, opinions and data contained in all publications are solely those of the individual author(s) and contributor(s) and not of MDPI and/or the editor(s). MDPI and/or the editor(s) disclaim responsibility for any injury to people or property resulting from any ideas, methods, instructions or products referred to in the content.

www.ingramcontent.com/pod-product-compliance
Lightning Source LLC
LaVergne TN
LVHW070727100526
838202LV00013B/1188